- Are there ways to prevent the disease? Can a change in diet help?
- Who is more likely to get breast cancer and why?
- How do I find the best doctor for *me*?
- What should I expect in the way of examinations and diagnostic tests?
- What can I do to be sure I get only the most effective and least damaging treatment, if I need it?
- Do benign breast lumps ever turn into real cancer? Can I tell the difference when I examine myself?
- When necessary, what are the newest, safest, and easiest methods of breast reconstruction?

ALTERNATIVES answers these questions . . . and more. It is dedicated to the idea that the most informed patient is the one most likely *not* to be victimized.

About the author: Presidential appointee to the National Cancer Advisory Board . . . consultant to numerous government and private agencies . . . breast cancer patient, journalist, and in the words of the *Baltimore Sun*, the woman who "has worked tirelessly to get reforms implemented, and although a layperson, is recognized as one of the nation's leading experts on breast cancer". . . . that is Rose Kushner. In 1979, she was a member of a National Institutes of Health panel that put an end to routine radical mastectomies. She is directly responsible for the "two step procedure" that gives women time after diagnosis to look into treatment alternatives. Today she spearheads the campaign against the indiscriminate use of toxic chemotherapy. Founder of the Breast Cancer Advisory Center, a nonprofit organization dedicated to collecting and disseminating information on breast cancer, Mrs. Kushner is so widely known that letters addressed simply to "Mrs. Breast Cancer, Kensington, Maryland," promptly reach her mailbox.

ALTERNATIVES:

New Developments in the War on Breast Cancer

Formerly published as *Why Me?*

ROSE KUSHNER

Foreword by Richard E. Wilson, M.D.

WARNER BOOKS

A Warner Communications Company

This Warner Books Edition is published by arrangement with the
Kensington Press, P.O. Box 643, Cambridge, Massachusetts 02139

Warner Books, Inc.
75 Rockefeller Plaza
New York, N.Y. 10019

 A Warner Communications Company

Printed in the United States of America

First Warner Books Printing: September, 1985

10 9 8 7 6 5 4 3 2 1

Alternatives is an update of the 1982 edition of *Why Me?*, a book that gave so much new, unpublished information about all aspects of the war against breast cancer that complete revision was unnecessary. In an introductory chapter, more recent developments are detailed; Kushner's search for alternative treatments for her recurrence is described in an "epilogue" to Chapter 1. To conserve space (and cost), technical terms explained in the text are not repeated in these pages. Readers can find definitions to unfamiliar jargon by consulting the Index.

In memory of Ann London Scott and the hundreds of thousands of other women who have died—too soon—from breast cancer.

To Harvey. . . for all he's done to help me and every woman. To Gantt and Karen, Todd and Lesley . . . for helping him. To my whole family . . . for putting up with a professional breast-cancer patient since 1975. It isn't easy!

> With much love and thanks!
> Momm

And, of course, with gratitude to everyone at the National Cancer Institute and to physicians, surgeons and scientists all over the world who have gladly shared their data and dreams.

> Rose Kushner

Contents

Foreword

This new edition of WHY ME? represents the stimulating and provocative style—but most of all the courageous personal dedication—of Rose Kushner. She has provided a service not only for all women, but for all physicians as well. Rose Kushner makes it clear that communication between doctor and patient at all levels must be the by-word for the best possible interactive relationship. WHY ME? is a highly authoritative, but understandably editorialized, view of the "State-of-the-Art" of breast disease and breast cancer viewed from the standpoint of the consumer. In this case, the consumer is clearly the woman with breast cancer, or one who is at risk to develop it.

I must admit that the depth of Mrs. Kushner's knowledge and the scope of this text could easily match the most comprehensive postgraduate course on the subject. Her role as a member of the *National Cancer Advisory Board* allows her special insight into most new investigative approaches that are under study in the United States today. She has interviewed experts from all over the world and intermingled their viewpoints with those of her own in a complex discussion of physical, psychological, biochemical and socioeconomic attitudes relating to the disease. There is no doubt that Rose Kushner has become a lay expert about oncology in general, and breast cancer in particular; this reader is deeply impressed with her ability to explain this disease in terms clearly understandable to all women.

In this new edition of WHY ME?, the author has placed particular emphasis on reviewing new forms of adjuvant therapy such as chemotherapy, anti-estrogens and hormones—taking special care to warn patients about their indiscriminate use. She has also carefully described those forms of benign breast disease which are more likely to be pre-malignant and precursors of breast cancer development. Likewise, she has tried to provide some explanation for the theories of carcinogenesis and their relationship to common medications and oral contraceptives. Her most enthusiastic efforts are directed toward helping women to cope not only with treatment for known breast cancer, but also with the process of diagnosing breast disease, either benign or malignant. She calls this "pre-clinical anxiety," and she is unquestionably correct. The number of women under significant emotional stress with concern about their potential to *develop* breast cancer is many times greater than the number of those patients who actually are found to *have* breast cancer. A realistic understanding of the methods of diagnosis, the reasons for these techniques and the ways in which patients should be evaluated for breast disease should go a long way to setting many minds at ease.

I must just take a moment to point out that, despite my praise for Rose Kushner's efforts, a note of caution must be sounded. Her personal saga and the techniques she developed for dealing with her disease have provided her with new insight and an enthusiasm to strike out and help other women with breast cancer. She is not a physician—a fact she clearly states—yet I feel the need to emphasize this point as well. The Surgical Oncologist must maintain an objective viewpoint when it comes to making decisions for management and providing a description of options for primary treatment of breast cancer. There are many important biologic concepts that still remain to be proved. It is just as dangerous to latch on to new approaches that have not stood the test of time for our patients as it is to persist doggedly with old shibboleths of conservatism.

These are very exciting times in the management of breast cancer because of the courage of many clinical investigators around the world, notably among them Dr. Bernard Fisher at the University of Pittsburgh (leader of the National Surgical Adjuvant Breast Cancer Project [NSAPB]) and Drs. Bonadonna and Veronesi of the National Cancer Institute of Milan, Italy. These clinicians have taken the leadership in defining important questions for patient management that can only be answered with appropriate clinical trials. These clinical trials must be brought to fruition, however, with adequate time for observation and careful statistical review of the data before the postulates that served to initiate the studies are to be accepted as fact!

The most pressing questions for which solutions are being sought with clinical trials in the treatment of breast cancer are: (1) Is a limited resection of the breast (partial mastectomy, lumpectomy, tylectomy) as effective in treating a primary breast cancer as removal of the entire breast? (2) If cancer recurs in a breast that has only been partially removed, can the life of that patient be salvaged with subsequent mastectomy in a manner equivalent to the chance for survival had mastectomy been performed as the initial treatment? (3) Is radiation therapy really necessary following partial mastectomy or lumpectomy? (4) What is the role of removal of lymph nodes in conjunction with resection of part or all of the breast? If lymph nodes involved with cancer are left behind in the axilla, does that change the outcome for the patient with primary breast cancer? (5) What are the requirements and advantages for adjuvant chemotherapy in postmenopausal women? Since more than 60% of patients with breast cancer are over 50, it is imperative that we identify how effective chemotherapy is in changing the recurrence rate and survival in these women. It is generally accepted that chemotherapy following breast cancer removal in premenopausal patients will extend disease-free survival, although the question of differences in ultimate survival is not yet settled; older women don't seem to fare as well following chemotherapy. New and better trials must be designed and tested to determine whether postmenopausal women should be subjected to the risk of chemotherapy in the face of questionable benefit. (6) What is the role of anti-estrogens in pre- and postmenopausal women with breast cancer? Rose Kushner is certainly correct in crusading for estrogen receptor determinations to be performed on all samples of breast cancer, and I might add that this applies not only for primary disease but for metastatic disease biopsies as well. Our ability to select patients for specific forms of treatment based on documented biochemical aberrations of the tumor cells is the hope of all oncologists.

When sound answers are available for these questions, then I think we will have solid evidence of improved survival and better quality of life for our patients. Unquestionably, the enthusiastic efforts of Rose Kushner will help bring these answers directly to the patients so that they, too, can participate in the decision-making process for their own management.

RICHARD E. WILSON, M.D.

Professor of Surgery
Harvard Medical School
Chief, Surgical Oncology
Brigham and Women's Hospital—Sidney Farber
    Cancer Institute
Boston, Massachusetts

Alternatives

It was almost eight years to the day.

On the evening of June 15, 1974, I had found a small cancer in my left breast; on the morning of June 14, 1982, a pathology lab reported that another tiny cancer had grown—far from the scar—in the skin over that amputated breast.

Tight cramps of fear again curdled by belly, bringing back memories of that terrifying Saturday night eight years earlier. Somehow, I had known that first lump was cancer as soon as I found it; this time, I had the same ominous feeling.

In my other books, Breast Cancer *and* Why Me?, *I described how hard it was to learn about alternatives in 1974. There was nothing in bookstores or in the public library, and I had to go to the library of the National Institutes of Health for help. This situation quickly changed, thanks to the wide publicity given to Betty Ford and Happy Rockefeller. Since their surgeries, dozens of articles, books and even television programs have told women about alternatives to mastectomy. But eight years later, there was a wider information gap than the one I found in 1974; even the NIH library had little about treating a late local skin recurrence.*

Details of my research to learn metastatic alternatives are described in an "epilogue" after Chapter I. But in these first pages of the 1984 update, Alternatives, *I want to introduce a new problem we women are facing: automatic "adjuvant" chemotherapy. It looks like indiscriminate use of toxic drugs for low-risk women has replaced the Halsted radical mastectomy as therapeutic overkill, when surgery is not enough.*

On February 19, 1976, the New England Journal of Medicine *published very early data from an Italian trial showing that a combination of cyclophosphamide, methotrexcte and 5-Fluorouracil (CMF), given after radical mastectomy, dramatically reduced recurrence rates in Stage II (one or more malignant axillary lymph nodes) patients of all ages.*

This study ushered us into a period (hopefully one that won't last a century!) in which almost every woman, regardless of age or other factors, who has even a few cancer cells in a single lymph node, can expect to be zapped by adjuvant "chemo." I've been told that doctors who don't offer Stage II breast-cancer patients this still-experimental treatment are subject to suit for malpractice. This is, apparently, a uniquely American phenomenon.

The only settings where women should allow any investigational treatment are controlled clinical trials where various anti-cancer agents are compared. Even here, since 1976, ethical and legal questions have made it almost impossible to test adjuvant therapies in a rigidly scientific manner. Clear, untainted results depend on having a "control group" of patients who either receive no treatment at all or one that has been proven to be safe and effective, over time. This is how most medicines and procedures become "standard" in the first place.

But even though followup data from Italy showed that estrogen-receptor (ER)-rich, postmenopausal women benefitted little from CMF, research trials were affected. For example, to test the value of the anti-estrogen tamoxifen, Dr. Charles Hubay in Cleveland had to give patients in the control group the suddenly-standard CMF while women in the study group got CMF + T (tamoxifen or Nolvadex).

"I wanted to compare Tam with a no-treatment control," he told members of NCI's Breast Cancer Task Force in March, 1983. "But my hospital's Institutional Review Board felt the Italian data made having a no-treatment group unethical."

In the summer of '82, of course, all this seemed irrelevant. I didn't know my ER status, and there were no clinical trials for women who recurred after eight disease-free years. As far as I know, there still is none. I had to guess my alternatives.

With approval from Tom Dao, my doctor, I chose only Nolvadex.

Sixteen months have passed, and I'm breathing easier, but I still watch and wait.

Of course, I've been doing that since 1974.

I was talking to Dr. Donald Henson.

"Any new breakthroughs for the new preface to my book?"

He answered quickly, as if he had already given the question a lot of thought. "I think we've learned most about what not to do, and this might be more important than any 'breakthrough'. We're not using high-dose radiation for mammography, and we're not doing diagnostic biopsies immediately before treatment. We do not rely on incisional biopsies anymore, either. It's been proven that all cancers, including breast, are made up of benign and malignant cells. Taking just a section could result in a 'false negative'."

Then we discussed his own turf: detection and diagnosis. A group at the University of Florida has developed a different way of teaching and learning breast self-examination (BSE). Known as Mammacare, the new method "educates" women's fingertips to feel lumps as small as a lentil by using a grid, like braille, instead of a circular BSE pattern. (For information about training centers around the country, there's a toll-free number: 1-800-MAM-CARE.)

Computerized ultrasound tomography (CUT) is just around the corner; thermography, diaphanography and nuclear magnetic resonance are still being studied. Digital mammography, a technique that exposes women to only one Roentgen of radiation over thirty years, is already in use at Harvard.

In May 1983, new guidelines for screening by mammography were issued by the American Cancer Society (ACS) and the American College of Radiology (ACR). These recommend that all women have baseline mammograms at some time between the ages of 35 and 39. Then, from their 40th to 49th birthdays, they should be screened at one or two year intervals, depending on their personal and family risk factors. National Cancer Institute (NCI) guidelines, in effect since 1977, restrict X-ray screening in this age group to women with strong family histories. After 50, all three agencies recommend annual mammograms.

Radiation levels have dropped because of better film and equipment, but there is still considerable opposition to exposing healthy, under-50 breasts to potentially harmful X-rays.

Dr. John Bailar, for one, insists there is no proven survival advantage from screening younger women. Since the under-50 group develops only about one-fifth of all breast cancers, he doesn't think mammography is cost-effective for them. But he agrees that women older than 50 should be screened.

"As long as they go where there are trained, qualified personnel and modern equipment that uses low-dose film," he told me, "the benefits do outweigh the risks for older women."

He stressed, however, that there is still a serious risk all women face from any type of screening: having a breast amputated because something abnormal or atypical is found.

"Atypical cells don't mean a woman has or will ever develop cancer," he said, "but they sure do scare doctors into surgery."

Of course, the reason for any screening is the hope of finding microscopic cancer cells before they have spread, and until the disease can be prevented, early-detection is all we have. But we can escape Dr. Bailar's terrifying scenario by refusing any surgery except a biopsy. If a mammogram (or any -gram) has a suspicious spot, women should give their informed consents (permission slips) only for diagnosis.

Or they can have the surgeon sign a contract (page 18).

Then, if abnormal or atypical cells are found, women can take their slides to breast pathologists for opinions about what to do. A superb (and free!) source of expertise is the Armed Forces Institute of Pathology in Washington, D.C. A tax-supported facility, the AFIP's services are available to everyone in the United States.

Scientists certainly know about this possible grim outcome of screening and are in hot pursuit of ways to identify those cells that are true precursors of cancer, so we can stop worrying about having mastectomies we don't really need.

One new "marker" for such identification may be the presence of or absence of proteins called laminin receptors—research being done at the NCI by Dr. Lance Liotta. On the more immediate horizon, monoclonal antibodies (MCAs) are being improved to home in only on cancer cells containing antigens they react with, either internally or externally. A professor of surgery at the Georgetown Medical School, Dr. William Feller, has combined two MCAs from the Netherlands with blood from women who have breast masses. By November 1983, the Dutch antibodies had accurately predicted cancer in 96 per cent of 84 patients. Maybe this will be the quick, easy and cheap "PAP Test" for breast cancer we have been waiting for.

The biotechnology industry has also jumped on the marker bandwagon, and hardly a week goes by without some new "cancer diagnostic" in the Wall Street Journal. *With economic incentives involved, an accurate marker should be available soon.*

But, at this time, markers are in The Future. We still must rely on some type of biopsy for diagnosis. And, until technological know-how improves, positive lymph nodes are only found surgically. As primitive as it is in our age of the space telescope, the condition of a woman's nodes can only be known by cutting them out.

Oncogenes upstaged MCAs as the hottest items in basic research in 1983. Genes are microscopic bits of DNA (deoxyribonucleic acid) that carry all information about living things from one generation to the next; onco-, of course, is the Greek prefix for cancer. Although oncogenes belong in The Future, I'll introduce them here, in early-detection, because they have been headlined in newspapers and magazines as the answers to everything. As a diagnostic, for example, if a gene for breast cancer is found (and some scientists are sure there is one for premenopausal, bilateral disease), a woman might be screened by having a few cells scraped from her skin or mouth.

Having oncogenes in most cells does not *mean everyone inevitably gets cancer. They can't transform cells to cancer without the help of environmental promotors like radiation, tobacco or asbestos. Without carcinogens to "turn on" oncogenes, they can lie forever dormant on their chromosomes and never cause any problems.*

For prevention, scientists hope to find a way to "turn off" the gene, so promotors won't have anything to activate. If an oncogene "antagonist" is found to deactivate the gene, this might then be made into a safe vaccination. For a cure, an antagonist may someday be injected to defuse oncogenes in advanced tumors.

But this is jumping into The Future too quickly. I'm describing the newest research "breakthrough" in these early pages, because women have already called and written me to ask where they can get "oncogene therapy." There isn't any yet.

What's new in the Who? When? Where? and Why? of breast cancer? A lot.

On the international front, Japanese, Finnish and Hungarian women still have lower breast-cancer incidences than American and northwestern European women do. But the rates are rising as politics and prosperity "improve" their lifestyles, especially diets.

And, according to a letter I received from Dr. George Wu, director of the National Cancer Institute of the Peoples' Republic of China, the same "improvement" is happening in his country.

Incidence for 1984 in the United States is estimated at 115,000 new cases, one of every eleven women living in this country, or nine per cent; about 37,300 will die of disease treated in earlier years.

These projections are made by the NCI's SEER Program (Surveillance, Epidemiology and End Results), our source of statistics about all cancers. Once upon a time, it was possible to estimate national data from only Connecticut, the first state to have a cancer registry. People living in the USA today, however, are too mixed and mobile to use one state's registry. Thousands of senior citizens develop cancer in the northeast, but their deaths occur in retirement areas of the Sun Belt; tens of thousands of blacks moved from the south during the 1950s and '60s only to return home in the 1970s and '80s; the past decades have brought Mexicans and Cuban, Haitian, Hungarian, Russian and Vietnamese refugees to our melting pot.

To cope with such volatile changes, SEER now collects data from Connecticut, Hawaii, Iowa, New Jersey, New Mexico, Puerto Rico and Utah; the metropolitan areas of Atlanta, Detroit, San Francisco/Oakland and Seattle/Puget Sound; ten counties of rural Georgia; and areas of Arizona with large Navajo populations.

An example of SEER's value to breast-cancer research are the statistical variations found between black and white women. In the past, it was automatically assumed that blacks had lower incidence rates because of poverty's effect on lifestyles; lower survivals were attributed to late diagnosis and poorer quality of care.

But SEER data have shown that regardless of the stage of disease at diagnosis, black women have higher death rates than white women do. Why?

Most black patients of all ages are ER-poor, and a lack of hormone *receptors predicts a grimmer prognosis. Yet SEER numbers show this can't be the only reason: stage-for-stage, ER-poor black women live fewer years after treatment than ER-poor white women. After getting these clues from SEER, the NCI initiated research to try to get the answers to this problem, work that is still ongoing.*

Incidence for American women under 35 has continued to rise, and oral contraceptives are still under suspicion. In October 1983, the Center for Disease Control (CDC), funded by the National Institute of Child Health and Human Development (NICHD), compared Pill-usage among more than 1,000 women who had cancer with 4,000 who did not. No link with breast cancer was found, and the CDC reported that OCs actually protect women against endometrial and ovarian cancers.

Only a few weeks later, research supported by the same Institute, showed far different results. This study involved 314 Los Angeles patients, younger than 37 when diagnosed, who were followed for ten years. According to these data, the women under 25 who used OCs having high levels of progestogens (synthetic hormones similar, but not identical, to natural progesterones) for five or more years had a quadrupled risk of developing breast cancer.

Two weeks after this article appeared, an international panel of experts met at the NICHD to try to make sense out of the conflicting reports. Their conclusion? The statistical methods used for analyzing Pill reports need to be standardized, so everyone evaluates data with the same equations and formulas.

What does this mean to women?

That the answers aren't in yet, and OCs should be taken with caution. Average-risk young women who believe The Pill's benefits outweigh its risks should ask their doctors to prescribe one that has as little of both hormones as possible to be an effective contraceptive. Some of these are Brevicon, Modicon, Loestrin-120 and Zorane-120 or 1.5-30. These women must be sure to practice regular BSE and see a breast expert for regular examinations.

However, I urge women who have strong family histories of breast cancer to investigate other ways for preventing a pregnancy.

The legacy of the wholesale use of diethylstilbestrol to prevent miscarriages in the 1950s and 1960s is still growing. In a new book, D.E.S.: The Bitter Pill, Robert Myers reports what many scientists have long suspected: that women who took the synthetic estrogen are developing "an excess of" breast cancer—more than were expected to develop in a specific number of women.

Another risk factor has become epidemic: a late-mother boom. In 1951, when Lucille Ball, then 40, was publicly pregnant on TV, everyone was shocked; in 1981, Ursula Andress, 44, was news only because she wasn't married to son Dimitri's dad.

The number of "elderly primiparas" is still growing, according to the

National Center for Health Statistics. There were almost twice as many women in their 30s and 40s who had their first children in 1980 than there were in 1975, and the trend continues. While toy makers may be delighted, scientists are afraid the late-mother boom will cause a sharp rise in breast-cancer incidence fifteen to twenty years from now.

Of course, women can't turn back their biological timeclocks and have first children earlier, but older first-time mothers should—like their sisters on The Pill—examine their breasts regularly and consult breast experts at least twice every year.

It may also be a good idea to cut down on fats. In 1982, a widely publicized National Academy of Sciences report, Diet, Nutrition, and Cancer, linked breast cancer to fatty diets. It suggested we reduce our daily dose of fat calories from the U.S. average of 40 to 30 percent, because of evidence that there is a "fat-estrogen connection." (Many studies have shown that some women's bodies convert cholesterol into estrogens. In another, breast-cancer patients who weighed less than 140 pounds lived longer than heavier women did. There are also data suggesting that cholesterol in breast fluid can cause damage. Many studies report an association between high-fat diets and low immunity.)

The report costs $13.50, prepaid, and can be obtained from: The National Academy Press; 2101 Constitution Ave., N.W.; Washington, D.C. 20418. Menus based on it are available from the Agricultural Research Service; Beltsville, MD 20705.

After the media blitz that followed publication of the report, the NCI designed two dietary trials to try to prevent breast cancer. One involves 2,000 Stage II patients, enrolled in adjuvant-therapy trials. They will be randomized into low-and average-fat diets to see if their recurrence rates differ; in the second, 6,000 healthy, but high-risk, women will be divided the same way to see if the disease can be prevented entirely by dietary modification.

Although results will be a long time coming, prevention research has to start somewhere, or we'll never have the answers.

Ten years ago, talk of using vitamins and minerals to avoid or delay cancer was medical heresy, almost kin to talking about laetrile. But now, I can come out of the nutritional closet and confess I take beta-carotene and vitamins C and E. (Selenium also slows cancer growth, but an effective does would probably destroy my liver first.)

And though I've cut down on fats, I do cheat occasionally.

This makes me worry about the women in the trial who will tumble off their 20% or 40% wagons once in a while. Obviously, some in each group will either recur or develop cancer, regardless of drugs and diets, and I worry that they'll believe their cheating made it happen. It's bad enough to have breast cancer without feeling guilty that you did something to cause it yourself.

This brings me to another shift in orthodox thinking: that there may be an association between cancer and emotions. For years, some reports have suggested that breast cancer might be linked with early losses of parents, spouses, children, etc. And there have always been stories of patients who managed to delay death until after an important family celebration.

But these were usually published in "soft science" journals, not in Cancer *or* Science. *Now that scientists have the technological know-how to measure miniscule amounts of substances released by the body when it is out-of-whack, even these prestigious publications have reported that extreme stress often reduces an animals's immune system, while a calm environment does the opposite.*

Paradoxically, some types of stress seem to be helpful!

A current NCI study is showing that women who are angry and fight their disease (and doctors) are making better progress than women who are passive and accepting.

We cancer patients have suspected this for a long time.

The "real controversy"—separate biopsies, ERA, PRA and staging—is an ex-controversy. More needle biopsies are being done because of a national trend toward hospital cost-containment, and needles are cheaper than knives. There may also be another reason: doctors entering clinical practice since 1981 are more likely to have been trained to do needle biopsies.

There have also been changes in the conservative American Cancer Society which has never "officially" backed the NIH's 1979 recommendation that biopsies be separated from further treatment. In the July/August, 1982 issue of Ca: A Journal for Clinicians, *the ACS printed a full-page article about the NCI's clinical trial comparing modified radical mastectomy to lumpectomy and radiation and asked its doctor-readers to refer patients. While it isn't a direct seal-of-approval, this is certainly implied. Unless a biopsy is separated from treatment, it would be impossible for a doctor to refer patients to clinical trials.*

In Why Me?, *the importance of the progesterone-receptor assay was still uncertain; now it's known that the PR assay is sometimes more significant than the ERA and* must *be done. Like markers, both assays are "diagnostics," and dozens of firms are in the race to find cheaper, quicker, easier and more accurate tests.*

By the way, I am now saying estrogen- and progesterone- "rich" and "poor," instead of "positive" and "negative." Both assays count how many receptors a tumor has in proportion to other things in it, and few women have no ERs at all (not so with PRs: see below).

Since 1981, the number of surgeons ordering ER assays routinely is almost at the 100% mark, but laboratories doing the tests for hospitals unable to do their own report high error rates for small community institutions. Because of poor packing and shipping, they claim specimens often arrive thawed instead of frozen at -73° Centigrade. Some samples don't even have enough cancer cells in them to do an accurate assay.

One way women can check on the reliability of their results is to compare the ER count with the PR count, because it is rare for a tumor to be rich in PRs and yet be ER-poor. Progesterone-receptors usually result from an interaction between estrogen receptors and molecules of estrogens entering a cell from the bloodstream. If an assay's result says a tumor is PR-rich but ER-poor, a mistake might have been made somewhere along the line.

This alone may be reason enough for women to go only to cancer specialists who work in excellent institutions. In 1974, this was easier said than done; by 1984, the situation is vastly improved. Thanks to the 1971 National Cancer Act, women can now turn to tax-supported Cancer Centers, Cooperative Oncology Groups and to dozens of hospitals for "state of the art" cancer care in communities where little, if any, care was available in the past.

"State of the art" for breast cancer, by the way, should include modern and monitored mammography equipment, the two-stage procedure and participation in clinical trials of surgery, radiation, adjuvant therapy and treatment for advanced disease. These programs are stringently quality-controlled, and those that don't comply with NCI standards will have trouble getting their grants or contracts renewed.

For information about an NCI center or program near your home, call the Institute's toll-free, hotlines, 800-638-6694 or 800-4-CANCER (You may have to dial "1-800.")

Or ask your doctor to "bring up" the PDQs on his/her personal computer. Protocol Data Query is a nationwide computerized information database that is organized geographically to help women (via their physicians) enroll in NCI-approved clinical trials. A special "user friendly" (most computer systems are "hostile") program gives instant access to explanations of treatment alternatives and lists of approved institutions and specialists trained and experienced in managing cancer.

The brainchild of Richard A. Bloch (of H&R Block), the PDQ system will be a lifesaver—if doctors use it.

Progress has been made toward giving women freedom of choice in primary treatment. By the end of 1983, there were laws in Massachusetts, California and Hawaii mandating that doctors tell women suspected of having breast cancer about alternatives to mastectomy. Similar laws were proposed in other states, but they never made it out of committee.

But legislation is not the answer. As anyone who has driven faster than 55 mph knows, a law is useless if it can't be enforced. Even in Massachusetts, probably the most enlightened state in the Union (the first "Patients' Bill of Rights" in May 1979), it's easy for doctors to convince panicky patients their favorite treatment is "best." ("If you were my wife...." is a popular line.)

So in the three states where there is a law, women referred to surgeons *will probably receive some kind of mastectomy; if they go to radiotherapists, they're more likely to have partial surgery and radiation. The solution may depend on obstetrician/gynecologists, usually women's primary-care physicians. They are the doctors who should tell their patients about treatment alternatives and then refer them to surgeons who will cooperate. A few paragraphs in a state's Annotated Code can't do it without help.*

To bring Chapter 10 up-to-date, the NCI's trial (begun in July, 1979) hasn't yet enrolled the 300 needed patients; data from the NSABP's Protocol B-06 (begun in April 1976) still show no significant differences in survival between patients who had either modified radical mastectomies, lumpectomies with radiation or lumpectomies without radition. In the two breast-preserving groups, the incidence of second tumors has, naturally, been higher than among the women who had mastectomies. (A breast that has been amputated will never grow another lump.) But no one yet knows whether this will affect their long-term survival rates.[1]

Happily, the Halsted radical mastectomy has become almost obsolete. The American College of Surgeons reported data from three surveys comparing the care of breast-cancer patients in 1972, 1976 and 1981. Only 3.4 per cent of them received Halsteds in 1981, compared with 27.5 per cent in 1976 and 48 per cent in 1972. While in absolute numbers, 3.4 per cent translates into more than 3,000 Halsteds, the modified is now the "U.S. standard."

This is as good a time as any to bring up some semantics: a "breast conservation procedure" is not a "conservative breast procedure." Most therapies that preserve the breast are "conservation," but exposing the gland and adjacent tissues to thousands of rads (radiation-absorbed dose) of X-ray is "radical radiation." Radical anything—surgery, radiation or chemotherapy—is, by definition, not a conservative procedure. The side- and after-effects of poorly done breast irradiation can be more devastating and disfiguring than a well done Halsted radical mastectomy.

Drs. Allen Lichter and Eli Glatstein of the NIH's Radiation Oncology Department kindly gave me some criteria women should know:

1. The radiotherapist must be certified by the American Society of Therapeutic Radiologists (ASTR).
2. He/she must have specific training to treat an intact breast.
3. The equipment should be a Cobalt, 4 or 6 MeV accelerator: isocentric (rotational).
4. The equipment should have a treatment-planning computer to program individual treatment, although it does not have to be located at the same site as the accelerator.
5. The therapist should compensate for breast shape with wedge filters or individual compensators.
6. The therapist should do a "cone-down boost" with irridium, cesium

(or other radioactive substance) or electron (or ortho-voltage) equipment to kill cells left in the tumor site.

7. *The therapist should not use "bolus" (a technical term).*
8. *The dose should be 4,500-5,000 rads, spread over 5-6 weeks, averaging 180-200 rads per day.*
9. *The areas to be irradiated (portals) should be custom-tailored for each woman.*

Women anxious to save their breasts must know that a diploma on the wall and an X-ray machine in the office do not an expert make. While the ASTR has about 2,000 certified members, only about twenty per cent, or 400, meet the above NCI criteria.

Caveat emptor: *buyer beware.* Check a radiotherapist's ability and equipment as carefully as you check your hairdresser's.

All of the NCI-supported clinical trials comparing mastectomy to lesser surgery require a complete removal of all axillary nodes, except for the apical nodes high in the armpit. Many surgeons who don't participate in trials remove only a sampling of eight or ten nodes to see if they are malignant. At a breast-cancer symposium in San Antonio in November 1983, oncologists agreed that this partial dissection is risky, because positive nodes are "skipped."

It's safer if as many axillary nodes as possible are removed.

Like most women who have recurred, I'm more anxious to know about drugs, hormones and immune therapies than I am about primary therapy now. Losing a breast was my all-consuming worry when I found the first lump....but no more.

For adjuvant therapy, women who have negative nodes, but who are ER-poor, are being called Stage II and are given adjuvant chemotherapy. NSABP's Protocol B-l3 was designed for them, but its informed consent statement tells women clearly that alkylating agents (e.g., Cytoxan, Alkeran) aren't used because these drugs can cause second cancers. Since most ER-poor women are pre-menopausal, they have many years ahead of them, and members of the Project believe the possible dangers of using such drugs for low-risk patients outweigh their possible benefits.

As I've said, clinical trials should be the only setting for such investigational treatment. Women must be sure their doctors take part in controlled programs, not free spirits who report their results only to insurance companies.

What else is new in adjuvant chemotherapy?

Some substances create drug-resistant cancer cells that may not respond to anything we now have, should a patient recur later: the drugs often damage DNA and mutate (change) the cancer cells they are instead of destroying them. The new cells differ from the "founding cell" and pass the mutated DNA on to the next generation. This phenomenon may account for the fact that adjuvant chemotherapy does cause a longer *disease-free interval after surgery but faster failure if the disease returns.*

The NCI will spend whatever it takes to find a way to resolve this dilemma, and I'm sure it will happen soon. But now, Stage II women who have a low risk of recurring should know that drug-resistance is a problem.

There is still no agreement about when to begin adjuvant chemotherapy, how long to give it and what to use.

At the beginning, adjuvant regimens were started after women recovered from surgery and were continued for two years. Later trial results suggested that treatment should begin immediately after surgery and that six months of cytotoxic drugs (not hormonal agents) are enough, because the first cycles kill almost all leftover cancer cells.

Now there are challenges, based on more recent clinical trials, that suggest 1) there is no difference if adjuvant therapy is delayed until patients are stronger and their wounds are healed, and 2) some groups of women may need more than six months to achieve a maximum cell-kill. There are still no answers to these two questions: only results from comparative trials will bring them.

What to use?

At this time, there is no combination that is "best" for every woman. ER/PR-poor women of any age usually receive some type of cytotoxic drug combination, depending on the one that's most popular in their communities. The reason for this, of course, is that there is still no way to evaluate a combination except by absence of disease, and it's literally six-one-way and half-dozen-the-other. Whatever keeps the cancer away is "best" for that woman.

ER/PR-rich premenopausal women also have a problem. While endocrine therapy should help them, except for removing their ovaries, most U.S. oncologists give younger women only cytotoxic chemotherapy. The reason is that—for reasons no one understands yet—data from the NSABP's Protocol B-09 (begun in 1979) show no benefit from tamoxifen, combined with L-Pam and 5-Fluorouracil (PFT), to this group of women. Since these results conflict with those from several large European trials (such as one directed by Dr. Michael Baum in Britain and Scandinavia) which have no-treatment controls, it has been suggested that tamoxifen may somehow interfere with the drugs' action.

Whatever the reason may be, this is the situation at the end of 1983. The trials will have to be filled and finished to have an answer.

For ER/PR-rich postmenopausal women, however, B-09's PFT and Case Western's CMFT are significantly better than PF and CMF alone.

In B-09, by the way, PFT seems to be so superior for over-60 women that future trials may use 60 as the accepted age of menopause.

Another finding from B-09 is that two years of tamoxifen may not be enough to prevent early recurrence in older women. Stage II postmenopausal ER-rich patients in the trial will be getting a third year of Nolvadex only.

What do community physicians do in the face of all these conflicting data? In San Antonio, a New York breast surgeon commented about current practice in the Big Apple.

"If a Stage II postmenopausal patient in New York city is referred to an oncologist," he said, "she'll get chemotherapy. If not, she won't. It's as simple as that."

Women with advanced breast cancer are treated by whatever works best. Since they have disease than can be measured, there isn't so much trial-and-error. No new substances have been approved for general use, but the drugs, hormones and anti-estrogens described in Chapter 11 are being combined in ingenious ways to increase their cancer-killing potential.

For example, women are being given estrogens to speed up and synchronize the growth of their cancer cells. When the rate of division is at a peak, they receive high doses of cytotoxic drugs to try to destroy a large proportion of cells when they are most vulnerable—during mitosis (Appendix).

These hormonal-chemotherapy trials are young and have been used in too few women for results. And since they involve only patients with very severe disease, their lives may not be affected at all. But all anti-cancer drugs begin by being used first in people who have failed everything else, and even small, short-term responses may mean future benefit for patients if given earlier.

Another hope is enhancing drugs and radiation by adding immune boosters like interferons, thymosin, Protein A and other biological response modifiers. These include beta- and gamma-interferons made by high, bio-tech, genetic-engineering firms.

As I write these lines, bisantrene, bromocriptine, mitotoxin, mitoxantrone (or DHAD) and platinum (or CBDCA) are winding through the long and tortuous process of Phases I and II. Only when Phase III is finally reached is a substance considered safe and effective enough to try as a "first line" therapy.

Progress in breast reconstruction?

While I'm delighted to write that most insurance firms now pay for plastic surgery to replace a lost breast, I'm unhappy to report that many are also paying for prophylactic mastectomies. As I wrote on page 293, there's a lot of feeling against amputating healthy breasts just because they might, someday, develop cancer.

Women whose close relatives had premenopausal, bilateral disease have reason to consider this drastic surgery, but the risks of the vast majority of women are being exaggerated and exploited.

Not long ago, a procedure in which the rectus abdominus *muscle and belly fat are removed from the abdomen to the chest for anchoring an implant received considerable publicity as a way to get a "tummy tuck" and reconstruction at the same time. Not long after, bone specialists began reporting that several patients who had this surgery later developed painful back problems, because their spines need the muscle for support. Women who are so allergic that they can't tolerate anything foreign may have no alternative. But for most, this free tummy tuck could wind up costing a very high price.*

Male Chauvinism? Politics?

We're a long way ahead of men in terms of media attention and education. Who has ever seen a TV ad teaching TSE (testicular self-exam)? How many men know the symptoms of prostate cancer? What publisher would print a book about alternatives for either disease?

And women are doing better on Capitol Hill too. The Breast cancer Task Force of the NCI is now an official "site" in the five-site Organ Systems Program. Its current $12 million annual research budget is bigger than the other four added together.

The Future?

The Imminent Future will bring customized therapies instead of a "current treatment standard" used for every woman. After all, the only thing "standard" about breast cancer is that every patient is so different, with a unique tumor (cell type, doubling time, ER/PR status) and personal factors (age, children, family history) that must be dealt with individually.

So tailored treatment is an idea whose time has come.

In general, primary therapy is already individualized in large metropolitan areas and even in many small cities and towns. A new generation of surgeons has taken over U.S. operating rooms, doctors who grew up with Ralph Nader, Women's Lib and consumers' rights. And they're still close enough to school books to keep up with current trends; they expect to give us alternatives.

In chemotherapy, tailoring the choice of drugs using a stem-cell assay is described in Chapter 11. A mathematical model called ONCOCIN is also being developed to try to match the right drug for a specific tumor in a computer. Another hope is an easy and inexpensive way to label a woman's cancer cells with radioactivity to count their doubling times. Then, the right drug could be given at the precise time and will be able to destroy them.

Individualized treatment is something we can expect tomorrow.

However, most of the Future relies on basic research. In Alternatives, *a constant theme is how dependent progress in oncology has been on the development of new technologies—from antibodies to zoetropes. I've already described a bit about the unknown potential of oncogene research; still to come are liposomes, bits of fat found in cells, that—like MCAs and oncogenes—may transport anti-cancer agents directly to tumors.*

Women with advanced disease who can't tolerate large doses of chemotherapy may soon be helped by marrow transplants. Their own cells would be removed, treated and frozen for reinjection, after intensive chemotherapy, so their immune systems will be restored.

In ending this introduction to the fourth edition of Breast Cancer, *now* Alternatives, *I sympathize with Congresspersons who are elected every two years; as soon as they win their seats, they have to begin campaigning for the next term.*

This is, happily, the way it has been writing about breast cancer: so much has happened so quickly that new and exciting progress is announced before a manuscript can be set into type.

I'm not complaining.

> *Rose Kushner*
> *Kensington, Maryland*
> *November, 1983*

---

[1] As reported on March 14, 1985 (New England Journal of Medicine 312: 665-73, 1985), the five year survival rates continued to be identical among the three groups. However, 28% of the women whose intact breasts were not irradiated had developed second tumors; only 8% of the women who were irradiated had developed second tumors at five years.

1

What Happened to Me

It was Saturday night, June 15, 1974, when I found the tiny bulge on the edge of my left nipple. The date will probably stay with me forever. Like all outstanding anniversaries, the precise time a malignant tumor is found has a way of sticking in one's memory.

I was in the tub, luxuriating in an unexpected reprieve from a business dinner party. The children were out, and Harvey and I had the house and the television all to ourselves. I wondered if there was a good movie on that night.

"Don't take too long," I remember his shouting from the living room. "It's a great night to be home—Archie Bunker, M*A*S*H, and a Humphrey Bogart oldie."

And then I found it.

I was not examining myself for suspected cancer. All I was doing was shaving under my arm.

Somehow the little finger of the hand that held the razor leapfrogged over something irregular, a minute hemisphere that curved ever so slightly above the firm strand of muscle. It was so small that I was not sure there was really anything different about the spot. But if my head pretended for a moment that nothing was there, my stomach knew immediately something was wrong. It coiled into a tight ball and stayed that way for weeks.

Until I was struck by cancer myself, the only women I had ever known personally who had the disease were all dead; several relatives on my husband's side of the family (no one on mine, so far as I knew), a dear friend, and friends of friends. Of course, everyone in Washington knew about Alice Longworth, Theodore Roosevelt's astonishing daughter. She had had both her breasts removed for cancer almost a half century ago and billed herself as

1

"the flattest-chested woman in the capital." Sometimes she joked that she was the only really topless woman in town.

But former presidents' daughters are legends; that's why she survived. Mere mortal women died from breast cancer. Betty Ford and Happy Rockefeller had not yet discovered their tumors. The flood of information and optimistic facts that filled newspapers and magazines after their operations had not yet appeared. There was nothing I had ever come across to show me anything but the shadow of imminent death.

On that awful Saturday night when I discovered the bump, I knew a great deal more about the history of the Arabs on the West Bank in Israel than I did about breast cancer. All I was sure of were the seven danger signals of cancer, and a lump in the breast was definitely one of them.

I can't remember how long I stayed rigid with fear in the tub. Finally Harvey came to remind me that Archie Bunker was about to begin. He opened the bathroom door and poked his head around it.

"What's keeping you?" he asked, annoyed. "Dinner is—"

I must have looked strange, because he stopped in mid-sentence. He came in, shut the door behind him, and forgot dinner and the Bunkers.

"Its cold in here." He reprimanded me gently. "You'll catch pneumonia."

I waved my hand in a weak shrug.

"Is anything wrong?"

"Feel this place," I said, pointing to the suspicious spot.

He leaned over. "I don't feel anything."

"Nothing much could hide in me, could it?" I smiled at our old family joke.

I reached for the bar of soap. "Try feeling the place with some soap on your finger," I said. "See if you can find it now."

Without a question, he did as I asked.

"There's something there," he said in a flat monotone. "You'd better call the doctor first thing Monday morning. Don't put it off."

The rest of the evening and all day Sunday stand out in my memory as hours of bizarre charades. I tried to read the *Washington Post*, cooked breakfast, and even had friends over for an early-summer barbecue—all done automatically. How did I do it?

What else was there to do? The children, of course, knew nothing, and I was reluctant to talk to Harvey about the possibility of having breast cancer. The epidemic that had flared through his family had claimed a cousin and two aunts. In his family, the disease was synonymous with death.

On Monday morning, I began calling my internist's office long before his secretary arrived. I was her first caller.

"I have a lump in my left breast," I told her.

Usually, to be squeezed into Bernie Heckman's busy schedule required at least a massive hemorrhage or a minimum temperature of 106. Perhaps it was his normal policy to examine breast lumps without delay, or maybe it was something urgent in my voice. There was no waiting this time.

"Can you be here at ten?" the secretary asked immediately.

"I'll be there, don't worry."

An hour to wait.

I had read somewhere about a new breast-cancer detection machine, the thermograph, that was being installed at a Washington hospital. I called the hospital and was referred to the American Cancer Society.

"This screening is a joint project of the American Cancer Society and the National Cancer Institute," I was told by a clerk there. "It is for women who have no symptoms at all. I'm afraid—"

"I am not interested in being part of the project," I explained. "I don't need anything to tell me if I have a lump. I can feel it. I just need to know if it's malignant or benign. Can the thermograph do that?"

"That's the whole point of the project," she answered impatiently. "This is what must be evaluated."

Giving up on the American Cancer Society, I called the hospital back. Couldn't they just slip me in? Yes, I'd come in as an outpatient. Yes, I'd be happy to be billed. No, I didn't need anything else.

"Come in Friday, June 21, at 10:00 A.M.," I was finally told. "But you will not be part of the ACS-NCI demonstration project."

That done, I drove off to my internist's office. Although the waiting room was crowded, his nurse escorted me into an examining room as soon as I arrived. Normally, when my doctor looked me over, his face was an expressionless mask that told me nothing. This time I read his signals loud and clear; he didn't like what he was feeling.

"You've never had lumps before, have you?" he queried.

"Never."

"Let's try to get some light on the subject," he joked feebly, turning off the switch. In the darkened room, he flashed a beam of powerful light in the direction of my lump.

"What's that?" I asked.

"Transillumination," he replied. "If it's a fluid-filled cyst or anything hollow, it will show up as a shadow."

"Is it?"

He shook his head. "It looks pretty solid to me."

The knot in my belly tightened and cramped. "What next? I've already made an appointment to get a thermogram at—"

He waved away any thought of the new detection machine. "That's not reliable enough. I'd like you to get a xeromammogram."

"A what?"

"A xeromammogram. It's a new way to take mammograms—pictures of the breasts. They've just installed the equipment at the hospital." Dr. Heckman explained that the full, official name of this new X-ray technique is xero-radiomammography. "But that's a mouthful to say. So most of us just call it xeromammography and xeromammograms. Some even cut it down more—to xerographs and xerograms."

He told me that the basic picture is taken by conventional X-ray machinery, but that the configuration of the breast is then reproduced on paper, instead of on film.

"Is it better than plain X-rays?"

"That's what I've been told," he answered matter-of-factly. "According to what radiologists say, it's more detailed and easier to read."

"Is it accurate?"

He shrugged. "Probably about as accurate as any picture can be. You know," he warned, "even if the reading is negative—which means the lump isn't malignant—the only way to be certain is to cut the thing out and look at it under a microscope."

I nodded.

"No matter what the pictures say, you've got something in that breast that doesn't belong there. It will have to come out."

Again I nodded, this time numbly.

The radiology department tried to set my appointment three weeks away, but with a magic word from Dr. Heckman, I had a slot at one o'clock that afternoon for a mammogram.

He led me to a chair in his office. "It will have to be biopsied," he said gently.

"I guess so."

"Is there anyone you have in mind for the surgery?"

"Just that I want a breast specialist."

"I don't know of anybody in this area who specializes in breasts," he said, surprised.

"I don't want any ordinary surgeon cutting into a possible cancer," I insisted. "It's got to be an oncologist."

He stared at me, amazed that I knew a cancer specialist is called an oncologist.

"I don't know of any oncologist in this area who specializes in breasts," he told me.

"I don't want any ordinary surgeon cutting into a possible cancer," I repeated. "It's got to be an oncologist."

"Why?"

"Well," I reminded him, "I use you—an internist—and not just a general practitioner. You must have learned something more in your two extra years of residency in internal medicine to make you a better doctor than just a GP. No?"

"Sure," he answered emphatically. "But any—"

"No, not *any* general surgeon can do a mastectomy, if I need one. It's got to be an oncologist. How can a person who knows a little bit about cutting everything know as much as someone who does only cancer surgery?"

"I guess you've got a point there," he conceded.

"After all"—I smiled weakly—"if I had a detached retina, you'd send me to an ophthalmologist, wouldn't you?"

"Naturally. I don't know a damned thing about detached retinas, except to recognize one when I see it."

"Then why send me to a general surgeon for cancer?"

He had no answer. For a minute or two, he said nothing. "I know a head, neck, and chest man in town, but no one who works only with breasts."

"There's a whole breast-cancer clinic out at NIH—the National Institutes of Health," I said. "There must be a specialist in breast cancer there."

"If you like a research setup . . ."

"What do you mean?"

"You might wind up being a random sample in some experiment."

"I don't believe that would happen at all," I argued. "I've seen enough clinical trials at Johns Hopkins, when I worked there in psychiatry, to know there's such a thing as 'informed consent'. "

"That's what they say. But some patient has to get the experimental treatment."

"I'll debate all that with you some other time." I waved my hand impatiently. "Right now, all I can say is that a research hospital is the best place for me. They've got the best."

Clearly, he didn't agree. "It's your body," he said. "Whatever you say."

"I'll need a letter to the National Institutes of Health," I told him, not even remembering how I knew. "The law says I'll have to be referred."

"If you know where to find a breast-cancer specialist, I'll write whatever letter you need," he promised.

"I'll find one, don't worry."

"First of all, you have to get that mammogram."

"All right."

"Then we'll worry about the surgeon. If the radiologist is sure it's nothing, all you need is a good general man."

It had been only about a half hour between the time I got to his office and the time I left, but it seemed as if a week had gone by.

The hospital was not far away; it made no sense to go all the way home and back for the xeromammogram. Stiff as a robot, not seeing or hearing anything along the route, I drove to Harvey's office to wait. Several of the people he works with told me afterward that I saw them in the elevator or the corridor without even nodding hello. I'm not surprised; I don't even remember getting there. Somehow, suddenly, I was standing in front of his desk.

"What did Bernie say?"

"He wants to do a xeromammogram."

"A what?"

As accurately as I could, I recited the definition of the new technique.

"What time?"

"One."

"Do you want to go out for some lunch?"

I shook my head. "I don't think anything would stay down—not even Maalox."

Harvey tried his best to be cheerful and nonchalant. "Well, it will just be nothing, and that'll be the end."

"No. Whatever the result is, the lump will have to come out."

"So why get the X-ray taken in the first place?"

"It's something to go on, I guess. And Bernie says it's right about 85 percent of the time. So I'd have some idea in advance about what I want to do."

"What do you mean, what you want to do?"

It was good to talk. I sat down on his visitor's chair. "Well, if it shows up a definite positive, I'm certainly not going to have any hack general surgeon operate on me. How can somebody who knows how to do hernias and gall bladders be an expert in breast cancer?"

After twenty-three years of marriage, Harvey knew my prejudices in favor of specialists well enough not to bother to ask for logic. We had already gone 'round that mulberry bush with miscellaneous children's crises; he had become a convert to specialization.

"It's probably nothing," he insisted. "Remember Joan? And

Nan and Gloria? They all went through the same scare, and it was just a cyst or something."

"But remember that they didn't know it in advance. Every one of them went to sleep on the operating table not knowing whether she'd wake up with one or two. It's only afterward that everything's—"

"Why do you always have to look at the worst side?" Harvey exploded angrily.

"The lump still has got to come out." I almost shouted across the desk. "You're the one who's always telling me about the unreliability of machinery. You're the one who keeps arguing about contingency planning. That's all I'm doing—trying to decide what to do *if*."

Harvey waved his reluctant concession to my attitude. "Okay, what if?"

"First of all, I've scheduled an appointment to have a thermogram."

I described what little I knew about this detection machine which measures heat patterns in the breast. Harvey, an engineer who had had lots of courses in thermodynamics, needed only a sketchy explanation.

"If that's either positive or negative, and if it agrees with the Xerox pictures from the mammogram, the statistics say the diagnosis would be 95 percent reliable."

"Then?"

I took a deep breath. "Well, if they are both negative, I'll go to that guy who did your hernias. He can do the biopsy."

"And if it's positive on both?"

I took a deeper breath. "I'll go to the National Cancer Institute. What's the point of living ten minutes from NIH, the top government medical-research center in the country and not using the place?"

"Can you get in?"

"With all the friends we've got who work there, somebody will have some influence."

"When do you get the thermogram?"

"Friday."

"That's a long time to wait."

"That's okay. There's a lot I've got to learn about breast cancer. I need the time."

Harvey's secretary came in. "There's a call from—"

"Is there a typewriter I can borrow somewhere?" I asked her, getting ready to leave the room.

She nodded. "Sure. Ev is in New York. You can use hers."

I turned back to Harvey. "One thing you can be sure of, nobody's hacking off my breast while I'm unconscious unless I'm convinced that that's the only thing there is to do."

He smiled weakly and picked up his telephone as I left.

In Ev's office, I called some friends, who gave me the names of their friends in the higher echelons of NCI—the cancer Institute of the National Institutes of Health. It was all set. Friday, June 21, at 2:00 P.M., I had an appointment in the breast-tumor clinic. Someone told me what had to be included in my doctor's referral letter, and I typed it out for his signature. I was as efficient and unemotional as the IBM computer clattering at the end of the hall.

"I've got an appointment at NCI right after the thermogram on Friday," I told Harvey. "It'll be a busy day."

"What are you going to do now?" he asked.

"I'm going to ride over and get Bernie Heckman to sign this referral letter," I told him, waving the paper. "Then I'm going to the X-ray clinic and then to the library."

"You'll call me as soon as the thing is done?" he asked.

I smiled. "I doubt that I'll know anything today, but I'll call."

I felt much better. Now that there were things to be done, the knot in my belly had relaxed somewhat. For me, nothing is worse than being pushed or pulled by events, with no gas pedal or brake I can operate myself. With appointments scheduled, a glimmer of plans made, books to read, at least I had my forefinger in my own destiny. I would be no slab of silly-putty to be manipulated helplessly by a pack of doctors.

The referral was signed in minutes, and I was soon waiting in the radiology department of the hospital. The technician was a round, jolly comedian.

"You should have seen the patient before you," she joked. "Hers were so huge I needed to use two plates for each one. It cost her, or her insurance company, twice as much as the regular price."

Her macabre humor was contagious. "Do I get a discount?" I wisecracked. "You're not even using half of each plate."

She thought I was hilarious. "I'll have to remember you too," she roared. "Between the two of you, I'll have a great story to tell in the staff dining room."

I watched her process the photographs of my breasts in the huge, conventional-looking Xerox machine in the corridor. The technique of taking the pictures in the darkened X-ray chamber had not seemed to be any different from old-fashioned mammography, but the rest of the procedure was new to me. The plates are treated with certain chemicals, I learned later, and are put into a specially built photocopier. The result is a carefully detailed blue-and-white image of the breast, showing the delicate network of blood vessels, ducts, and glands, as well as muscle and fat.

To the trained eye, both kinds of mammograms can predict the presence of cancer in about 85 percent of the cases. However, the xeromammogram, according to experts in the detection field, has several advantages. There is more detailed illustration of the structure, and a more objective opinion can be given; the previous experience of the "reader" in interpreting shadows, hollows, and densities is not as vital. Also, the processing takes much less time, and xeromammograms can be available quickly, if needed.

"But is the thing accurate?"

She was defensive about her machine toy. "It's every bit as good as film," she lectured, "and a heck of a lot faster and easier to read. You don't have to wait hours for these things to dry."

Pictures of my breast were sliding from the slot, as quickly as copies of an ordinary letter. I stared at my innards. On one marked with an *L*, I noticed an odd bluish spot that seemed to coincide with my lump's geography. But there was also an odd bluish spot on one marked *R*. There were lots of funny bluish spots on both.

"How does the left one look to you?" I asked anxiously. "I can't see much of a difference."

"That's the boss's job." She grinned, getting back her good humor. "If I could do it, he'd be out of work."

"How long does it take?"

"He usually comes in about two every day to read them," she said. "I'll put yours up front, so he'll be sure to get to it today. Tell your doctor to call about ten tomorrow morning."

"Thanks," I said gratefully. "It's hard to wait."

"Well, you're the only one with a real symptom today. The rest are just routine examinations. They're not as worried."

The session over, I drove to our public library and looked up breast cancer in the card catalogue. There was a listing for just one book—*What Women Should Know About the Breast Cancer Controversy,* by Dr. George Crile, Jr.

I hadn't even known, then, that there *was* a breast-cancer controversy!

Back home, I still had an hour or so before I had to face the chores of dinner. I scooped a hole for myself in my favorite beanbag chair and had finished the book before the dogs began to whimper for their chow. Harvey found me at the can opener.

"You didn't call," he scolded.

"I'm sorry. I guess I forgot, because there was nothing to say except to tell you about the new machine they're using." Knowing his consuming interest in any and all gadgetry, I described the Xerox technique.

"Amazing!" he said, and paused. "But what about you?"

"The technician said to tell Bernie to call about ten tomorrow morning."

"Did you find anything in the library?"

"Mainly that there's a big fight going on over what to do about breast cancer," I told him. "What was done to everybody we know is not necessarily the only way to go."

"There never is an only way to go with anything," he said scientifically. "Everything has an alternative if you look for it."

"I've never heard of doing anything but cutting off the breast and then drying yourself out with X-ray," I replied. "But now there's this Dr. Crile, in Cleveland, who says that sometimes taking out the lump is enough. He's also violently against having X-ray treatments afterward. Besides that, there's more than one operation for taking off—"

"Now, wait a minute, honey," cautioned Harvey, always the scientist. "*His* way may be no good, either. You're going from one extreme to the other. There must be things in the middle. There always are."

By then it was time to eat. We had decided still not to say anything to the children, and the subject was dropped. Later, while I cleaned up the kitchen, Harvey skimmed through Crile's book.

"He's got a great pedigree," he commented, after everyone had disappeared from the immediate vicinity of the kitchen sink. "But he doesn't write like a scientist. He sounds as if he's on some kind of a vendetta because his wife died even though she had her breast taken off."

"He does sound bitter about that," I agreed, "because it was done for nothing. She went through all the pain and mutilation of a mastectomy, and the cancer had already been spreading."

"But when they operated there was no way to know that," he reminded me. "It took five years. Maybe she could have been saved. Maybe it was a freak. You really have got to find out more about it and not go by one man's opinion."

I nodded. "I'll go over to the NIH medical library tomorrow. This is all there was in the public library."

The next day, as soon as the family had left, I drove to the National Institutes of Health and installed myself in a quiet corner of the library (which is open to the public), on a comfortable

leather couch piled high with everything I thought I could deci-
pher on mammary carcinoma—the medical term for breast
cancer.

Before leaving, I had called my internist with the message from
the X-ray technician, and I read with one eye on the clock. My
first question was answered right away: the thing had to come out.
Every scientist was emphatic that even if every possible external
test indicates a lump is nothing to worry about, the only way to
know for sure is to cut it out and look at it under a microscope.
The exceptions are in the cases of young women who grow breast
cysts just as teenagers grow acne. While eighty-five out of every
hundred diagnoses from mammograms are accurate, the other
fifteen are not. How could I know I wasn't one of those fifteen?

I took time out to call about my result. "Everything is fine," Dr.
Heckman's nurse told me. "The radiology department says it's
just benign fibrocystic disease—nothing to worry about."

With the information about "false negatives" fresh in my mind,
however, the news did not fill me with optimism. I was convinced
by now that I would have to undergo a biopsy no matter what the
mammography result was. (As it turned out, I was indeed one of
the fifteen—a "false negative." "It happens," the radiologist told
me casually afterward. "Nothing's perfect. The only way to be
sure is on biopsy.")

According to the literature I was reading in June 1974, two
kinds of biopsies were most popular in the United States. One
was the excisional biopsy. The entire lump, or tumor, is removed
intact, surrounded by some insulating tissue. The other was the
incisional biopsy. Only a part of the tumor is removed. Most
surgeons routinely cut out the whole mass, unless it was very
large. This is still true today.

Afterward, the common practice was to send everything to the
pathology laboratory for fast-freezing—the procedure called a
frozen section—while the patient lay unconscious on the operating table. A slice of the lump was put under the microscope, and
within minutes the surgeon was given the diagnosis. If the tumor
was benign, the incision was closed, and the patient was up and
around in a few hours. However, if it was malignant, most surgeons in the United States performed a radical mastectomy then
and there.

So, in most instances, a woman going to sleep for a simple
biopsy did not know whether she would wake up with two breasts
or one.

(Incidentally, I also learned that the plural—breasts—is not
strictly accurate. The breast is actually a single organ with an

internal crossover between its two segments. For the sake of clarity, however, I have decided not to pay too much attention to this nicety of medical syntax.)

Sometimes, of course, for medical reasons, the biopsy and mastectomy as a single procedure is imperative. For example, if a local anesthetic cannot deaden all pain, necessitating the use of a general anesthetic and the patient has something else wrong that makes her a high surgical risk, one operation is better than two. Certainly, there are women who do not want to go through two surgical procedures and "want to get it all over with" in one. They have the right to chose a single operation.

Under ordinary circumstances, however, I learned that there are advantages to the patient in having a two-stage procedure instead of the one-stage. To me, at that time, the psychological part was the most important. Not to know beforehand what was going to happen was unthinkable. Needing to have a mastectomy would be bad enough, but not to have time to adjust to the idea in advance seemed absolutely barbaric!

Separating the diagnostic biopsy from the mastectomy has benefits for the patient in addition to preventing psychic trauma. The surgeon does not have to make the critical decision on the basis of a quick-frozen section pathological examination but can wait for the more trustworthy permanent section. Although it is rare for the fast method to be inaccurate, it has happened.

Also, the patient can do some research into the various alternatives and decide for herself what she wants to do about the tumor. While anything short of mastectomy was considered very risky in 1974, why should the doctor, husband, father, brother, or whoever make the choice? It is, after all, the woman's life—not someone else's.

Once a decision is made, the woman can shop around for a surgeon. Although a competent general surgeon may do an excellent biopsy, this skill does not mean he will do an excellent—and thorough—piece of cancer surgery. Someone who performs ten mastectomies in the course of a year cannot, understandably, be as experienced as a surgeon who does the operation every day.

These were my reasons for insisting on an interval between the diagnosis and treatment. But later, after my mastectomy, as I learned more and more about "the breast-cancer controversy," I also learned more and more reasons for separating the biopsy from the removal of the breast: the need for staging. But that is getting ahead of my story, and it will be explained in detail in Chapter 8.

What I already had learned made it easy for me to decide about the one-stage versus the two-stage procedure. My lump was tiny, and I was no surgical risk. I made up my mind to have the biopsy first and then wait. After all, the one diagnostic test I had had said it was benign anyhow. (At the time, I was naïve enough to believe that any surgeon would do as I asked. This, I discovered, was more naïve than to believe a radiologist's report is always accurate.)

I read on, anxious to know what oncologists thought about the opinions of their colleague Dr. George Crile.

Apparently, not too much—for some reasons that made sense to me and others that did not. First, there is what is called the multicentricity of breast cancer. Pathologists, specialists in the study of cells and tissues, have proven that many breasts with a cancerous tumor that can be felt or seen also have microscopic clusters of cancer cells that may (or may not) grow to be large cancers. This condition was found in Happy Rockefeller's right breast, for example.

Therefore, oncologists argued, how could Dr. Crile or any surgeon following his theories know that the single lump he removes is all the cancer there is in the breast without examining the organ under a microscope? How could he be sure no cancerous cells were hiding in the hundreds of lobules that make up the breast? How could he tell that no stray cancer cells have escaped from the primary tumor to metastasize, or spread, without removing all or some of the under arm lymph nodes (or glands)?

There was no way then and there still isn't today.

Another of Dr. Crile's arguments against mastectomy was his belief that the lymph nodes of the armpit—a part of the body's first line of defense against infection and other diseases—must *not* be removed.

Dr. Crile argued that if the cancerous lump alone was removed, the immunological apparatus of the lymphatic system is set free to fight stray, malignant cells, and even the invasion of a node or two. He felt that in some patients with early cancer leaving these immunological factories in place might permit the woman's own body to fight any remnants of the cancer that were left behind.

A growing body of evidence, back in 1974, indicated that the immune system does indeed play a major role in preventing cancer and stopping its spread, and perhaps even in causing cancer (by breaking down or becoming weak.) But at that time, this evidence was based on animal models and not humans. Therefore, Dr. Crile's thesis that removing the nodes might do harm to the immune system was not generally accepted. Moreover, some immunologists believe that, as with veins and arteries, the hundreds of other nodes of the lymphatic system throughout the body begin to work harder—within a matter of hours—to compensate for the ones removed from the armpit. However, this also had been shown only in animal models by 1974.*

Of course, these were "preliminary opinions." But all the opinions, including Dr. Crile's, were then too preliminary for me to risk my life on.

And even if I had wanted to go along with his "lumpectomy," I discovered, this kind of surgery was out for me; Dr. Crile himself would not have recommended it in 1974. He wrote: "Cancers that are large in relation to the size of the breast, cancers that are located near the center of the breast . . . are *not* well adapted to treatment by partial mastectomy." Since my unwanted lump bordered the nipple of my left breast, I could not have been a candidate for less than total removal, if I had cancer, even by Dr. Crile's standards.

The problem I would have to face then was not whether to have a mastectomy or not, but what kind of mastectomy, and all mastectomies involve the amputation of that part of our bodies we women know as our breasts. In the one called the simple, or—as doctors now prefer—the total, mastectomy, I learned that only the breast is removed, leaving the nodes intact.

The radical mastectomy is more extensive. In one operation, known as the Halsted or "standard radical," the pectoral muscles of the chest are also removed. In the modified radical mastectomy, (now, total mastectomy with axillary dissection) these are left in place. There are several ways to accomplish this so that any nodes lying under the pectorals can be seen and removed. In the usual modified radical, both of the pectoral muscles, the pectoralis major and minor, are retracted (held back by special instruments); another version, the Patey modified radical, developed in England, requires the muscles to be cut and restitched, if necessary. In all radical mastectomies the nodes in the armpit are cut out.

I absorbed all this with what seems now to have been an almost insane clearheadedness I never could muster while cramming for final exams during my college days.

As I have said, I recognized immediately that anything less than removing the entire breast was out for me, because my lump was located on the edge of the nipple.

---

*This has since been proven in humans, and Dr. Crile now advocates removal of axillary nodes to see if a woman needs further adjuvant treatment, explained in Chapter 11.

Frankly, I could not understand why there was so much medical fuss about leaving the nodes, via the simple (or total) mastectomy, if there was any chance that some of them might be cancerous. The important parts of me, I thought, were the external breast and the internal chest muscles—in that order—yet surgeons and researchers kept arguing about taking out or leaving in the axillary lymph nodes. To me, looking as normal as possible minus the breast, having as little scarring as possible, and getting out all of the cancer were the important issues—not the invisible nodes. Later, I was to learn about the importance of the nodes in avoiding unnecessary "frozen shoulder" and lymphedema— swelling of the arm.

After reading the literature and telephoning some friends at the National Cancer Institute, I made my choice: a modified radical mastectomy, if my lump turned out to be cancer. My breast and lymph nodes would be removed; the chest muscles controlling my left arm would stay with me.

Although 90 percent of the surgeons in the United States who performed mastectomies, in 1974, did the Halsted radical, I could find no cancer expert—in books or by personal questioning—who thought it was necessary to take out the pectoral muscles.

"But it depends on what the surgeon learned in school and during his training," a friend warned. "Don't let any inexperienced guy do you a favor by leaving your muscles alone if all he's ever done in his life are Halsteds. You don't want to be his guinea pig."

Another friend at the NCI agreed. "The Halsted's easier. It's like being a barber. You don't need to be as expert just to shave all the hair off as to give somebody a good-looking cut. And if a surgeon is used to having a clear field of vision, with no muscles in his way," he continued, "he could easily miss a couple of positive nodes."

So I decided it was to be a modified radical mastectomy for me, provided I needed one, even if I had to go to Timbuktu to find an experienced surgeon to do it.

Friday morning came, and the thermogram was taken. In spite of my pleas of urgency, I could get no promise of an early reading. When the result was finally called in to Dr. Heckman weeks later—while I was already recuperating from the mastectomy—it was: "Mildly suspicious neovascularization of the left breast around the areola." This was a bit more accurate than the mammogram, I agree. But my cancerous tumor had been a full-blown, palpable lump, hardly a microscopic discovery. The thermogram, obviously, was not something that could be trusted, either.

I spent the time between the thermogram and my two-o'clock appointment at the breast-tumor clinic of the National Cancer Institute shopping for a new wardrobe of underwear. I had no superstitious premonition; I just had two hours to kill, with Lord & Taylor on my way from the Georgetown University Hospital to NIH. Besides, even an overnight stay in the hospital for a biopsy deserved better than the raggedy old nightgowns I had been wearing. Some wild bikini panties also went into my shopping bag. And I bought two new-style bras that latched in the front, for easier opening and closing.

After a long wait in the breast clinic, I unhappily discovered that becoming a patient in a federal facility means a lot of rigmarole and red tape—even when you have friends working there. Because of certain inflexible rules, no surgeon could put a scalpel to my lump unless and until I underwent considerable preoperative testing and examination, which took about ten days to two weeks. They were also redecorating the operating rooms.

"I thought we weren't supposed to wait," I complained to Dr. Ernest V. deMoss, who examined my lump. "They always say, 'Rush to your physician'."

He smiled. "Don't wait six months," he said. "But ten days won't matter. The tests and scans have to be done in advance."

Dr. deMoss explained that if all the preoperative tests were negative, then an operation would be scheduled. However, if they turned up any sign of existing spread of a malignancy into bones, stomach, or other organs, there was no point in operating at all. "A mastectomy is done to arrest the carcinoma," he said. "If the disease has already metastasized beyond the regional nodes—in your case, the ones in the left axilla—there's no reason to put you through the ordeal at all. We'd go right to chemotherapy."

"But I don't even know that it *is* cancer," I wailed. "The mammogram said benign fibrocystic disease. Do the biopsy, and then we'll worry about your scans and tests."

"What you say makes a lot of sense from an ordinary medical point of view," he conceded. "But this is a research hospital, established by law to conduct clinical trials under certain rather rigid rules. One of these is that every patient must have a complete work-up before anything at all is done, so that we have base-line data on everything." He smiled apologetically. "A good many of the tests might be helpful in other areas of NIH research."

Maybe this was what Dr. Heckman had meant when he so scornfully said "if you like a research setup."

"I don't know if my mind can stand the wait, even if my body can," I said.

Dr. deMoss nodded his agreement. "I understand. If it were my wife, I'd tell her to have the tumor biopsied immediately. Then, if it was diagnosed as carcinoma, she could have the mastectomy without worrying about being in a protocol. That's what we call a clinical trial," he explained, "a protocol. Every one has its own guidelines and requirements here."

Suddenly the almost forgotten cramp in my belly was back. His face, his tone of voice, his attitude, all shouted that, negative mammogram or not, his fingers told him a mastectomy would be needed. For two days I had been unpanicked; now I was again gripped by dread.

"Do you have any friends in private practice?" I asked him.

Dr. deMoss took a pad and wrote down the names of some surgeons he knew in the area who had had considerable cancer training.

"I don't know if they're involved with breasts," he said. "But I've trained with them all in oncology in various places around the country."

My clothes flew on, and I cashed two dollars into dimes. Locking myself into a public phone booth, I started on his list.

"No patient is going to tell me how to do my surgery," one of them growled when I asked for a two-stage operation—biopsy now, mastectomy later. "I've never heard of such a thing."

"You're absolutely ridiculous!" another exploded. "If the diagnosis is positive on frozen section, the breast must come off immediately."

And so it went. It was Friday afternoon; the weekend would be lost!

Frantically, I called Dr. Heckman at 4:50 and outlined what had happened.

"Calm down," he urged. "If you want just the biopsy without a mastectomy, you don't need a cancer specialist. I told you before, any competent surgeon can do that. What about the man who did Harvey's herniorrhaphy?"

He was right, of course. And I had a better chance of getting things done my way with a long-time family surgeon, who had stitched many a child's cut in addition to that hernia.

"Don't be so pessimistic," the surgeon soothed, when I reached him by phone. "You're probably making a mountain out of a molehill. After all, nine out of ten breast lumps are benign. Take it easy." He did want to know why I was so insistent on having the operation done in two stages.

"If the thing is cancer," I told him honestly, "I'm going to NCI or to Sloan-Kettering in New York to find a breast-cancer specialist."

"But the mammogram diagnosed it as benign?"

"Yes," I said. "Otherwise I'd be on a plane up there for the biopsy, too."

He sounded offended. "What do you mean?"

"I'd feel like an idiot, running off to a cancer hospital when the only test there is says it's nothing."

"I think you're being unnecessarily gloomy," he said. "But I'll go along with you. I'm sure it's probably a cyst or something benign."

He kindly met me long after his regular office hours, examined the tumor, tried to aspirate the contents with a hypodermic needle (nothing aspirated), and said he would schedule the biopsy as soon as possible, because hospital beds were in short supply.

"Fine," I agreed.

With the help of a lawyer, I drafted a legal document, to be countersigned by the surgeon before my operation, refusing to authorize him or the hospital to do anything more than a biopsy.

24 June, 1974

Under no circumstance is   or anyone else in the operating room of   to perform the procedure known as mastectomy (removal of either breast).

I hereby release   and all other parties connected with the above consented-to procedure from any liability for damage sustained by me due to my refusal to consent to the performance of mastectomy (removal of either breast).

ROSE KUSHNER

On admission to the hospital the following Tuesday, I scratched lines through the part of the routine form every new patient must sign that gives blanket permission to the doctor and the hospital to do anything "deemed necessary." I also blacked out the part that gives permission to dispose of "the tissue removed." Nobody objected at the time. My surgeon treated the contract as a huge joke, signing it with a flourish as I watched from my stretcher.

"Ready to be put to sleep now, worrywart?" he scolded when I finished rereading it.

Afterward, he was not so flippant. He seemed to take my refusal to let him do the mastectomy as a personal insult, although I had told him more than once that I planned to find a breast-cancer specialist to do it. He must have forgotten; or perhaps he hadn't understood me in the first place.

I was still drifting in and out of anesthetic euphoria when his face appeared, grim and angry, over the rail of my crib.

"I've got bad news," he said. "It's cancer."

Without another word, my noble healer turned away and went to the anteroom with the same message for my worried husband.

One of the nurses told me I had hurt his feelings badly. "He's considered one of the best general surgeons around," she explained.

"I know," I recall telling her sleepily. "But for cancer I want more than a general surgeon."

She patted my hand. "I'd do the same thing in your shoes, Mrs. Kushner," she assured me. "Exactly the same thing."

Since I had not entered a protocol at the National Cancer Institute for the biopsy, it would have taken the intervention of friends to have the mastectomy done there. Besides, July 1 (and the beginning of a new medical and fiscal year) was only a week away, and not even the most influential of friends could get space for me on an operating room schedule upset by vacations, rotating staffs, and new budgets.

"It's almost impossible to expect any action from any government agency at the end of June," one of them told me sadly. "There's nothing I can do now until July 1." Because the biopsy had already been performed, he suggested I not wait. "Nobody's sure about anything, you understand," he explained. "But most experts think a woman shouldn't play around once the tumor is cut out. Something could have been nicked."

I needed no encouragement from anyone. I was ready to run. The day after the biopsy, Harvey and I left for New York, pathology slides and tumor (pickled in formaldehyde) in hand.

Unlike the National Cancer Institute, Memorial Sloan-Kettering Cancer Center is a private institution. A friend at NIH had arranged an appointment for me that same afternoon with one of its top breast-cancer specialists, and before any surgery could be scheduled, I first had to be examined by him in his office. Of course, I already knew the diagnosis was carcinoma. I was still groggy from the general anesthetic as I listened to the surgeon tell me what he would do.

"There will be a diagonal incision. I'll excise the breast, axillary nodes, pectoral muscles, and pectoral nodes," he said in a monotone. "You will have some numbness for a variable period of time. There will be some temporary muscular disability, which can be overcome with proper exercise, but some permanent disability in your left arm may remain. There may also be some permanent swelling. This varies."

The room was quiet and his voice was soft. In the state I was in, his words barely penetrated. The only things I remember hearing were "Fourth of July . . . shortage of staff . . . new interns and residents . . . no beds."

The important words, "Halsted radical," were never mentioned, and so I never heard them.

We left the office, with the nurse promising to get me a bed as soon as possible. It was not until I had had two sips of a very strong Scotch back in our hotel that the full meaning of what the doctor had said entered my befuddled brain.

"He wants to do a Halsted," I told Harvey weakly. "That's what he meant by the pectoral muscles and permanent disability. It didn't sink in."

"I've been calling all over to see if anybody I know has influence with Sloan-Kettering, so we can get you in right away," he said.

"Forget it! I'm not having a Halsted. We've got to find out where I can get a modified."

I was so terrified by the surgeon's quiet description of the Halsted he proposed to do that it never occurred to me to ask if someone at Sloan-Kettering would do a modified radical mastectomy instead. In my panicky state, I assumed it was standard hospital policy to do Halsteds, not a matter of a surgeon's personal preference.

After some frantic telephoning, a business associate in the New York office of Harvey's firm gave me the name of an internist in Manhattan, who referred me to the Roswell Park Memorial Institute, in Buffalo, where, he told me, Halsteds are never done. Roswell Park, a New York State hospital, is the oldest cancer hospital in the world, dating back to 1895—and, as I was to learn, is one of the best there is. We flew up to Buffalo that same evening, and I was examined the next morning by Dr. Thomas L. Dao.

Under the direction of Dr. Dao, who is chief of both breast-cancer surgery and breast-cancer research, I was X-rayed and tested in advance, as the National Cancer Institute surgeon had told me I should be. That took two days. By the time Dr. Dao came in to announce that I "could be scheduled for surgery," that "everything was clear and clean," being a suitable candidate for mastectomy was the best news anyone could have given me.

Unfortunately, the importance of doing an estrogen-receptor assay for my tumor's hormone dependency had not yet filtered down to suburban Maryland in 1974. I still do not know if it was estrogen-positive or negative—an omission that distressed Dr. Dao very much.

But he did many tests to be sure the lump was the only cancer present. As I had learned all too well by then, breast-cancer experts do not perform any mastectomy if there are signs that the malignancy has metastasized beyond the regional nodes, since it is pointless to put a woman through major surgery when the cancer has already spread. So my good test results meant that—as far as any mortal could determine in advance—the little centimeter-long tumor removed in the biopsy had been all there was. It had been caught in time. But, in 1974, Dr. Dao felt a mastectomy still had to be done, in the event I had any multicentricles—those microscopic scattered cancers that often grow, along with the big one, in other parts of the breast. And the radical part of the mastectomy—removing the lymph nodes in the armpit—was necessary, to know if the nodes had been invaded.

Suddenly, surprisingly, hilariously, being able to have a mastectomy had become good news! As they say, everything is relative.

Harvey bought a bottle, and we had a party in the "cancer ward" to celebrate my eligibility for mastectomy!

The operation was long and tedious for Dr. Dao, but uneventful for the rest of the twelve-man team. None of my nodes was malignant on gross examination—to the naked eye, without a microscope—and there weren't any visible pieces of tumor that could be retrieved to do the estrogen-receptor assay. Dr. Dao came into my room grinning as I woke up. "I couldn't even find a little bit. There was absolutely nothing. If anything has spread to the nodes, it was microscopic."

My physical recovery is described in another chapter, and the psychological details are elsewhere, too. But I am going to talk here about one aspect of my experience as a cancer patient, because going to a research hospital is so frowned upon by many doctors, and because these institutions so often are thought of as last resorts for hopeless cases.

I admit that my first half day in Roswell Park was a difficult adjustment. All I could think of was Alexander Solzhenitsyn's *Cancer Ward;* I didn't belong with all these people. Although few had any visible signs of being cancerous, *I* knew they were. Why was I here?

It took a while to accept the fact that I did belong. In retrospect, it was only a few hours before I began to realize the benefits of being in a cancer ward. The first advantage was the incredibly sensitive care everyone gave every patient. From the cleaning staff up to the top physicians, all were specially trained to deal with patients who have a potentially fatal disease. The treatment was a combination of intensive attention to the most insignificant symptom and the almost pitiless realism that "Everyone has to die sometime." The entire staff had been taught how to live with the prospect of death, and the patients were the beneficiaries.

Second, I had the support and comfort of people who had lived with cancer as long as twelve years. A plumber who had been brought in as terminal years before puffed on his cigar while he described the advanced treatments—available only at places like Roswell Park, treatments that had kept him alive, reasonably well, and still plumbing more than a decade after that diagnosis. In the course of his years of intermittent care at Roswell Park, he told me, he had developed and regressed at least sixteen cancerous tumors throughout his body.

It is a personal decision whether or not to go to a research hospital. Institutions like Roswell Park do make certain demands on patients that non-research hospitals do not. Physicians, nurses, psychologists, and social workers often interview and question patients. Members of the medical staff may want to examine their wounds; many people object to being handled, except for emergency care, by anyone but their private physicians. For all I know, I may have been part of a "random sample." My operation may have been done using a new type of scalpel, while samples of other women were cut by a standard-type instrument. I honestly don't know. But what difference does it make?

If anything untried and unproven—and with possibly serious consequences—is to be done, patients or their families must give what is called "informed consent." The experimental procedure must be explained, as well as the reasons the physician feels it should be done. Papers are signed by the patient or the family to authorize any extraordinary treatments. This was not necessary in my case; the mastectomy was quite humdrum.

I also want to stress the value of breast self-examination (BSE) and mammography. Although the technique did not diagnose my own cancer accurately, the mammogram (xero- or conventional) is the best external detection technique available today. Even the best mammography can give a "false negative" diagnosis, and that is why I say—as strongly as possible—that all strange lumps should be removed, no matter what the tests show. (A woman who is constantly "lumpy" or "cystic" is one of the few exceptions to this rule.)

I do not doubt now that there were surgical treatments available in 1974, other than the modified radical mastectomy, that would probably have been just as effective in treating my own cancer. But these less-than-mastectomy procedures had simply not been done long enough with large enough numbers of women to have yielded the kind of long-term survival rates that might have tempted me to risk my life. Now that more data have been accumulated from more women over more years, I believe that removing my breast and axillary nodes may well have been "over-treatment." There is no point in looking back, however, to dwell on what-might-have-been, "if only . . ."

There are still thousands of polio victims living paralyzed lives, in and out of iron-lung machines, because they contracted the disease before the Salk vaccine was developed. Medicine and science must progress, and there will always be advances that will make former treatments obsolete. The important thing is that what I chose was my own decision.

I must add here, for women's liberationists who see an evil plot to mutilate women by mastectomy, that I found none—anywhere. There has definitely been male chauvinism—enough to warrant a separate chapter later. But I found no one like Dr. Towers, the sadistic surgeon Henry Bellaman describes in his novel *King's Row*. I found no surgeons, male or female, who had any doubts that radical mastectomy offered women their best chance to survive breast cancer. This—not male chauvinism—is why mastectomies were recommended by almost all surgeons. In 1974, the controversial issues were separating the diagnostic biopsy from mastectomy, what kind of mastectomy should be performed, and who should decide. In my case, the choices were my own.

My ideas may differ from those of other women, but the point of this book is to show that we women should be free, knowledgeable, and completely conscious when the time comes for a decision, so that we can make it for ourselves. *Our* lives are at stake, not a surgeon's.

My experience is no model of what to do or not to do. It is only one example of what women can do—if they have some information to go on.

It also does no harm to have a streak of stubbornness, and a loud voice as well.

Epilogue to
Chapter 1

"It's far away from the incision," Dr. Teunis assured me, "and it's soft and rubbery, like putty. Cancer never feels like this."

My doubts must have shown on my face.

"It's only a little infection, Rose," he insisted, "and I wouldn't even dignify this zitz by calling it a complication. You know this kind of thing can happen after any surgery. I'll drain it and give you an antibiotic. It'll be gone in a couple of days."

It was almost Hallowe'en, 1981. A month earlier, I looked at my nude self in the mirror one morning and saw bony ribs where a curved, saline-filled hemisphere had been the night before.

The implant had sprung a leak.

"It happens," Dr. Scott Teunis, the plastic surgeon who had sculpted the soft mound on the flat half of my chest four years earlier, said. He answered my frantic telephone call calmly, as if he'd done it many times before.

"The deflation rate on those all-saline implants is just too damned high, and that's why we're using bi-lumens now."

He told me bi-lumen implants are still covered with the same material, Silastic, but that their innards contain cores of silicone floating in saline. While a bi-lumen's fluid could conceivably dribble into my body, as the saline of the first one had done, it couldn't suddenly become a thin crepe. The silicone helps the implant stay shapely.

"And we've added some steroids to the salt water to keep the contracture rate lower than it was with all-silicone implants," he explained. "So far, they've been pretty good."

I made an appointment with his secretary to have a new implant inserted and the flat flaps of Silastic taken out.

"What a mess," I complained to Harvey. "I don't even remember where I put the old dingbat I wore inside my brassiere."

24

Finally, I found it under a pile of unused boxes of soap I'd brought back from hotels and motels around the world.

The whole business was an inconvenient nuisance, coming as it did during the Jewish High Holidays. All our plans would have to be changed while I convalesced from another operation.

I scheduled the replacement surgery to be done in Dr. Teunis' office, not in a hospital where my original reconstruction mammoplasty had been done.

"This isn't any big deal," he told me. "Slipping a second implant under the muscle is easy. It only takes about an hour."

I wondered how Dr. Teunis could do a surgical procedure in the cubicle where I had always been checked. On operation day, however, I discovered that—like many plastic surgeons—he had a completely equipped operating room in his suite for patients who don't want hospital records to tell anyone their cosmetic secrets.

As he predicted, it was no big deal. My pectoral muscles were well stretched and accustomed to a 450 gm bag of water tucked underneath them. Within a week I was back at work, and the external prosthesis went back to its hiding place under Hyatt and Mariott bars of soap. When Dr. Teunis took out the last of the sutures, I saw that the incision was less apparent than it had been. He used my disaster to trim some extra scar tissue and narrow the edges.

I found the pimple the way I found the first lump, when I was taking an early evening bath (Maybe I should switch to showers?), and that's all it was: a common, ordinary adolescent-skin-type zitz glowing bright red about four inches southwest of my adam's apple. I smothered it with Bacitracin, covered it and tried to forget it. But even protected by the Sheer-Strip, the thing was exquisitely tender. Even the slight, light touch of a sheer nightgown made it hurt. It wouldn't let me forget.

By the time the adhesive was washed off by a week's worth of baths, the zitz had developed a white head, and the rest of it was bigger and brighter. Although it wasn't in the incision, an ominous place to have anything after any cancer surgery, I worried about it and decided to take the thing back to Dr. Teunis.

He did his best to convince me, and, of course, I wanted to believe him.

"Honest," he said, "it just can't be anything serious."

And, I reminded myself, it hurts. Everyone knows early cancer doesn't hurt.

I took the capsules he prescribed, and as Dr. Teunis predicted, the glowing red and white pimple was gone by the end of the week. But a colorless, sore knot stayed behind.

"How about taking it out," I asked him when I returned to be checked. "It's bothering me."

"You're over-reacting, Rose. If it wasn't tender, I wouldn't hestitate. But I'm sure it'll go away by itself, and doing a biopsy right there over

your sternum could leave you with a hell of a scar right in the middle of your trademark. How would that look on TV?"

During my visit to Buffalo the following January, Dr. Dao examined the spot, and he also thought it was nothing.

"I'm sure it's a sebaceous cyst caused by an internal suture you got when you had the implant replaced," he said. "All your test results were negative, so forget about it. And keep your fingers off it. If you keep rubbing it, it will never get better."

But I couldn't stop thinking about the knot even though I was busy planning for the April publication of Why Me? In the back of my mind, I decided that if it was still there when the book's promotion tour was over, I'd order Dr. Teunis to take it out if I had to.

The last TV show was taped on May 25th, and the thing was still in the skin of my chest. I called him to insist on a biopsy, but I got no argument. Immediately, Dr. Teunis scheduled surgery to be done on June 10th in the same facelift operating room in his suite.

"This will take about an hour," he told Harvey. "I want to be real careful with that fine-line incision and make it pretty."

The local anesthetic froze me immediately, and Dr. Teunis delicately tipped the scapel into my skin. I felt only slight pressure as he first cut two curves, like parentheses, and then scooped something from the ellipse in the cleavage he had given me four years earlier. He put a gray dab of jelly on a towel-covered tray near the operating table. I sensed he didn't like what he saw.

"I'll get this right over to the lab and have an answer tomorrow," he said, closing the incision with a needle as slender as a hair. "I don't want you to go through a weekend of waiting."

But his face had already given me the diagnosis.

Although he sent the specimen by courier, I had to wait a day and a weekend for the pathology report. On Monday, June 14, 1982, Dr. Teunis called with the devastating diagnosis.

"I'm sorry to have to tell you this, Rose," he told me softly. "I could've sworn it was a sebaceous cyst....just a 'zitz'. Something must have kicked up a dormant cell that's been around on your skin for eight years."

He paused. "But I knew the minute I cut into it. It was too hard and gritty to be anything but cancer."

I grabbed for a slim shred of a straw.

"What lab did you send it to? Maybe they made a mistake."

But, somehow, I knew it was cancer and had known it ever since the thing had sprouted eight months earlier.

How could it be?

Five years means cure: everyone knows that. After five years, I—like most women who develop breast cancer—was sure I was out-of-the-woods; after seven years; I had stopped counting. Yet it had come back: "Mammary adenocarcinoma, consistent with metastatic breast cancer."

I had been sure it was malignant, but it never occurred to me that it was a metastasis—a spread from the original tumor that had been removed in a mastectomy in 1974.

Harvey had heard the report on the kitchen extension and quickly came into my office to wrap his arms around me. "They can't know," he said. "You didn't believe the first path report. Why believe this one? We've got to get some other opinions."

Still numb, I nodded. "Scott was so sure it was nothing that I didn't think to ask him to send the thing to the NCI. I didn't tell him to have dry ice to freeze it for estrogen-receptors either."

Harvey had gotten the lab's telephone number from Dr. Teunis.

"Call up and tell them we're coming for the slides," he ordered. "It might be a mistake." After thirty years, he knew the best medicine for me is to give me something to do.

The drive to the lab in Virginia seemed to take us to the end of the planet.

"I hope we're wrong," the nurse-receptionist said kindly. "It can happen, even with the best, you know."

I thanked her for her optimism but doubted it. Errors are often made with rare cancers, but mine was a "common garden variety" duct-cell adenocarcinoma. It was unlikely that a pathology freshman could miss it. A more realistic hope was that it wasn't a metastasis but a second primary made up of entirely different cells. After all, this pathologist had never seen the original cancer. As Harvey said, how could he know?

I felt better: there were places to go and things to do. With the slides and report firmly in my hands, Harvey started the car.

"Where to now?"

Unlike 1974, I wasn't just a medical writer who was lucky to live near the NIH library anymore. By 1982, I knew almost everyone involved in breast cancer at the NCI and had lots of experts to turn to.

"Bethesda."

Without a word, Harvey made a U-turn, and we drove north to Maryland.

I called Dr. Pietro Gullino, Chief of the Institute's Department of Pathophysiology, from a lobby telephone, and he took the small box from me as soon as we appeared at his office door. With both of us trailing behind, he charged down two flights of backstairs to his favorite microscope.

"Well-differentiated," he commented, "and incompletely surrounded by lymphocytes. Look and see."

"Is it a metastasis or a new primary?" I asked.

"It's impossible to say without seeing tissue from the original tumor," he answered, exactly as we'd hoped. "I must see slides from the blocks of your first biopsy to make a comparison."

Harvey was right. How could a small surburban lab have been so positive when an NCI expert needed the blocks to be sure?

Specimens of surgically removed tissue are put into wax (hence the term, "paraffin section") and kept in backrooms and basements of hospitals for years, often decades. Required by law in some states, most institutions keep them for research or, as in my case, to make new slides for future comparisons. These tissue tombs are, in medical/surgical jargon, called "blocks," and as a rule, they're not released to patients.

Again I was lucky. A friend, Dr. Cecil Fox at the Armed Forces Institute of Pathology, called the hospital where I had had the 1974 biopsy and requested that the block be sent to the AFIP—probably the best pathology lab in the world.

After it arrived, Dr. Fox and Dr. Henry Norris, the AFIP's Chief of Breast Pathology, made new slides from sections of the first cancer, coloring the tissue with special stains to see each cell in detail.

"Your surgeon sure did a thorough job," Dr. Norris said. "He didn't leave a bit of breast tissue for a new cancer to grow in."

He looked up from his microscope. "The new cells look just like the ones in your first tumor."

Instantly, the cramp came back. The Virginia lab's diagnosis had been right after all: it was a metastasis.

Dr. Norris didn't let me panic. Instead, he talked to us as if we were seeing him about a bad cold.

"I guess you'd better get some exams now to be sure this little thing is all there is. If this is it, a little sprinkle of X-ray over your chest should be all you need."

The exams he recommended are the same tests used for "staging" (Chapter 8), and in medicalese, they're usually called "work-ups." Since I was a subject in some NCI studies, I had many of my scans done in Bethesda, saving me an overnight stay in Buffalo. But now it was critical, not just convenient, to use the same equipment so a comparison with my previous scans was as accurate as possible.

In spite of hearing from Dr. Norris that this cancer had, indeed, spread from the first, we got the feeling from his calm voice that it wasn't so dire after all. And Dr. Dao, who had more than 35 years of breast-cancer experience, had told us by telephone that a skin metastasis, after eight disease-free years, isn't the same grim omen as a recurrence found after only a year or two.

So three days later, by the time my appointment in Nuclear Medicine for the scans was scheduled, my nerves had settled down. Harvey, like most husbands, reflected my mood, and we were sure the gamma photos wouldn't show anything.

We had decided to leave the "sprinkle of X-ray" up to Dr. Dao. To believe there was only one lone cancer cell on the skin of my chest, waiting to spring into action after eight years, was as unlikely as thinking our planet Earth has the only life in the universe. This is why Dr. Norris sug-

*gested radiation: to make sure any other cells lying in wait would be zap-
ped to death. But Dr. Dao, I knew, had fought against unnecessary X-ray
therapy as long ago as the 1950s. If he thought I needed radiation, then I
really had to have it.*

*My scans were, as doctors say, "unremarkable," and I spent the rest of
the day cooking a celebration dinner. Before Harvey came home from
work, Dr. Gerald Johnston, who had recently retired from being chief of
the NIH Nuclear Medicine Department, telephoned.*

*"You know that funny little hot-spot you've had on your sternum all
these years?" he said.*

I froze.

*"Well, it's been sitting on your breastbone right under the place where
that new lump grew."*

Harvey still hadn't come home; I was alone in the house.

"What does that mean?"

*"Well," he answered matter-of-factly, "maybe you ought to have Tom
go in there and see what's going on. It's too close for comfort."*

"Do you think the skin cancer could have come from the bone?"

*"With breast cancer, anything's possible, Rose," he said. "I just think
Tom ought to take a look-see."*

*Until 1979, the hot-spot had not appeared on any of the scans I'd had at
the NCI. Then an ultra-modern scanner was put into Nuclear Medicine, a
scanner so sensitive it showed a hole in my shin left by a dart thrown by my
brother when I was five years old. When the spot on the sternum was seen
the first time, Dr. Dao ordered X-rays, and these were all clear. Everyone
then decided that, like the tiny scar from the dart, it had always been there
but the old machine wasn't sophisticated enough to show it.*

*The skin metastasis suddenly made the hot-spot suspicious, because it
could mean there was a cancer in my breastbone that was growing upward.*

*Anxiously, I waited for the busy signal to end. I finally sneaked past Dr.
Dao's teenagers and told him about Jerry's fear. He remembered the wor-
risome spot.*

*"That place is too small for a needle biopsy," he said. "I'm sure it
would be missed. If you want a surgical biopsy, I'll do it, but I don't see
how it could be cancer. You have had no pain, and that place has been
there for years without growing or spreading. That doesn't sound like
breast cancer metastatic to the bone."*

*He also told me he saw no point in doing any diagnostic procedure
unless it affected the way a patient's treatment is decided.*

*"The most I would give you is some radiation, no matter what a bone
biopsy says," Dr. Dao told me. "So why take the risk of giving you
another infection? That operation to reinsert the implant is probably what
caused the skin tumor in the first place. Cancer thrives on infectious tissue,
you know."*

As I knew from past experiences, he was right. I'd read papers im-

plicating infections in the growth of cancer, and a friend, Dr. Isaiah Fidler, whose work is studying metastases, had suggested that the second surgery might have triggered the recurrence.

How could I know what that hot-spot was without a biopsy? After talking to Drs. Dao and Fidler, I knew another operation and possible infection (and possible recurrence) was out of the question.

Maybe a three-dimensional X-ray, a CAT scan, could tell?

Drs. Eli Glatstein and Allen Lichter in the NCI's Radiation Oncology section didn't think so.

"A CAT might give you a definite diagnosis," Dr. Lichter said. "Or it might not show anything an ordinary X-ray wouldn't show."

"You'd probably be right back where you are now," Dr. Glatstein added, "needing a biopsy to be sure."

Both agreed that "a sprinkle" of X-ray was a good idea.

"What's a sprinkle?" I asked Dr. Lichter

"Four to five thousand rads over six _____ ess might do more harm than good by damaging cancer cells inste _____ stroying them."

"Will X-ray help if there's cancer in my sternum?"

"If it hurts, radiation would shrink the tumor and palliate the pain, but you might need systemic treatment. Why don't you talk to a medical oncologist?"

A visit to a chemotherapist showed me that treatment for a late skin recurrence is still a mystery, and there's a tangled snarl of medical opinion about what to do. If all the drugs, hormones, anti-estrogens and immune boosters—in varying combinations, doses and schedules—now being used are spread on a chart, the permutations and combinations of possible regimens would have to be calculated by a fourth-generation computer.

While the three medical oncologists I asked all agreed that I needed chemotherapy, they didn't agree on what drugs to use.

One conversation went like this.

"You definitely need aggressive chemo. That's the whole point of adjuvant therapy—to hit cancer cells hard when the primary tumor burden is very small."

"But I don't need adjuvant therapy," I protested, "I've gone eight years without anything."

"When drugs are given to women who recur," he said, "we call it 'pseudo-adjuvant' therapy. We're giving patients FAC."

FAC is oncological shorthand for 5-Fluorouracil Adriamycin and Cytoxan—a combination guaranteed to make me bald and nauseous.

"That's hitting a mosquito with a Sherman tank," I joked feebly. "What's left if this concoction doesn't work?"

"There are other effective drugs that can be used."

"Is FAC working as a pseudo-adjuvant?"

"It's too soon to know."

"How long have you been using it?"

"About three or four months."

"On women that had no trouble for eight years?"

"No one in the study has been disease-free that long."

"I'm not going to take FAC for a four-millimeter skin cancer that's already been cut out and a hot-spot that's been on my scan for three years without causing any trouble," I cried.

"Look Rose," he said gently, *"even if the spot on the bone is nothing, you're Stage IV metastatic now, because the skin is another organ. What has always been called a 'local recurrence' is really a signal that there are micrometastases somewhere else."*

"Are you giving FAC to postmenopausal women who are ER-rich?"

"Right now, we're not stratifying women according to their receptor status," he said, *"and patients who recur are being randomized into either FAC or observation only."*

Of course, I hadn't had an ERA in 1974. And the second tumor was so small there wouldn't have been enough tissue for the test, even if Dr. Teunis had had dry ice in his operating room.

"I don't know my ERs," I said, *"but Tom Dao thinks going eight years with no problem must mean my tumor had a lot of receptors."*

"If you're wondering about tamoxifen," he continued patiently, *"data predict TAM would hold you for, maybe, fourteen months and then you'd relapse. By getting FAC now, when so few cancer cells are in your body that there are no symptoms, you might get a 100 per cent cell kill."*

"What about the studies showing that drugs change DNA and start a drug-resistant strain that no other drug can kill?"

"There are such data, but they're preliminary."

"So I'm between a rock and a hard place."

"I've told you all there is to know."

It was all there was to know. He was using FAC; most oncologists would have suggested the "standard" CMF combination; others CMFVP (Vincristine and Prednisone added). Some added immune boosters like BCG (bacillus calmette guerin); there's also levamisole and chlorambucil, ad infinitum. *The same substances used as adjuvant therapy are used for advanced disease, and there are tons of data from clinical trials about various dosages, schedules and durations of therapy.*

For treating recurrences, however, there was no study that had any long-term (i.e., five-year) data. This was especially true about late, local-regional recurrences. While almost every doctor had some patients who were "cured" only to have their disease return after five or ten years, I found no data about any therapy except radiation. There were none about the value of chemotherapy for "long-term survivors."

Even a name for the thing on my chest was controversial. Was it a Stage IV metastasis? Technically, yes, because it was in the skin—another organ. Then what is a "local-regional recurrence?" Does the time between primary treatment and recurrence change a woman's prognosis? Is sur-

vival different if it's a local-regional recurrence and not a metastasis?

This wasn't the first time I'd asked these questions. Long before the thing on my chest was finally diagnosed, I had been worried about the rush to routine radical adjuvant chemotherapy for all women. Science magazine, a respected weekly journal, published an article as early as March 12, 1976 cautioning readers about being too optimistic about such drug use. The title, "Breast Cancer: Reports of New Therapy are Greatly Exaggerated," is self-explanatory.

After the Bonadonna et al *study in Milan was reported in early 1976, its results were challenged by many breast-cancer experts. The trial's data were based on an average of fourteen months of treatment, and—according to too many critics to list—this wasn't enough time to draw any conclusions.

Dr. Antonio Rodriguez-Antunez, of the Cleveland Clinic, began a still-ongoing literary battle against indiscriminate chemotherapy by writing a paper, "The Triumphalistic Oncologist," that appeared in the April, 1978 issue of *Surgery. From England, I read articles by Drs. Trevor Powles and Michael Baum challenging U.S. doctors' immediate adoption of CMF as standard treatment for all Stage II breast-cancer patients. Dr. Stephen Carter—an associate director at the NCI when the Milan trial was initially funded—wrote an article, "Adjuvant Chemotherapy of Breast Cancer," with a disappointed tone, for a January, 1981 issue of the* New England Journal of Medicine.

As much as I wanted to believe adjuvant chemotherapy would cure breast cancer, all of this was enough to make me think the high-flying balloon of optimism about it would eventually pop—just as my saline-filled implant eventually popped.

But, of course, I had no data to back writing negatively about adjuvant therapy for the same reason no one should have been so positive: there had simply not been enough time. This is why, when I wrote Chapter 11 in December 1981, I merely mentioned two clinical trials (NSABP and Hubay) where cytotoxic adjuvant chemotherapy was being compared with the same drugs plus tamoxifen. Data from both suggested it was the tamoxifen that was delaying recurrences in ER-rich postmenopausal women, and not the cytotoxic drugs.

Since these data were also too raw, I wrote only that adjuvant chemotherapy for postmenopausal women was controversial.

Then I began to get letters. In early 1982, Dr. Dao wrote me "officially" as a member of the National Cancer Advisory Board to ask that something be done about automatic adjuvant chemotherapy. Women referred to Roswell Park, he said, weren't responding to anything, and he blamed adjuvant chemo for making them drug-resistant.

I took Dr. Dao's letter to the next Board meeting to help slow down an NCI program that might have hurried premature use of the drugs by doctors in general practice. (This program was tamed, by the way, because no member of the NCAB wanted to take experimental therapies to community settings before they were proven to be as safe and effective as possible by controlled clinical trials.)

By then, the American College of Surgeons' hospital survey reported that 22 per cent of all breast-cancer patients had received adjuvant chemotherapy in 1981, up from seven per cent in 1976. The use of drugs in the United States had risen quickly.

But not in other countries.

Thanks to Dr. Robert Keating of the International Cancer Research Data Bank (who still sends me regular packages of computer print-outs on the subject), I've been able to follow results from trials going on in other countries as well as in the United States.

There has been a continuing war in foreign journals about the premature use of the Milan data in this country. More recently, eminent U.S. cancer biostatisticians like Drs. Marvin Zelen of Harvard, David Byar of the NCI and Alvin Feinstein of Yale have become critical of our doctors' unusually hasty acceptance of the Italian results.

I might have written these off as everyday American chauvinism, except that The Lancet, on July 31, 1982, published a paper from the Instituto de Ricerche Farmacologiche 'Mario Negri' in Milan. In the article, "Quality of Breast-Cancer Care in Italian General Hospitals," the authors (A. Liberati, F. Columbo et al) described medical record-keeping for 2,406 women in 31 hospitals and wrote that the situation they found showed, "Careless organisation and documentation of clinical activity...."

From the beginning of the brouhaha about the Milan data, I had trouble understanding how they could have such high "overall" survival rates from such a young trial. In breast cancer, five years are nothing; ten may be significant. But probably fifteen or even twenty years will have to pass before a genuine survival advantage from anything can be determined.

In the past, two clinical trials proved the inaccuracy of projecting 10-year survivals from 5-year data: the NSABP's studies to evaluate adjuvant ovariectomy and radiation. Both showed that more treated women lived five years than those who had no treatment. But at ten years, the benefit was lost. The 10-year survival rates of the women who got adjuvant radiation were actually worse.

Since the Italian Cancer Institute, like the NCI, has patients from the entire country, it was hard to believe that all women who recurred went back to Milan for treatment. In the U.S. trials, this is a common problem: patients who recur blame whatever therapy they were given and don't want to use the same doctors. Why should it be different in Italy? And, if so, how do the scientists in Milan know what was done afterward? It might have been a "second-line therapy," like ovariectomy, that was responsible for patients' longer survivals, and not the drugs they received in the adjuvant trial in Milan.

After reading The Lancet *paper by Italian doctors about their own hospitals, the old adage, "You can make statistics say whatever you want them to say," answered my questions.*

Everyone who has gotten this far in Alternatives *knows I was prejudiced against adjuvant chemo for ER-rich, post-menopausal patients long before I had to weigh alternatives for myself. Followup data from most adjuvant trials, including CMF, showed that drugs just don't help postmenopausal women very much. Older, Stage II women do just as well, if not better, by taking tamoxifen.*

Why?

Since the beginning of chemotherapy, certain second cancers, especially leukemia, have been linked with alkylating drugs like cyclophosphamide and phenylalanine mustard. While benefit must always be weighed against risk (It makes no sense to be afraid of developing leukemia in ten years if a woman has a fast-growing, life-threatening tumor.), postmenopausal, ER-rich women with 1-3 nodes are at relatively low risk of recurring. Why subject them to the side-effects of adjuvant chemotherapy with an added risk of another cancer if drugs are only "of marginal benefit?"

And Dr. Dao's belief that the chemicals themselves create mutant strains of new drug-resistant cells has been proven by research of Drs. James Goldie, Andrew Coldman and Victor Ling in Canada. In the 1940's and 1950s, bacteria developed such resistance because of the indiscriminate use of antibiotics, and this discovery earned Drs. Salvador Luria and Max Delbruck Nobel Prizes in 1969. Nowadays, these powerful weapons against infections are used for serious problems and not for colds and flu.

Again, why should low-risk women take the chance? They may need FAC someday, and it might not work.

All of this information went into my mental equation about what to do for my own problem.

Dr. Dao wanted only careful followup, but I'm not equipped temperamentally to watch and wait for an ax to fall without doing something. If there had been a clinical trial for late recurrers, I would have signed up. But there wasn't.

In August, 1982, I decided to gamble (That's what all breast-cancer patients must do today.) on taking only tamoxifen. A month later, the XIIIth International Cancer Congress was held in Seattle and was followed by a special breast-cancer symposium in Jasper, in the Canadian Rockies. I re-met Dr. Trevor Powles, met Dr. Michael Baum and other experts from abroad. Although I admit they told me what I wanted to hear (that I made the right decision), it was good to have their statistics as well as their moral support.

At the Jasper meeting, Dr. Diana Brinkley, a radiotherapist at the King's College Hospital in London, listened to several U.S. medical on-cologists recite remarkable results from regimens in certain subsets of women. She stood patiently, waiting her turn at the microphone, during the discussion period. Then quietly, she made her comment.

"It appears to me that in America, many women are suffering for the possible benefit of a very few."

Her remark sums up the situation in this country.

Postmenopausal, ER-rich women who received adjuvant chemotherapy must understand that doctors follow standards set by experts in a field, and adjuvant chemo was routine after 1976. But thanks to clinical trials, standards change; no-treatment controls are again "ethical." I urge women in this category, who are referred for adjuvant therapy, to call the NCI (Ms. Betty MacVicar: 301-496-5583) for information about clinical trials near their homes.

In October 1982, I visited Dr. Michael Shimkin, a Founding Father of the NCI, in San Diego. He was annoyed with me and Why Me?

"Why didn't you tell the chemotherapy story like it is? You could have done women a lot of good."

"There weren't enough data yet in 1981."

"You'd better be sure to do it when you revise the book next time," he ordered. *"There will be plenty of data by then."*

I hope I have.

2

What Is Cancer?
What Is Breast Cancer?

Vung Tau, South Vietnam, October 22, 1967: The short, square-faced Vietnamese major, wearing the black pajamas of the Revolutionary Development Cadré, was briefing the press (me).

"Mao Tsé-tung has written that the insurgent guerrilla is a fish, and the people are the water that nourishes the fish," Major Nguyen Bé chanted. "I would like to change Chairman Mao's quotation." He smiled.

"To me, an insurgent is like a fragment of cancer in a healthy body—invading, destroying, and drawing its nourishment from the healthy organs around it. The goal of this fragment of cancer is not to live peacefully side by side; its goal is to replace all the healthy organs with the disease. Its aim is the total destruction of the body—in the case of a nation, the government."

It was hot and the small room was not air-conditioned. To keep out Vung Tau's gargantuan mosquitoes, the windows were tightly closed. The ancient French ceiling fan droned lazily around, so slowly that each of its four blades could be clearly defined. I was the only reporter to attend the briefing that beautiful Sunday afternoon; everyone else was romping on the silken white sands of the resort's famous beach.

Major Bé doggedly pursued his analogy. "A healthy stomach, for example, does not voluntarily give to the fragment of cancer the vitamins, minerals, and other substances it needs to live," he explained. "The malignancy takes these materials from the healthy stomach against its will. The cancer forces the healthy stomach to bring about its own death."

His physiology was bad, but his English was excellent. And his parallel between what he thought the rebellious insurgents were doing in Vietnam and what a cancer does when it invades an organ was a novel approach to me. I made a note to remember it when I tried to describe the Vietnam war to my readers back home. Everybody, of course, knows what cancer is, I thought to myself. That will make it easier to describe what this crazy civil war in Vietnam is all about.

The idea that within a few years I would be trying to define cancer via the Vietnam-war analogy never occurred to me. But here I am doing exactly that.

A human body invaded by cancer is like a country battling a small guerrilla insurgency. If the government (the body) is strong and healthy, if there are no weak spots in its society (possible genetic predisposing factors), if there are no traitors within the government to help the enemy (chemical, viral, or radiation carcinogens), and if the defense machinery (the immunological system) is strong, then the insurgency can be put down with a minimum of over-all damage. However, bodies and governments are rarely fault-free. A microscopic cancerous rebellion, started in the proper environment and supported and nourished by various contributing factors, can grow and grow, until—like the war in Vietnam—it endangers the very life of the whole body. Without the right kind of outside treatment, the malignancy will inevitably cause the body's death.

Cancer cells do absolutely nothing to benefit the body. They do not supply energy or support the functions of the tissues or organs they are part of; they only use up nutrients to make more and more cancer cells. As Major Bé said, in comparing them with the Vietcong guerrillas, they help themselves to what they need from surrounding healthy tissue, turning an entire organ—if unchecked—into a cancerous one.

Cancer is also very species-specific. That is, each type has an affinity only for certain animals. The mouse gets almost every kind of cancer there is; the monkey gets few. Injecting a monkey with tissue taken from a cancerous cat would probably not give the monkey the disease. Dogs get breast cancer, but not the same kind that thrives in mice or in humans.

This selectivity of cancer is one of the major obstacles to research. Experimentation cannot be done on humans, of course, but with many diseases it is often possible to extrapolate, or apply to humans, information from experiments on lower animals. The species-specificity of cancer, according to many authorities, makes extrapolation unreliable for investigating this disease.

These, then, are the characteristics that all kinds of cancers have in common: They are caused by something that upsets the segment of DNA in a particular cell that controls its growth and reproduction. They never stop growing, but appear to proliferate wildly and invade other parts of the body helter-skelter. They contribute nothing whatsoever toward the functioning of the organism. The disease is highly species-specific.

Here the nature of cancer changes, and every kind seems to go its own way.

Cancer is actually a blanket term that covers more than a hundred different types of invasive diseases, which are very different from each other except for the factors just mentioned. For example, all animals—including women and men—are made up of three basic cell layers that originally formed their embryonic bodies: the ectoderm, the mesoderm, and the endoderm. A cancer called a "carcinoma" is one that originates in either ectodermal (covering tissue, like the skin) or endodermal (lining tissue) layers. A malignancy that is formed in bone, muscle, or any connecting or supporting tissues (mesoderm) is called a "sarcoma." The organ site where a carcinoma or sarcoma is growing is translated into either Latin or Greek, and the prefix describes where that particular cancer is. For example, the prefix, "osteo" means bone, and an osteosarcoma means that there is a malignant tumor in a bone somewhere in that animal's body.

In the breast, virtually every type of tissue found in a body is also present—even bone, if a woman develops calcifications. However, most breast cancers are adenocarcinomas, because they begin to grow in ectodermal or endodermal tissues, and the prefix, "adeno," is the medical term describing a gland. There are sarcomas of the chest wall, ligaments, and other connective tissue of the breast, but these are relatively rare.

Metastasis, a word that means spread of the original cancer from one organ or part of the body to another, complicates the problem of defining breast cancer even more. If a breast cancer metastasizes to the lung, this secondary tumor will be composed of the same kind of cells as those in the breast growth. But a primary lung cancer—one originating in the lung—will be composed of a different kind of cell. Some cancers, particularly the leukemias, afflict young people; prostatic carcinoma mainly attacks older men. Some organs are seldom, if ever, invaded; cancer of the heart is a medical rarity. In other words, while anything that is malignant and invasive can be called cancer, "cancer" is really many different diseases, with different causes, victims, and treatments.

When scientists speak of cancer's "wild, uncontrolled proliferation," they are comparing the malignant cells with the normal ones around them. In fact, the disease's growth is rigidly controlled by certain rules that are seldom broken.

Neoplastic, or tumor, cells reproduce rapidly or slowly, depending on the reproduction rate of the normal cells of the same organ. Healthy liver cells reproduce slowly, and so do cancerous ones; healthy blood cells reproduce rapidly, and so do cancerous ones.

Of course, if an organ is damaged or injured, the trauma triggers the dormant growth gene back into immediate reproduction. If one kidney is removed, for example, the normally slow-growing cells in the remaining organ begin reproduction to take over the work of its missing twin. A damaged liver—whose cells normally reproduce slowly—will regenerate quickly. Adults whose bones have stopped growing will suddenly get new bone cells if a limb is broken and needs repair. Also, once a malignant invasion begins in a slow-reproducing organ like the liver, the presence of cancer cells can itself foul up the growth genes of neighboring normal cells and trigger cancer, just as trauma does. This phenomenon is not well understood, but it does occur.

The important thing, though, is that cancerous cells never *stop* reproducing and soon outstrip the growth of the healthy tissue surrounding them.

The second rule that governs cancer growth is more complicated, but when it is explained, one of the puzzles of cancer becomes easier to understand. This is the phenomenon of doubling time.

Often a person with cancer will say, "I just had a checkup a couple of months ago, and then the lump was only a little thing to keep an eye on. It is the size of a marble now." The reason is doubling time.

By the time any neoplasm—not only one in the breast—is large enough to be palpable, or felt, it has gone through at least thirty "generations" of doubling in size. (This assumes that a lump can be palpated when it weighs one gram.) Thirty doublings can take anywhere from weeks to many years; the length of time depends on the kind of cell it is. Doubling is not haphazard, but is a steady, exponential growth that one writer has described as obeying "the compound-interest law": each increase in size is added in before the next increase is calculated.

There is a big difference between cancer and a bank account, however. An especially high-yield bank might pay a depositor 25 percent in interest every year. Cancer's interest rate is 100 percent, compounded more frequently. One cell becomes two, two become four, then eight, sixteen, thirty-two, and so on, until after some twenty generations there are about 1 million cells, weighing approximately one milligram (one-thousandth of a gram). The tumor is still in its "preclinical" stage, invisible to the human eye and not palpable by even very sensitive and experienced fingers.

Then the compound-interest law that brought a single cell to 1 million cells in twenty generations will take the milligram of cancer and multiply it by a thousand in just ten more generations. After thirty doublings, there will be 1 billion cells, weighing one gram. A tumor this size can easily be palpated.

Bear in mind that it grew a thousand times larger in half the time required for it to reach a thousandth of a gram. If the gram-size cancer is not detected and removed at this stage, one more generation will increase it to two grams. Another single generation will make it four grams. (Of course, cancer cells, like other cells, do die. Unfortunately, their death rates are far lower than their birth rates.)

To put doubling into another kind of time frame, a tumor having a 100-day cycle, which took nine years to grow from a single cell to a one-gram lump—the size at which it can be felt—would take only about fifteen months longer to become a tumor weighing about sixteen grams—about half an ounce. In just another fifteen months, it would weigh about a pound. Thus, in exactly the same length of time, the size of the neoplasm would increase thirty-two times!

The same exponential rules of doubling apply to metastases. If, when a primary cancer is discovered, a secondary one is also found somewhere else in the body, it is a sign that the metastasis began very early in the life of the first malignancy. Otherwise, it would not be palpable. Advanced cancers, however, seem to double more slowly.

President Gerald Ford, in an announcement about his wife's breast cancer, wondered aloud how a tumor an inch in diameter could have developed in the seven months since her last physical examination. Cancer's laws of proliferation and doubling time are the explanation. It almost seems like an optical illusion, this business of having nothing and then something relatively enormous within a few short months. But that is the nature of the growth of cancer. It is very important to understand this doubling-time rule, because the best hope of curing breast cancer today is to find ways to diagnose it during those first twenty generations of preclinical life, long before a lump can be felt.

Although doubling time applies to all cancers, palpability of a mass is useless as a test for tumors of the ovary, pancreas, liver,

Doubling Time "Atomic Explosion"

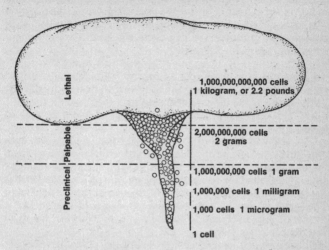

Lethal

1,000,000,000,000 cells
1 kilogram, or 2.2 pounds

Preclinical | Palpable

2,000,000,000 cells
2 grams

1,000,000,000 cells 1 gram

1,000,000 cells 1 milligram

1,000 cells 1 microgram

1 cell

Reproduced with permission from *Scientific Foundations
of Oncology* by T. Symington and R. L. Carter.
William Heinemann Medical Books Ltd., London.

or other deep-seated organs. By the time such cancers cause
symptoms, it is usually too late for anything.

Benign lumps, by the way, are caused by somewhat the same
kind of disturbance of the growth gene that makes a cell cancerous. The difference is that benign masses usually grow more
slowly and, in due course, stop growing; they remain localized,
do not metastasize, and do not destroy normal cells while they are
growing. Benign cells live peacefully side by side with healthy
ones. There are differing opinions about when a benign mass
eventually becomes malignant. Many experts think that while a
benign growth in the breast may not be dangerous in itself it
should be removed, because it could be masking or hiding a
cancer. On the other hand, there is also evidence that the development of cancer—from normal to malignant—is a "continuum."
This means that change is gradual, that a healthy cell goes through
many stages before it becomes cancerous. If these data should
turn out to be correct, they might mean that an atypical cell—anything not identical with its neighbors—is a "precursor," or premalignant, cell.

In the brain, this is nothing to worry about, because no one looks for cancers in that organ unless a person is suffering from some kind of symptom. But in the case of the breast, the question of what is and what is not a true precursor to cancer has become a hot scientific controversy. This issue will be discussed in more detail in Chapter 10: Surgery.

I once met a veteran sports reporter who constantly griped about the trials and tribulations of having to deal with athletes. "Why in the world did you decide to be a sportswriter, then?" I asked him. "You don't seem to like the people you have to cover."

"I'll tell you why, honey." The old man grinned. His eyes crinkled closed and he chuckled. "It's the only kind of journalism there is where a guy doesn't have to start every new piece by saying, 'Baseball is a game with nine players on each side. One is the pitcher, a second the catcher. The other seven are field men. The game is played with two teams on a field shaped like a diamond.' And so on and so on, the way everybody else has to do in a regular news piece."

I have a similar advantage now. I certainly do not have to say, "Female breasts are two globular organs located on a woman's chest in the area between her shoulders and her waistline." But it may well be necessary to add the reminder that the primary function of the breasts, the reason they are there, is to make milk for feeding the young. Although they have been sex symbols from the beginning of time, the mammary glands were *not* created for the purpose of attracting males.

From the day a teen-age girl begins to menstruate, her breasts regularly prepare themselves, month after month, for a possible pregnancy. Organs like the heart and lungs may work harder twenty-four hours a day, but the breasts have many more, and more varied, jobs to perform. Their continual cyclical change of function is accompanied by changes in the tissues and cells, and this is the main reason the female breast is especially vulnerable to cellular damage. Any routine that is constantly being upset by one interruption or another—even if it is perfectly natural for it to be upset—is subject to a greater risk of errors. The overworked breast cell is always being bathed in some hormone that orders, "Stop doing that. Start doing this." No wonder so many of the daughter cells go haywire.

The largest number of breast cancers occurs in the milk ducts, where the cells are most subject to being annoyed by hormonal or chemical agitators. Relatively few start in the fatty tissues, which have considerably less work to do.

Not only does the breast perform an enormous number of jobs and contain every kind of tissue found in the body, except for bone, each tissue—skin, duct, fiber, fat, and the rest—has a different vulnerability. As if this were not enough, cancers of the nipple, in or between the lobes, of the smooth muscle, and so on, all have their own doubling times and other individual peculiarities.

All the apparatus of the mammary gland is enclosed by a membrane called the fascia. The fascia immediately under the skin and over the breast tissue is the superficial fascia; the membrane that separates the breast tissue from the muscles of the chest wall is the deep fascia. There are two muscles under the breast, the pectoralis major and the pectoralis minor, which cover the ribs and control much of the mobility of the arms. The Cooper's ligaments (named for the anatomist-surgeon who discovered them) are attached to the pectoral muscles, and these are what keep the breasts attractively tilted upward. (So all those pectoral-muscle exercises we do are absolutely no good for improving uplift; it's the Cooper's ligaments that count.)

In each breast, scattered within, among, and beneath protective layers of fat, are twenty or more lobes, further subdivided into lobules, ending finally in tiny bulbs called acini. These are the milk-producing factories, and they are all connected to the nipple by a network of very fine ductules, leading into larger ducts, which finally merge as they enter the nipple into a single main tube, the lactiferous sinus. The external opening of the tube consists of a number of pin-sized holes in the nipple that secrete milk when it is needed.

The nipple is made of a sturdy, pigmented, corrugated kind of skin tissue and is filled with tiny glands that lubricate the area during breast feeding. It is surrounded by the areola, a pink or brownish circle of skin. The nipple and areola also contain many nerve endings and blood vessels, which come from larger connections in the breast itself.

Along with an extensive network of arteries, veins, and their capillary subdivisions, each breast has a network of lymphatic vessels that drain into the lymph nodes in the armpit. Each breast also has an internal mammary chain of nodes which runs down the center of the chest alongside the breastbone. Knowing something about what the lymphatic system and axillary lymph nodes do is especially important to an understanding of breast cancer.

The lymphatic vessels, which are found throughout the body, are primarily involved in removing wastes from the tissues. But they also carry many of the components of the immune system. Every organism is endowed with a self-defense force to keep it healthy and help it fight off any invaders that might injure or destroy it. This immunological system is so sophisticated and complex that scientists—even with today's technical know-how—have barely begun to penetrate its mysteries. (Immunology is one of the youngest of the medical sciences.)

The regional lymph nodes are the first defense outposts in the human immunological system. These vital little fortresses, often misnamed glands, are scattered in critical spots throughout the body. The nodes under the cheeks in the upper neck are the ones we are most familiar with; they ward off and destroy harmful substances that enter the body through the nose or mouth. When these nodes are busy attacking an invader, a case of "swollen glands" results. All the nodes in the body are constantly manufacturing lymphocytes—cells that go out into the blood stream and attack anything that doesn't belong there. Usually they succeed. But sometimes they need help from other elements of the immune system, which will be described in more detail later.

The nodes and the lymphatic vessels—the channels connecting the nodes—play a part in the metastasis of cancer from a single localized spot to another organ of the body. The lymphatics are the usual invasion route a cancer cell takes when it breaks away from the primary tumor. Luckily, it is not an express route. The highways have many barricades—those trusty guardians, the lymph nodes—which block the channels and try to filter out and destroy the wandering malignant invader. But sometimes the nodes themselves are conquered. Until relatively recently surgeons believed (and some still do) that removing malignant axillary lymph nodes during a mastectomy is imperative to "get the cancer all out." However, meticulous scientific studies carried out since the 1950s have proven that malignant lymph nodes are nothing more than indicators, or sign posts, showing that the cancer is not localized to the breast but may have already spread throughout the woman's body as micrometastases. Before anticancer drugs were developed, women who had malignant (or positive) axillary nodes were given X-ray (usually cobalt) treatments in an often futile effort to destroy any cancer cells that were left behind. Now, with an arsenal of agents to fight micrometastases available, oncologists use the presence or absence of cancer in the nodes as clues to tell them whether or not a woman needs systemic (whole body) treatment by some kind of chemotherapy.

Most women have about twenty-five or thirty nodes in each axilla, and when they are removed, each one is carefully examined under the microscope by a pathologist, who is looking for a sign that the node has been invaded. If a node is cancerous, it is diagnosed as "positive"; if it is normal, it is called "negative." Even with more than a century of experience to rely on, surgeons and statisticians are still unable to predict the relative risk of metastasis elsewhere in the body except by counting the number of involved nodes found.

The very best report a pathologist can give, of course, is that all the nodes are negative. This means that the disease has been caught while still localized in the breast itself—even if, as in Happy Rockefeller's case, there was not one but multiple tumors in both breasts. Doctors have different rules of thumb regarding what to do about how many positive nodes. Nodal status and its implications for further therapies of all kinds will be treated elsewhere in this book.

Some surgeons believe that the internal mammary chain of nodes, the ones lying along the breastbone, should also be removed during a mastectomy. However, it has been found that these nodes are rarely involved if the primary cancer is in the outer half of the breast. Since that is where most of the tumors do appear, removing the internal mammary chain is usually unnecessary. There is some argument about this, but the consensus seems to be that the surgery required is too extensive to be performed routinely.

Cancer cells trapped in the lymph system are more likely to be destroyed than those in the blood stream, which lacks the nodal filters and screens. The blood stream, however, does have its own kinds of cancer killers floating around in it, as will be made clear in the later discussion of the immune system.

The location of a tumor can affect its seriousness and potential invasiveness. A relatively slow-growing neoplasm can metastasize quickly if it is near a lymph channel or near a blood vessel. Cases have been recorded in which a stray cell floating in the lymphatic system caused a cancer to grow to palpable size in the axillary nodes, although the original malignancy in the breast itself remained microscopic. No examination of the breast, by palpation, mammography, or thermography, would be able to detect such a cancer.

Furthermore, the lymphatic system links the two breasts, under the breastbone. That is why, if a breast cancer reappears, the most frequent site for the recurrence is in the other breast.

Although the words metastasis and recurrence are frequently used interchangeably, they are not synonymous, even though both refer to second cancers. Metastases are certainly recurrences of the cancer, but they are usually tumors that have spread, or metastasized, to other—often quite distant—parts of the body via the bloodstream or lymphatic system. Recurrences are new cancers that appear in the immediate area of the first, such as in the incision itself or around it, or in the adjacent chest-wall. A cancer discovered in the second breast is usually—although *not* always—a tumor known as "second primary." This happens because breast cancer is a multicentric disease, and women who develop a tumor in one breast may have others scattered in the same or second breast. Such new primaries are not recurrences or metastases, but are considered to be completely independent of the first. For this reason, the discovery of a cancer in the other breast is neither a sign that the disease has spread nor that widespread disease is inevitable.

Metastases, on the other hand, are dangerous and insidious, because there is no way to know where a circulating cancer cell may decide to stop and colonize. The lungs, liver, and bone are the most common sites for breast-cancer metastases, but they can begin to grow anywhere and be far advanced before their discovery by even the most careful examination after surgery. Recurrences are more likely to be found early, when treatment can be effective, since even a superficial follow-up includes careful scrutiny of the operative area, the second breast, and the axillas.

The cyclical changes in the breasts and the nature of the regional nodes are enough to show how breast cancer spreads but pregnancy and lactation (breast feeding) may worsen a woman's condition if she has cancer.

During ovulation, the breasts begin to get ready for the conception of a baby. They become enlarged and engorged as the milk glands grow. If there is no pregnancy, the swelling disappears, and for the rest of the cycle the breasts are in their normal state. This is the reason for the perfectly normal periodic lumpiness and soreness women experience.

However, if pregnancy does occur, the glandular system keeps on growing, so that it will be able to provide a good milk supply; more lobules are produced and the duct system expands. Then, if the mother breast-feeds her baby, all these additional assets continue to be used to make milk. If she does not breast-feed, or as her milk supply dries up, the breasts gradually return to their prepregnancy state.

All of these changes are triggered by a variety of hormones, some of which aid and abet neoplastic growth. More about these later.

The work of the hormones leaves permanent changes in the mammary gland after a pregnancy. It will never again be a "virgin" breast. Even though external shapeliness might not have been affected, the breasts have undergone changes of internal structure, which will remain forever. The changes may not be visible to the eye, but they often show on mammograms as areas of less density, leaving light spaces and gaps on the film. Nulliparous—never pregnant—breasts have a dark, compact firmness.

There are many different kinds of breast cancers, all blanketed under the label mammary carcinoma. The specific name of each generally identifies the kind of breast tissue that has become malignant. A favorite starting place for a cancer—almost three-fourths of all—is in one of the hundreds of milk ducts, and these are known as intraductal carcinomas.

Although all breast cancers are technically classified as soft-tissue tumors, some feel hard and can assume various shapes; others are gelatinous and mushy. Still others feel fibrous. Some cancers of the breast have no lump or thickening at all.

The uncommon Paget's disease (named after the doctor who first described it) is one of these. At the beginning, the nipple and areola look as if they had a slight case of eczema. Then the nipple begins to crack and to leak what sometimes looks like milk or sometimes a greenish or bluish fluid. Even though there is no lump, Paget's disease is a cancer, and a mastectomy must be performed. However, when Paget's disease spreads and invades a duct, there is a lump.

Another one of these is a generalized (in medical parlance, the opposite of localized) breast cancer, a relatively rare type that gives as its first symptom only pain and soreness; there is no lump that can be seen or felt. Since a certain amount of breast tenderness is a regular part of every woman's life, this cancer can be very dangerous—especially in premenopausal women—because the symptoms may be ignored and the cancer go undetected until after it has already metastasized. However, it can be caught in time if the woman is alert and not bashful about seeing her doctor for what could turn out to be an insignificant symptom (and insisting that he do an examination and, perhaps, order a mammogram). When it is found early, the outlook for this kind of non-lumpy, nonthickening cancer is as good as for any other malignancy diagnosed at an early stage. But it must be found early for successful treatment, because it may be the onset of inflammatory carcinoma.

Inflammatory carcinoma is very virulent, and usually by the time it is diagnosed, the skin and lymphatics are severely inflamed, and the breast is swollen, hot, red, puffy, and excruciatingly painful.

Not too long ago, doctors were so pessimistic about the outlook for women with this kind of cancer that many simply declared it to be inoperable. However, those surgeons who refused to give these women an automatic death sentence tried various procedures of irradiating the breast to shrink the tumor and reduce the inflammation before doing a mastectomy. The results of such treatment have been good, especially when followed by some kind of systemic drug or hormone therapy, and inflammatory carcinoma is now routinely treated this way. Of course, if there is visible evidence that the cancer has already metastasized to other organs, the breast is not removed, and systemic treatment is begun immediately. While these women, at this time, have no chance of being cured, the treatment does give them more years to live.

A rare kind of breast cancer—mammary sarcoma—attacks the connective tissue of the muscles, ligaments, and tendons that back up and support the breasts. For a variety of reasons, connective tissues are among the last parts of the body to be invaded by cancer. In other words, the pectoral muscles—routinely cut out during the Halsted radical mastectomy—are very low-risk targets of malignant invasion. Many experts, in fact, have told me that by the time a woman's pectorals are invaded, she probably has so many other metastases in her body that any kind of mastectomy would be an unnecessary ordeal.

Cancers in the large milk glands are called lobular carcinomas, and they are often found *in situ*. This is the term used to describe a noninvasive, microscopic cancer that may stay in the same spot, without spreading. *In situ* cells look different from invasive carcinomas. In addition, when looking at a biopsy specimen under the microscope, the pathologist looks for a band of healthy cells completely circumscribing and insulating the cancerous ones, and also for membranes with solid, unbroken perimeters enclosing the cancerous cells. If both these conditions exist, the pathologist will diagnose it as an *in situ* cancer and will predict that metastasis to the axillary nodes is highly unlikely.

As I said earlier, some surgeons do a mastectomy in such cases, and some do not.

Whether the breast should be amputated for an *in situ* cancer is, I think, also a decision the woman really must make for herself. To do so, however, she should know that follow-up studies have shown that a large proportion of these carcinomas do change and become invasive within ten or twenty years.

Each of these mammary carcinomas, then, is quite different from the others. It has been estimated by cell kineticists (experts in cell-growth speed) that doubling times for human breast cancers vary widely, too, ranging from twenty-three days to 209 days. Depending on the kind, it can take anywhere from two to seventeen years for the cancer to reach a size that can be felt. Stated another way, the twenty-three-day carcinoma—the one with the shortest doubling time—could not be palpated for two years at the earliest.

Actually, the doubling times of the various breast cancers follow no known hard-and-fast rules. The interval varies with the reproductive rate of the part of the breast from which the cancerous tumor came, since the proliferating malignant cells follow the same relative speed of division as the tissue from which they grew. Skin, blood, and other fast-growing tissues, for example, would have faster growing malignancies; connective tissue, slow ones; nerve and muscle cells would never become malignant.

This explains why there are no cancers of the heart, an organ composed almost entirely of muscle cells. If these cancers exist at all, they are so rare I could find no one who had ever heard or read of one. Muscle sarcomas are suspected of arising from epithelial or other cells nearby, not from the muscle cells themselves, which never divide, and brain tumors such as gliomas are thought to develop in the same way. The reason scientists hedge by saying "suspected" or "thought to be" is that once a cell becomes malignant, its cellular origin cannot always be determined. Therefore, these are assumptions based on the firm knowledge that nerve and muscle cells never reproduce and, theoretically, would never have a synthesis or twinning period when they can be transformed.

All the tissues found in the breast, except for those of the nipple, are scattered throughout the organ. Therefore, the various kinds of cancers, aside from Paget's disease and others of the nipple, can begin anywhere. Statistically, however, the upper outer quadrant—the quarter of the breast closest to the armpit— is the birthplace of about half of all breast cancers. Another one-fourth begin in the nipple. The other three quadrants account for the remaining 25 percent.

For reasons unknown, it is far more common for breast cancers to develop in the left breast first.

An interesting opinion I learned during a tour of European cancer centers is that premenopausal and postmenopausal breast cancer are two completely different diseases, having different causes and requiring different treatments. This theory has been supported by recent studies in the United States, and it explains many age-related differences and paradoxes about breast cancer that had puzzled me throughout my research. For example, I learned that breast-cancer statistics show a very distinctive pattern of incidence according to age groups, and statisticians told me that this kind of age-specific incidence rate is uncommon in cancers of other organs. I will go into this in greater detail later and just say now that the many opinions about the reasons for this phenomenon all revolve around the menopause and the reduction of estrogens in the body of an older woman.

A word must be said about breast cancer in men. Although it is extremely rare—less than 1 percent of all breast cancers—it does exist. It is by and large a disease that hits men who are in middle and old age and who, in the United States, are predominantly foreign-born or of Jewish backgrounds. For some unknown reason, black men have a somewhat higher incidence of breast cancer than white men do. Another interesting aspect of the male disease is that older men being treated for prostatic cancer with estrogens have developed breast cancers from taking the female hormones. However, many of these are also metastases from the prostatic cancer.

One oddity of masculine breast cancer might someday help in finding the cause of breast cancer in women. Men who have Klinefelter's syndrome—a rare genetic defect that gives their sex-bearing chromosome two X genes and a single Y gene, rather than the normal X and Y—have a much higher incidence of breast cancer than do men in the rest of the population. Many scientists believe this is evidence that breast cancer is genetic and anticipate that the technical know-how to find a specific breast-cancer gene on a chromosome will be developed.

Whatever the cause, cancer of the breast in men is treated in the same way as it is in women: by mastectomy, preferably a modified radical, which leaves the muscles intact. Also, if the tumor developed from taking female hormones, they would probably be discontinued. Since the disease usually occurs in older men, and since it makes up such a tiny percentage of all breast cancers, male mastectomy is not a burning issue. When the day comes that female breast cancer can be cured, male breast cancer will also disappear.

Although *Why Me?* is a book for women (and men) about breast cancer, no manual or text about the disease can really be useful unless it also discusses benign breast problems, disorders, and diseases. As we women are constantly being told, ninety percent of all breast symptoms are symptoms of harmless conditions— *not* of cancer. The reason I have separated these nonmalignant "conditions" into three categories—problems, disorders, and diseases—is that the natural and normal reproductive processes all adult women experience, like menstruation, are usually the cause. Therefore, in my opinion, these problems are as normal and natural as menstruation, pregnancy, and childbirth. Just because they happen to make women's breasts tender, enlarged, and lumpy is no reason to label them "diseases."

By the same token, there are certain operational mixups that can occur—malfunctions of some type—that may need repair, just as a broken arm would need to be set and splinted. An injury, for example, might cause a bruise or a blood clot. These are certainly problems; they may be temporary disorders.

However, there are real benign diseases of the breasts that must be treated and cured, or they may get worse. Many doctors consider a woman who has chronically cystic breasts to have a disease. Mastitis is also usually considered to be a disease, even though it is short-term after breastfeeding (as a rule) and is often self-limiting without any treatment at all. Certain harmless, but abnormal, growths that seem to take root in women's breasts are also real diseases in the sense that they may interfere with function, cause pain, and require treatment.

The reason for my spending so many words on these semantic nuances that may seem totally unimportant is that there has been a great deal of publicity within the past months that having "a history of benign breast disease" is a "high risk factor" for developing cancer. This publicity has set off a wave of unjustified terror, especially among young women who routinely and quite naturally are having cyclical lumpiness and pain—problems that are *not* any more "diseases" than the menstrual period. To make matters worse, there is a trend in the land toward doctors practicing "defensive medicine," and this has forced some fine surgeons into filing pre-biopsy diagnoses of "suspected breast disease" for hospital records. Women who may then have biopsies because of their surgeons' fears of malpractice suits, believe they actually had some kind of benign breast disease, when all they had were uncertain surgeons who might have been doing unnecessary biopsies for legal reasons.

Obviously, these women are not at higher risk because of the biopsies *per se*; the pathological report must clearly state that something abnormal was found. Dr. David Page, a pathologist at Vanderbilt Medical School in Tennessee, emphatically told an NCI conference in March, 1980 that "having a surgical biopsy is not proof that a woman had a disease of the breast. Only the path report can give that kind of proof."

Often, we women need this sort of reassurance from an expert.

In the rest of this chapter, I will describe the most common benign breast conditions women encounter. Some are diseases and some are disorders. But most of them—like fluid-filled cysts—are simply problems. Normal worries about breast cancer are being turned into needless terror as women are continually being warned about cyclical problems. Some women grow masses in their breasts the way teenagers sprout pimples on their foreheads, and knowing something about these non-malignant lumps and bumps will, I hope, also prevent the "fear of feeling"— women's stubborn refusal to examine their breasts regularly enough to know what is normal *for them*.

Earlier in this chapter, I explained how long and hard women's breasts work. Only the heart and lungs have longer hours, and only the liver has more jobs to do. When a baby girl is born, there is already breast tissue on her tiny chest, and—because some of her mother's hormones were transferred from the placenta during pregnancy—the tissue is already responsive to their instructions. Female infants' breasts may even be enlarged at birth, and milky fluid is frequently secreted by both newborn females and males.

Before puberty, there is usually some development of girls' primary breast ducts, although nothing may be visible as far as their actual breast size is concerned. By the time puberty begins, the hypothalamus region of their brains has already begun to stimulate production of many hormones involved in the reproductive process. These speed up the growth of the ducts and lobes in the breast. Fat deposits elevate the areola and nipple, and when a girl finally starts to menstruate (i.e., begins her "reproductive years"), her breasts change monthly because of these hormones.

Without going into more detail about the luteal phase, follicular stimulation, various rises and falls of one substance or another, I will say only that the breasts of menstruating women are constantly stopping and starting in response to batteries of instructions from hormones triggered by the master conductor—the hypothalamus. All this frenzied, frenetic activity, of course, is aimed at organizing the dairy factories for milk production.

But it is usually all for naught. Except for a few fertilizations in a lifetime, there will be no pregnancy, and the extra hormones, blood, and fluid pumped into the breasts usually disappear until the next cycle. Since the average woman's reproductive life lasts about thirty years, this means her breasts will go through such hormonal machinations about 360 times before she finishes her menopause. And most of these hormonal changes cause enlargement of both lobes and ducts, as well as accumulation of fluids, that may or may not go away. As a result, most women spend most of their lives with "lumpy" breasts. Obviously, the vast majority of these are normal cyclical masses and are nothing to worry about, even if they hurt so much that the touch of a flimsy nylon nightgown may be excruciating.

As a rule, such problems last only a few days, because cyclical engorgement goes away. But some fluid may persist and be surrounded by a hardened membrane. When this happens, a cyst has been formed, and it may or may not eventually be absorbed by the body.

In addition to these fluid-filled cysts, some young women develop solid masses known as fibroadenomas and papillomas. A fibroadenoma is made up of a combination of fibrous and glandular tissue. It is usually movable, does not hurt, and is most often found in women between the ages of 17 and 35. Fibroadenomas feel like marbles or peas with curved, clearly defined boundaries, and these, as well as cysts can be found in any part of the breast.

On the other hand, papillomas are small, wart-like masses that usually grow inside a duct, near the nipple. Papillomas are especially scary to women—young and old—because they often cause a nipple discharge which may be bloody. Certainly, these benign growths should be removed to be sure they are really benign and are not hiding or "masking" a malignancy. But cysts, fibroadenomas, and papillomas do not become cancerous.

There are also harmless breast problems that can occur at any time in a woman's life as a result of infection or injury. Mastitis, for example, is an umbrella name that is used to cover any inflammation in the mammary gland and—although it results most often from bacteria entering nipple-openings during breast-feeding—mastitis can be caused by overly vigorous lovemaking or an injury. Should a simple infection get out of hand, an abscess may form, and a breast abscess is no different from a pocket of infection that develops anywhere in the body. The area around it may swell, become sore and tender, hot to the touch, and the skin may redden. Lumps caused by trauma or injury may abscess or they may be hematomas (blood clots). An injury may also trigger formation of a mass called "fat necrosis."

Most common benign breast conditions are usually grouped under the general term: "fibrocystic disease." There are objections—especially from pathologists—to the use of this term, because it has almost become a "garbage can" for all benign breast masses found during surgical biopsies. More precise terminology, they insist (e.g., in situ, dysplasia, ectasia, hyperplasia, etc.) would be helpful in identifying certain cell "markers" to predict which benign lesions are signs that those women will someday develop true, invasive breast cancer. Once the vague term "fibrocystic disease" is abandoned, many pathologists feel, it will be possible to look back into a breast-cancer patient's past records to see exactly what kind of harmless mass had been removed in an earlier biopsy. Since the issue of "precursor cells" will be discussed in Chapters 4 and 10, I am mentioning the matter here only briefly to illustrate its importance. A change in surgeons' terminology has not yet occurred, so all women should know that this business of "fibrocystic disease" covers a great deal of benign territory. Few women will go through their lives without being told, at some time or another, that they have such a condition.

Later, I will discuss various treatments for breast cancer in detail. A list of ways to reduce or even to prevent most benign breast problems may be lost in those pages. For this reason, I would like to mention here—where benign conditions are the major issue—that thousands of women have found eliminating caffeine from their diets (in coffee, cola drinks, and in chocolate) seems to relieve breast pain and lumpiness. There are scientific data showing that a daily intake of Vitamin E may also help many women. In addition, there are now various preparations containing progesterone, danazol, and bromocriptine on drugstore shelves. These, of course, should not be used without a physician's advice.

These drugs are relatively new (for this use), and the only reports I have been able to find about their effectiveness are the pharmaceutical companies' own public-relations brochures. Interested women may want to do their own sleuthing about their value and safety.

A discussion of benign breast problems is a good place to explain what seems to be a statistical discrepancy concerning the incidence of such harmless growths in relation to the number of malignant lesions found. Most leaflets, brochures, manuals about breast self-examination and even *Why Me?* repeat the litany that "nine out of ten lumps are benign." Yet women also often read that eighty percent of all possible symptoms turn out to be benign and not cancerous—eight out of ten.

The reason for this difference is that some statisticians use the ratio based on women-found lumps, while others describe the proportions determined by a doctor's examination or a biopsy. This means that women often find lumps and bumps that a doctor's experienced hands can identify as harmless cysts and/or normal thickenings. However, of those suspicious enough to warrant a biopsy, some are found to be benign. Thus, on the average, nine of ten that reach the operating room are harmless. Writers of leaflets, brochures, and books use the statistic that happens to be most suitable to the point being made in that piece of text.

There are about 120 million women in the United States today—more than 60 million older than thirty. Estimates are that about 110,000 diagnoses of breast cancer will be made in 1981. This is, of course, a terrifying number. However, women should not let the fear of breast cancer prevent them from doing something about a problem. So I insist—like most leaflets and brochures—that "nine out of ten breast lumps are harmless." Don't ever forget that.

3

History, Myths, and Quackery

HISTORY

The first known reference to breast cancer in medical history is found in the "Edwin Smith Surgical Papyrus," written during the time of the Old Kingdom in Egypt, which extended from around 3000 to 2500 B.C. (No one knows who wrote these ancient scrolls; Smith was the archeologist who discovered them.)

I was curious about the omission of breast cancer from the cave and wall scratchings of primitive man, and most of the authorities I asked about this said that it was probably because women died of other causes long before they reached the vulnerable breast-cancer age. "Few women lived past thirty in those days," one expert at the National Cancer Institute told me. "They just didn't live long enough to get breast cancer." Another specialist suggested that early man wouldn't have known it was the actual cause of death. "A woman doesn't die of the breast disease itself," he explained, "but from its spread to a vital organ. So if a woman died of metastatic liver or lung disease, who would think the problem had originated in the breast?"

For whatever reason, the Smith papyrus has the earliest known mention of breast cancer—male or female—in medical history. Even the eight cases the papyrus describes are called not breast cancer, but cases of "bulging tumors," and all were found in males. This first doctors' manual says, with straightforward honesty, "There is no treatment." In another Egyptian medical papyrus, written about 1,500 years later (this one named for Georg Ebers), no cases of "bulging tumors" are mentioned, but prescriptions are given for healing fatty tumors and abscesses "with the knife" and by fire.

There are also recorded references to breast cancer in ancient Mesopotamia. Here (where poppyheads were used to relieve pain), cutting out breast tumors was routine procedure—and presumably the noble poppy was used as a painkiller during the surgery.

Then, in the chronicles of ancient Greece, the historian Herodotus tells the case history of Atossa, the daughter of the Persian king Cyrus the Great and the wife of Darius I. She had a breast tumor, which she attempted to conceal from everyone, until finally, according to Herodotus, it ulcerated and spread, and she could no longer hide the problem. Atossa then sent for the court physician, Democedes, and he cured her. No details are given about this legendary successful treatment. However, one thing hasn't changed much: even in those long-ago days, women delayed before seeing a doctor.

As a matter of fact, Dr. Edward Lewison, of the Johns Hopkins Hospital, in his textbook *Breast Cancer and Its Diagnosis and Treatment*, complains that Atossa's attitude is typical of all women through the ages everywhere.

> It is a revealing commentary to note that throughout the annals of history women have never outlived their vanity. Cosmetic considerations and false modesty have hindered the early diagnosis and timely treatment of breast cancer from the dawn of humanity until today. Since the breast has always been an esthetic symbol of fertility and womanhood, amputation of the breast provoked mutilation of the mind as well as the body. Women have taken great pride in their breasts and formerly wore décolleté dresses with disarming propriety. Indeed, it was a customary and respectful form of salutation up until the seventeenth century to touch the breasts in a warm and friendly greeting. Thus, through the ages, vanity has always been the death-trap of reason in the struggle toward the early diagnosis and treatment of breast cancer.

So much for critics who say American culture is mammary-mad.

Hippocrates, the "Father of Medicine," who was born about 460 B.C. and was roughly a contemporary of Herodotus, made his opinion about all cancers perfectly clear: they were incurable. In his monumental seventy-volume medical encyclopedia, he wrote, "Those diseases that medicines do not cure are cured by the knife. Those that the knife does not cure are cured by fire. Those that fire does not cure must be considered incurable." The extreme nature of the cures is probably why Hippocrates did not try to do much for his cancer patients. As he said, "It is better to omit treatment altogether: for, if treated, the patients soon die, whereas if let alone, they may last a long time."

In defense of Hippocrates, it must be remembered that he had no anesthesias (apparently, he knew nothing about the Mesopotamian use of the poppy), no antiseptics, and no effective way to stop hemorrhage except by searing the wound with fire (called then, as now, cautery).

For 500 years Hippocrates' theories reigned supreme and unchallenged in the known medical world. Then, in the first century A.D., a Roman dilettante, Aulus Cornelius Celsus, switched his attention from agriculture, military science, law, and philosophy to medicine, particularly the study of cancer. According to his contemporaries, Celsus wrote many volumes about medicine, although only eight are still in existence. But those few indicate that he may have known more about the natural history of cancer than Hippocrates did. Celsus's writings also imply that not all of Hippocrates' successors had followed their master's warning to leave cancers alone; some of them must have been performing surgery, including breast amputations, because Celsus emphasized that "irritation of cancer by the imprudent intervention of a physician could put the patient into danger."

Interestingly, almost 2,000 years ago Celsus came out strongly against removing the pectoral muscles if a mastectomy was attempted. His influence apparently was great enough that throughout the so-called "dark ages of medicine" surgeons left the pectoral muscles intact. It took the bright age of modern medicine to make excision of these chest muscles a routine practice. By and large, Celsus was against treating any but very early cases of breast cancer. He felt that to use "caustics . . . burning irons . . . or [to] remove the growth with the scalpel never cured a patient." In particular, "burning exasperates and the growth spreads rapidly until it proves fatal."

Not that Celsus believed in doing nothing. His treatment seems to have been based on the idea—one still wrongly held by many— that there is some turning point after which benign masses (which he called *cacoethe*) become malignant. Since he had no way to know exactly when the change would occur, Celsus's rule of thumb was to put caustic, burning medications on the breast as soon as a symptom was noticed. If the symptom disappeared and the patient's condition improved, he assumed that the *cacoethe* had been caught in time. He then proceeded to do whatever surgery or cautery he felt was indicated. However, if there was no change or if the patient's condition worsened, Celsus believed this meant that the lump had already become malignant, and he did nothing more.

A century after Celsus, the famous Roman physician Galen (who was born in Greece) appeared on the scene and captured the imaginations of his colleagues with his four-humor theory of health and disease.

The human body, he said, was governed by the four humors of black bile, yellow bile, phlegm, and blood, and in a person who was healthy all four were in perfect balance. Minor imbalances shaped temperament and personality. Too much black bile produced melancholia or depression; excitable people had a shade too much yellow bile; lazy folk suffered from an excess of phlegm, and nice people inclined toward too much blood. The presence of a disease, however, meant that the humors were seriously out of kilter—the implication being that all physical ailments were generalized diseases of the whole body, with none confined to a single organ.

And what did the great Galen have to say about cancer? That the disease was caused by an overload of black bile and should be treated by special diets and purges. But there were exceptions. A breast tumor, for example, was usually cut out if it moved around easily and was not in a fixed position. In addition to surgery, a variety of medicines was used during that period. The most common were caustics, which, it was hoped, would burn out the cancer. It was Galen, by the way, who named the disease *cancer*—the Latin for "crab"—because most malignant tumors looked so much like this crustacean.

There were also prayers and incantations, for medicine then was as much religion, superstition, and mysticism as empirical knowledge. Indeed, such practitioners might be considered the forerunners of today's quacks. Even in those far-off times, victims of cancer were exploited by healers who promised a sure cure for a fast fee. Along with feminine vanity, crooks and quacks seem to permeate the entire history of breast cancer.

Although Galen's humoral theory traveled only as far as the borders of the Roman world, this was a considerable realm. His opinions were also perpetuated for centuries. In medieval times, Galen's views were accepted everywhere as "God-ordained," and his own words became his epitaph. "Never as yet have I gone astray," he wrote, "whether in treatment or in prognosis." For his apostles, he prophesied, "If anyone wishes to gain fame . . . all that he needs is to accept what I have been able to establish."

Galen was certainly ahead of his time, but not ahead by more than a thousand years. Yet his authority, supported by the Roman

Catholic Church, was so incredible that it was not challenged until 1543, by a young anatomist, Andreas Vesalius. In that year, he proved, by the dissection of cadavers, that the human thigh bone was straight, not curved, as Galen had stated—and he was severely attacked for contradicting medical doctrine. "To question Galen was unorthodox heresy," medical historians have written, in describing those dark ages of medicine.

In the age we live in now, when every new medical theory has to be experimentally and clinically verified by independent researchers before it becomes scientific gospel, it is hard to believe that Galen's ideas, however brilliant, could have controlled medicine so completely in the sixteenth century. Yet Vesalius was told that, in spite of what his cadavers showed about straight thigh bones, Galen had been right. The femur had changed, because, since his time, men had begun wearing tight-fitting clothes instead of togas!

We really should not be too hard on Galen. He was, after all, far ahead of his time as a physician. Until the first microscope was put together, in about 1590, it was impossible to know much about the actual nature of health or disease. All that could be done was to observe, classify, and theorize. Treatment was either the repetition of what had worked before in a similar case, sheer guesswork, or, more likely, the combination of both.

This was especially true for cancer. By definition, it is a disorder that involves cellular growth and reproduction, and no one could begin to understand it until the microscope permitted scientists to peer into the mysteries of cells and learn something of how they worked. Quite literally, all progress in learning about cancer has been directly related to the development of better microscopes. In the last quarter of the twentieth century, this is still the story I frequently hear from frustrated cancer researchers: "We don't have the technical know-how to see that yet."

I don't mean to imply that there were no changes in the way breast cancer was managed between Galen's time and that of Vesalius. When tumors were small, cutting them out and cauterizing were often successful. Leading physicians and surgeons began to believe, correctly, that if the cancer could be caught before it had spread into the armpit, there was a good chance of a cure. There were medical as well as surgical attacks, including the use of arsenic, zinc-chloride pastes, and other caustics to try to burn out the tumor; doctors thought that if the skin over the growth began to corrode or blister, the tumor would somehow pop out of the diseased breast.

Even without anesthesia or antiseptics, enough mastectomies

were apparently being done to justify a section in a medical book giving detailed instructions for performing the operation. Except for the poppyheads of ancient Mesopotamia, I found no mention of a painkiller for any surgery. Split-second speed seems to have been the only way agony could be alleviated. Organs were pinched, sawed, or hacked off, and burning irons were put directly on the wounds to stop the bleeding. There are no data on the mortality rates from infection and massive hemorrhage, but these, like the torment, must have been horrendous.

By the mid-1500s, Galen's medical authority was clearly on the wane. Vesalius had been the first to undermine that authority, and his *De Humani Corporis Fabrica* is considered to mark the beginning of the modern study of anatomy. Soon a wholesale exodus from Galen's dark ages into a medical renaissance was under way. One of the foremost leaders of the movement was William Harvey who, in the early 1600s, discovered the principles of the circulation of blood. Between laboratory advances in the study of the nature of cells with the microscope and advances in the knowledge of anatomy and physiology, a great deal was soon learned about cancer in general, as well as about breast cancer.

Unfortunately, all the new knowledge did not make much difference in the outcome. Breast cancer was almost invariably fatal. But now doctors understood why. Once the malignancy had reached into and beyond the lymph nodes of the armpit, it was no longer breast cancer; it was spreading through the whole body. For successful treatment, the malignancy had to be cut out before this happened.

The most thoughtful surgeons of those early centuries of modern medicine theorized, accurately, that careful removal of the entire breast and the lymph nodes gave the best chance for a cure. But who could bear such excruciating, lengthy surgery while remaining fully conscious? Also, any kind of surgery was perilous. Although techniques had been developed to ligate—tie off—arteries and veins, so that massive hemorrhage could be controlled, there was still infection to battle. So, even though by at least 1800 it was known that the breast should be removed and the armpit cleared of nodes, medicine lacked the technical know-how to do this safely and without hours of wakeful agony.

Then, in 1846, a dentist named William Morton successfully used a painkilling drug during an operation at Massachusetts General Hospital in Boston. His creation was an early ether. In 1865, Dr. Louis Pasteur developed his germ theory of disease, and soon afterward Joseph Lister presented the world with a compound he named an antiseptic. These advances changed the nature of surgery, and a new era opened up for breast-cancer patients.

At the time, a long-term cancer survivor was a clinical curiosity. But in 1867, Mr. Charles H. Moore, a surgeon at the Middlesex Hospital in England,* began to perform, with a good deal of success, what we would now consider a very extended radical mastectomy. (He removed the breast, neck, chest, and axillary nodes, some muscles, and even rib-cage bones.) More important than his survival rate, however, was what he learned—and wrote—regarding the nature of breast cancer. "Local recurrence of cancer is due to the continuous growth of fragments of the principal tumor," he said. "It is not sufficient to remove the tumor, or any portion only of the breast in which it is situated; mammary cancer requires the careful extrication of the entire organ." Moore also insisted that the surgeon must not cut into the tumor at all and should be careful to remove the axillary nodes with the breast itself in a single, continuous operation.

Before anesthesia or antiseptics, surgeons tore into a woman's chest with all the precision of an amateur demolition freak planting dynamite. They had no choice—if they didn't work as fast as possible, she would die on the operating table. According to Moore's lectures to his colleagues, even after anesthesia was introduced, these practices were still going on. He called them "barbarous, not to mention dangerous," and his operations and his statistics were convincing. By 1889, Moore's technique had been refined into the operation that remains more or less the standard procedure in the United States today—the Halsted radical mastectomy. It was first performed, in Baltimore, by one of The Johns Hopkins Hospital's greats, William Stewart Halsted.

Halsted was one of the first surgeons in the world to use gloves and a mask routinely. By the time he did his first mastectomy he already had an international reputation as a skilled surgeon, inventive genius, and inspiring teacher. His original radical mastectomy removed a great deal: the breast, the lymph nodes and all their surrounding tissue in the armpit, a lot of skin, and the large pectoral muscle with all its connecting ligaments and tendons. He grafted skin to cover the resulting hole in the chest wall. It was a mutilating operation, but it seemed to give survival rates that surpassed anything else ever done.

The frozen-section technique for quick pathological examination of a biopsied specimen had been introduced in 1818 by a

---

*In Great Britain, then as now, surgeons are not called "doctors," but just plain "mister"—perhaps a leftover from the day when barbers did all surgery.

Dutch physician, Pieter de Riemer, and after anesthetics came into use, it became a godsend in treating breast cancer. (A biopsy diagnostic technique had long been used for uterine and cervical cancers, but it was not too helpful for breast tumors, since the microscope slide took about a week to prepare.) Now, being able to freeze a bit of tissue and examine it within minutes meant that the tissue specimen could be diagnosed while the patient waited unconscious on the operating table. (Though surgeons, no doubt, applaud this as a clear advance, I see it as a mixed blessing. Without the frozen sections, they would have to delay their mastectomies, giving their patients time to think.)

After 1889, the technological know-how began to come quickly. X-ray was discovered, and it did not take long for doctors to realize that this strange, powerful, but invisible force was lethal to cancer cells. By 1913, it was routine to give a "shot" of X-ray after cancer surgery, just to be sure any remaining stray malignant patches were destroyed.

Surgical pioneers—Dr. George Crile Sr. in the United States and David Patey in England—developed mastectomies that did not require the disfiguring and disabling excision of the pectoral muscles. The Patey modified radical became popular in Europe after its introduction in 1930. Unfortunately, Dr. Crile was not as successful in defeating the Halsted in this country, and until the late 1970s, it was still most surgeon's first choice here.

In the late 1800s, a search had begun for a drug that would kill cancer. Talk—and hope—intensified after Dr. Paul Ehrlich developed his "magic bullet" against syphilis. But nothing came of it then.

It took World War II and the research that produced nitrogen mustard to bring on the era of chemotherapy. Mustard gas was known in World War I, but it was outlawed by international agreement after the war because it was so poisonous. However, because it poisoned cells, research chemists quickly recognized that this quality might make mustards effective anti-cancer drugs. Thus the "alkylating" mustards became the first important members of medicine's arsenal of chemical weapons against the disease, and trials with various combinations of such compounds went on for years. Some were so potent that they killed the patients before their cancers were affected; others had hardly any effect. Finally, during World War II, a nitrogen-mustard combination was developed, which proved to be both effective and relatively safe.

Another big advance in cancer research resulted from that war, one that had more to do with learning about a cause of breast cancer than about its treatment. Part of the fallout from the atomic bombs dropped on Hiroshima and Nagasaki and the release of their intensely powerful X-ray-like force, was new knowledge of the relationship between irradiation and cancer. While it was already known that the mysterious force could cure or arrest cancer, the A-bomb also caused much malignant disease.

A high incidence of leukemia diagnosed in the Japanese survivors of the atomic raids within the first five years after World War II created scientific interest in the possible relationship between nuclear radiation and cancer. The Atomic Energy Commission and the National Academy of Sciences were given the job of studying the problem, in both animals and humans. Since the end of World War II, survivors have been carefully studied by international teams of experts. In 1970, a special group known as the BEIR Commission* (the initials stand for Biological Effects of Ionizing Radiation) issued a report giving the latest data about the victims. Within a few years of the atomic explosions, it became apparent that the incidence of leukemia was increasing. Later, data showed breast-cancer incidence was also higher.

Leukemia was reported earlier because its latent period (the length of time between the birth of a cancer and its appearance) is so much shorter than that for mammary carcinoma. Blood cells reproduce quickly, have frequent twinning periods, and any cell damage resulting in leukemia is diagnosed earlier. On the other hand, breast cells reproduce slowly, and transformation from healthy to malignant can take decades.

As in the sixteenth century, further advances on the basic cellular level had to wait for further technical know-how. Finally, the mid-twentieth century brought the electron microscope, and, quite literally, endless new vistas were opened up to curious,

---

*An interesting piece of information in the 1980 BEIR report was that the Japanese survivors most likely to develop breast cancer are women who were either just beginning to menstruate or who were pregnant when the atomic bombs fell on Hiroshima and Nagasaki in August, 1945. Women who were older than 50 years of age at the time did not develop any more breast cancers in later years than Japanese women who were *not* exposed to The Bomb. Nor has there been any significant excess of breast cancer in women who were exposed to the atomic radiation when they were at other ages.

The implications of this information are still not completely understood, but breast-cancer experts generally believe there is some kind of interaction between ionizing radiation and the massive quantities of female hormones, especially estrogens, present in women's bodies during puberty and pregnancy. The phenomenon is being carefully studied, and the BEIR Commission's follow-up will continue. The high incidence of these two cancers (i.e., leukemia and breast) in the Japanese survivors, however, has been accepted as proof that X-ray of any kind should not be used indiscriminately for either diagnosis or treatment.

probing scientific eyes. Now they could see what was going on inside cells!

Meanwhile, the unraveling of the code of DNA—that microscopic programmer in the nucleus of every living cell—was triggering molecular research on cancer in laboratories all over the world. Perhaps DNA carried a gene for it, making the disease hereditary?

Immunology was brought into the act, through organ transplants and the accompanying use of heavy quantities of certain drugs. A disproportionate number of transplanted kidneys became malignant. Other kinds of cancers also appeared in these patients. "Why?" scientists wondered. "Because of the drugs used to prevent the body's rejection of the foreign organ," some answered. "These immunosuppressant drugs are also lowering resistance to other things." Other experts said these cancers were not due to the drugs at all but to stimulation of the body's immune system by something in the alien kidney.

Using this bit of knowledge about immunology, some irradiation here, chemotherapy there, doctors found they could cure most skin cancers. Some of the leukemias (there are many types) are now also long-term chronic diseases, instead of being immediate death sentences. Advances in immunology for detection, as well as treatment, have been so dramatic that these will be detailed later.

On another front, the American Cancer Society (founded in 1913) made public education a top priority. Massive publicity about the seven danger signals began to bring cancer out of the closet it had shared with syphilis and gonorrhea. With financial support from the ACS, Dr. George M. Papanicolaou developed the "Pap test" for detecting cervical cancer, and this once lethal women's disease can now be entirely cured if caught in time.

And breast-cancer progress?

The success of the Pap test led scientists to believe that a similar technique could be developed to detect early breast cancer, and the search to find it became an international project. The most successful method seemed to be the use of mammography—breast X-rays—and these early efforts were pioneered by Dr. Jacob Gershon-Cohen of Philadelphia. (Remember, the dangers of ionizing radiation to the female breast were not known until long after World War II.) As I will describe later, mammography has come a long way since then.

As far as saying anything to challenge the continuing litany, "There has been no change in survival rates since 1930," there is still no concrete evidence that more women are being cured of breast cancer than they were a half-century ago. However, adjuvant therapy—prophylactic treatment with drugs, hormones, and anti-estrogens immediately after surgery for high-risk women—was not widely used until 1976. Because data collection and analysis take such a long time, the numbers people at the National Cancer Institute usually do not even get them for two or three years.

As a result, the current SEER (Surveillance, Epidemiology, and End Results) Report's latest survival rates are for the years 1973-1976. The SEER data for 1976 to 1979 are not yet available, and until the statistics through 1981 have been analyzed, it is a matter of faith. I believe the use of adjuvant therapy will be reflected in the next SEER Report by a dramatic upward shift in survival rates, especially of premenopausal women. (Adjuvant therapy is so important that it too will be discussed in detail elsewhere.)

But even without these anticancer agents, more women are living now with breast cancer, because surgical and operating-room improvements have reduced the number of deaths resulting from mastectomy itself, and techniques for earlier detection have extended the time from diagnosis to death. Yet, since these general improvements in surgery have occurred, the mortality rate seems to be unchanged: in the countries of the world from which data are available, half of the women who develop breast cancer die of it sooner or later. The number of deaths each year from breast cancers diagnosed in previous years equals about one-third of that year's incidence rate (the latter is estimated at about 110,000 cases in the United States in 1981).

However, the actual number of years women can live with breast cancer is longer today. In other words, while I may ultimately be a breast-cancer statistic at ninety instead of at sixty, I will still be listed as a breast-cancer mortality statistic. The extra years of life are not reflected in overall mortality data.

There have been two ominous changes in the incidence statistics since 1930, however. Incidence rates (the number of cases per 100,000 of the population) have been rising, and the average age of onset is dropping—more and more women under thirty are becoming victims.

But in the awful first moments after a diagnosis of breast cancer is confirmed, there has been little change in her treatment.

"Unfortunately," Dr. Paul Carbone, of the National Cancer Institute, told me, "the first course of action is still some kind of radical mastectomy. The best treatment to produce a cure first requires removal of the breast and the axillary nodes."

That is exactly what Mr. Charles Moore was saying in 1867—more than a century ago.

MYTHS

No history of any disease is complete without telling some of the myths about its causes and cures that have accumulated over the centuries. There are probably more myths about cancer than about any other disease except, perhaps, epilepsy or leprosy. Only these three have been so enshrouded in an aura of fear and mystery through the ages. Some of the most persistent—and most easily refuted—myths concern breast cancer.

To get right to one of the more prevalent of these, breast cancer is not contagious and neither are any other cancers. Viruses are under investigation as a possible cause of these diseases, and this viral research will be described in a later chapter. But even if every laboratory in the world should prove beyond a shadow of a doubt that a virus is the cause, it would not be the kind that can pass along the flu, a cold, or any other contagious disease. There has never been any indication—and certainly no hard evidence—that anyone ever caught breast cancer from someone else.

And no kind of cancer can be caught from a sick animal, either. I recently read of a woman who was convinced that her breast tumor was somehow caused by contamination from cleaning up after her cancerous dog. When I asked scientists about this, I was laughed at so many times that I finally stopped from embarrassment. It is nonsense.

The idea that "cancer germs" can enter the breasts either through the ducts of the nipple or through a cut or scratch is also without scientific foundation.

Many women say they were hit or bumped on the spot where a tumor later grew. An ordinary injury will not develop into a malignancy. But it is true that a woman is more likely to develop a neoplasm if she has a prior history of breast disease—by which doctors generally mean benign growths, breast abscesses, mastitis, inflammations of the milk ducts when nursing, and the like. So it might be that certain kinds of breast injuries could be classified as prior diseases. This, then, may not be altogether a myth, after all.

It is also true that a trauma can call attention to an already existing cancer that had simply not been noticed before. In any case, soreness or a lump caused by a fall or blow should be reported to a doctor if it does not go away within a reasonable period of time.

I interviewed two patients, in two different countries, who blamed their breast cancers on their husband's overeager manipulations while making love. A radiologist laughed when I told him this story. "It was probably the husbands' constant attention to their wives' breasts that led to the early discovery of cancers that were already there," he said. As a matter of fact, I had asked the women who first discovered the lumps, and both admitted it had been their husbands.

I also interviewed several women who blamed malignancies on their babies for having sucked too hard and painfully during breast-feeding. If the baby caused real damage to the breast, would this qualify as a prior breast disease? I asked, and was told, "Nature provides for the skin of the nipple to become very tough during breast-feeding days, making it unlikely for a child to inflict serious trauma." But if that does happen, a woman should follow the rule for any injury: report it to her doctor.

Pregnancy does not cause breast cancer either. Unfortunately, the myth that it does has some factual underpinnings. If a woman has a cancer at the time she becomes pregnant and it remains undetected or untreated, her outlook is not good. The body sends a flood of estrogens, the female hormone, into the blood stream to prepare first for the nine months of creating the baby and then for feeding it. This hormonal overload is fine for the baby, but it also feeds the developing cancer, which spreads like weeds after rain.

One woman I interviewed thought her cancer came from having too many chest X-rays to detect tuberculosis. She was a restaurant cook, and the law required that she be X-rayed every six months. A radiologist told me that, while it was possible, he doubted her tumor was caused by the semiannual examination. "The average chest X-ray gives so very little irradiation," he explained, "that the chances of its happening are almost zero. A mammogram can expose a woman to several Roentgens of irradiation per breast, for example, and yet we recommend it annually for older women. A TB examination is measured in milli-Rs—thousandths of a Roentgen."

Possibly one of the hardest myths to die—it isn't dead yet!—is the notion of "implantation by knife." The myth persists because often patients do die soon after a mastectomy or other cancer surgery. The reason, however, is not that the surgeon spread the cancer into the blood stream with his scalpel. While this may sound plausible, scientific evidence does not support it. For one thing, after a biopsy of a cancerous breast, malignant cells are frequently left at the site of the surgery, but they usually die or are killed by the body's defense system. It is also now known that all malignant tumors constantly shed living cells into the blood stream, in the same way that healthy tissues do. While these could travel on and start new cancer colonies somewhere else, most die. Random blood tests of cancer patients show that about 70 percent of the test samples contain either living or dead cancer cells that did not metastasize. But they were not put there by the surgeon's knife; they were "sloughed off" by the tumor.

Then why do some cancer patients indeed seem to fade and slip away from life so quickly after surgery? Is it a false illusion? Is it a bizarre coincidence? One doctor told me his theory. "Some kinds of cancer cells are hypoxic, that is, they require very little oxygen. So long as they are tightly enclosed in the body, they grow slowly but steadily and could probably stay that way for a long time before causing death. Then surgery exposes the internal tissue to air, and that shot of fresh oxygen might make the cells grow faster." This is but one man's theory, however; nothing more. I could find no evidence to support it.

Originally, I had planned to put into the myth category the statement that lactation—the production of milk for breast-feeding—is a protection against breast cancer, because some renowned epidemiologists in the United States had announced that nursing does not give a mother protection. However, I found that most European, Japanese, and South American experts I interviewed disagreed strongly with the new view. Further inquiry showed that many American authorities share the European opinion that a woman *is* protected *while* she is breast-feeding. So I have moved lactation out of the myths and back where it had rested comfortably for decades—among the epidemiological aspects of breast cancer, which are discussed in the next chapter.

Does going bra-less cause breast cancer? Dr. Dao did not think there could be any connection, and everyone else I questioned agreed. "Too many cultures that have never seen a brassiere have very low incidences," he explained. Immediately, a mental picture of the legendary "topless" women of Bali came into mind. "But no woman should think that, just because of these data, being bra-less gives any protection against breast cancer," an epidemiologist cautioned. "it's just one of those statistical coincidences."

Does being amply endowed make a woman a higher breast-cancer risk than one who cannot fill a size-32AA bra? No, but it makes lumps harder to find. For this reason, large-breasted women should be careful to examine their breasts every month and, after the age of fifty, have an annual checkup that includes a mammogram. Mammograms are much more accurate in finding cancers in large, fatty breasts than in small, dense ones, by the way. Fat, the major component of a 40DDD cup, provides what the technicians call "good contrast material," and even small tumors are easily picked up.

What about silicone implants used to enlarge the breasts? Studies done by members of the Breast Cancer Task Force of the National Cancer Institute have produced no evidence that the added filler *causes* cancer, but any extra padding inside may make a tumor more difficult to find. Also, those under-the-skin stitches feel like tiny growths themselves, and can therefore lull a woman into neglecting a malignant growth. Women whose breasts have been enlarged by surgery should take the same precautions as naturally large-breasted women.

The Pill?

To me, and to many others, there was proof-positive in 1975 that the hormones in birth control medications caused breast cancer. Since then, scientists have published conflicting data, and many believe the Pill may actually prevent breast cancer. The newer data have muddied and muddled the situation to the point where most women are even more confused than they already were. This data will be discussed in Chapter 5.

QUACKERY

"Cures" for breast cancer over the ages have included exorcism, the laying on of hands, concoctions to drink or apply, and even fire. In the Middle Ages, when herbs were virtually the only medicines for any disease, a mixture of herbaproserpinaca (knotgrass) and butter was prescribed to make tumors disappear. Sweet butter was in almost all the medicinal ointments, mixed with other ingredients, such as milk or vinegar. Burning out a suspected cancer was another favorite treatment. This was done either with red-hot irons or with instruments called "fire drills."

In the Arab world, external applications of caustics were popular, because the Moslem religion forbade any kind of mutilating surgery. But Christian doctors also used caustics for chemical burning. French physicians of the thirteenth century applied arsenic and zinc-chloride pastes. In Germany, in the fourteenth century, the breasts were squeezed between heavy lead plates.

In England, Queen Elizabeth's personal physician, William Clowes, decided that the laying on of the royal hands was the perfect treatment, although there is no record of any cures being effected by Elizabeth's "divine, royal touch" or by the ring she wore between her breasts. If Elizabeth had her ring, the common people had amulets and talismans of their own—preventives that are probably still worn in many places around the world today.

Lourdes and many other religious shrines have always had their share of breast-cancer patients seeking a miracle cure, and no doubt, in the United States today, faith healers like Oral Roberts have a good many visits from them.

Shortly after my own mastectomy, I began to receive in the mail literature about three substances—laetrile, hydrazine sulfate, and abscissic acid—that were described as being able to prevent a recurrence of cancer. Every authority I questioned, if he had heard of them at all, felt they were a waste of money, and a biochemist who examined the formulas thought they might even be dangerous.

When I wrote about laetrile (amygdalin) before, I was able to tell all about it in a single paragraph. I said it was "nothing more than ground-up apricot pits," and that it was an ancient Chinese cancer remedy, according to a friend who was born in Shanghai. The only reason I gave for my being skeptical about laetrile was that it contained cyanide. So I shrugged "vitamin B_{17}," out of *Why Me?* by simply saying it was nothing to consider seriously.

Since that time, laetrile—alias amygdalin, alias vitamin B_{17}—has become a political, not a scientific, issue all over the world. The reason it has now catapulted into the limelight is that a cancer patient (Glen Rutherford of Conway Springs, Kansas) brought suit against the FDA to let him import the illegal substance to treat his curable (with conventional methods) rectal cancer. When he was first diagnosed in 1971, Rutherford decided to go to Mexico for laetrile therapy instead of having his surgeon remove the polyp—an operation a Mexican surgeon performed about two weeks after his laetrile treatments began. When he came back, he brought a smuggled supply that lasted for several years. After he ran out, he filed the initial suit, and the legal battles continued for years. Finally, in October 1976, the 10th U.S. Circuit Court of Appeals in Denver ruled that the FDA had "insufficient information" about laetrile to ban its use. The higher court sent the case back to a District Court in western Oklahoma and told the FDA "to develop a record supportive of the agency's determination."

This was the beginning of a national movement to turn laetrile's legality into a civil rights issue. Advocates said the ban was an invasion of cancer patients' freedom-of-choice. The cause had been taken up as a political issue by the John Birch Society and then several national organizations were formed for the purpose of promoting laetrile. These included the Committee for Freedom of Choice in Cancer Therapy, the International Association of Cancer Victims and Friends, and the Cancer Control Society. Even before Rutherford, laetrile had already had a staunch friend in the National Health Federation, an advocate (since 1955) of many unproven or worthless medical treatments of all kinds.

Actually, laetrile has been around since Prohibition when someone thought the apricot flavor might make bootleg whisky more salable. I have not been able to find any record of how laetrile went from cognac to cancer, but, somehow, it emerged in a "purified" form in 1952 as a miraculous, new "magic bullet." In the years since, laetrile has been attacked by almost all cancer experts as being an ineffective and potentially unsafe substance. Its supporters continually changed their tactics to avoid and evade the stringent standards required by the FDA. They even began to call it a food supplement: vitamin B_{17}.

The loud voices of its supporters managed to get laetrile tested again and again. In 1953, the Cancer Commission of the California Medical Association investigated it and found it ineffective; in 1965, scientists in Canada tested two kinds of laetrile, and both were found to be useless. Between 1957 and 1976, the National Cancer Institute tested the substance in animals at least five times, and there were four other studies in various cancer centers—including the prestigious Memorial Sloan-Kettering Institute in New York—that resulted in the same conclusion: laetrile had neither prolonged life, reduced the size of tumors, or stopped any cancer from spreading.

The pro-laetrile forces, apparently, finally decided that it was not only a civil rights issue, but a states' rights issue. By the summer of 1977, amygdalin had been legalized in eleven states in the United States, and bills to legitimize it were waiting for some kind of action in several others. Under these circumstances, the FDA, a federal agency, has no right to intervene and cannot prevent individual legislatures from permitting laetrile's manufacture, import, or sale.

In 1980, advocates claimed that about 70,000 American cancer patients were benefitting from laetrile, but when the NCI spent $152,000 to review the medical records of cancer patients who used the substance, only 22 could be obtained. Of these, six patients had shown improvement, nine stayed the same, and seven had gotten worse.

Above all, however, laetrile and other ineffective treatments—even nonsensical electronic gadgets like the "Spectrochrome"—have emotional overtones. How can any Congressman, Senator, or judge deny dying cancer victims any flimsy straw they can clutch?

This moral and ethical dilemma finally convinced Congress to order the National Cancer Institute to set up impeccable trials to answer the question.

In October 1978, *Science Magazine* reported: "In an attempt to clear up the 200-year-old 'laetrile controversy' once and for all, National Cancer Institute (NCI) Director, Arthur C. Upton, on the 27th of September called for an NCI clinical trial of the apricot-pit derivative. Between 150 and 300 terminal cancer patients are expected to begin receiving the drug before January, with the first results coming in by next spring."

That would have been the spring of 1979. Why didn't this happen?

Unfortunately, what may seem simple on Capitol Hill is not so simple in the clinic. First of all, because laetrile has been illegal, the FDA had no standards for measuring its quality. As every user of marijuana knows well, all contraband materials have different strengths, contaminants, and are often just plain fraud. No scientific tests can be done legally with any substance that does not meet certain criteria of cleanliness, purity, and potency. So before the NCI could obey its Congressional mandate, various types of laetrile had to be evaluated. Then standards had to be set by the FDA. Even though one of laetrile's major claims has always been that it has no side effects, the toxicity of purified amygdalin turned out to be a serious problem during the preliminary animal tests required by law. Advocates insisted that the FDA did something deliberately to cause it, and it is possible that contaminants in impure laetrile did, somehow, prevent the toxicity the FDA found. Nevertheless, the NCI's trials were delayed and did not even begin until June and July 1980.

The studies were conducted at the Mayo Clinic, the UCLA Cancer Center, the University of Arizona Health Sciences Center and at Memorial Sloan-Kettering Cancer Center. The results were reported on April 30, 1981 and were based on 156 patients, because 22 were not eligible for a variety of reasons. Testing methods were the same ones used by the NCI to evaluate other anti-cancer agents. The cancer patients included in the trial were those for whom no other treatment had been effective or for whom no proven treatment existed. Many different cancers were involved, and the treatment design followed current laetrile use: the substance was given intravenously for 21 days and was accompanied by a diet rich in fresh fruits, vegetables and whole grains. Refined flour and sugar, meat, other animal products and alcohol were restricted, and patients were also given the vitamins and enzymes recommended by laetrile advocates.

There was a serious obstacle in the way before testing an

"unproven method": getting enough of the right people. The law and medical ethics prohibits any doctor from using any treatment in humans that he/she considers unsafe and ineffective, if there are safe and effective treatments available. This meant that the only patients scientists could recruit for the laetrile trial were those who have already tried everything else without success.

Under these circumstances, if these patients were given laetrile and *did* get better, it is impossible for anyone to know whether they improved because of the laetrile or because the conventional treatment had a delayed reaction. To add to the confusion, there are documented cases of people—told they have only weeks or even days to live—who go into spontaneous remissions. Such phenomena may be the result of a sudden strengthening of the immune system or to a God-given miracle in answer to a prayer. But they do happen. A third factor that clouded the trials' results was something known as the "placebo effect." Studies of hundreds of substances tested to treat virtually every disease under the sun have proven that people often feel better and actually seem to be better even if they are given "medicine" made of sugar or salt water.

On the other hand, advocates argued that the patients who really received laetrile but got worse and died, were given the apricot-pit extract too late, that the patients were already at death's door when they finally got the medicine that might have saved their lives.

So, all in all, it looks like the expensive, Congressionally-mandated NCI trials of laetrile were a no-win battle for all sides—including the patients.

The laetrile trial finally got underway and was concluded in April, 1981. On April 30, the final results were given to the press.

In spite of reports that laetrile has no toxicity, patients experienced nausea, vomiting, headaches, dizziness, mental confusion and skin rash. As patients' cancers worsened, they were withdrawn from the trial. Based on the data from 156 patients:

1. Within one month, 50 per cent of the patients' conditions worsened;
2. Within three months, 90 percent of the patients' conditions worsened;
3. Fifty percent of the patients died before 5 months;
4. Only 20 per cent were alive at the end of 8 months;
5. Only one patient showed a partial improvement, but his lasted only 10 weeks.

The official NCI report stated: "The findings of the laetrile tests with cancer patients present public evidence of laetrile's failure as a cancer treatment. The question of laetrile's effectiveness has been a significant public health issue for years. The hollow promise of this drug has led thousands of Americans away from potentially helpful therapy of scientific validity. Now the facts speak for themselves. Laetrile (or amygdalin) in combination with so-called metabolic therapy does not produce any substantive benefit in terms of cure or improvement of cancer . . . slowing the advance of cancer, improving symptoms or (the) general condition of the cancer patient, or in terms of extension of life span."

Perhaps laetrile will soon be a memory like krebiozen, a drug that caused a furor just a few years ago. Apparently, this substance has been dropped by the promoters of quack cures entirely, because the only mention I found of it involved the dispute between the "cancer establishment"—The American Cancer Society (ACS), the FDA, the NCI, and the American Medical Association—and people who were clamoring to have this horse-serum derivative legalized. For some reason, the issue has since disappeared from the news.

This is a good time for me to give my definition of "quack cures." The ACS and the NCI have both—for legal reasons, I've been told—stopped using the term "quack cures" and are now calling them "unproven methods." But "unproven methods" are not the accurate words to use, because there are many drugs and other therapies being used by reputable physicians in respected institutions, therapies that have yet to be "proven" as a cure for cancer. If this weren't true, no one receiving any orthodox treatment would ever die of the disease. Obviously, then, virtually every drug, procedure, technique, or combination being used today is "unproven." Certainly, interferons and most immunological treatments (discussed in Chapter 12) would be covered by the same term. Then, what is the difference between these and quackery?

One difference is simply that quacks usually defraud cancer patients, bilking and bankrupting them while also depriving them of possible life-prolonging treatment. (A government investigation in the late 1970s showed that almost all of the top people in the laetrile business had multi-million-dollar bank accounts stashed away in various countries.) Another definition could be that a quack cure is something that does not permit any conventional treatment during or after its use. For example, a doctor in Switzerland advertises, via the grapevine, that his special blend of an extract of mistletoe cures breast cancer. The vital—or should I say fatal?—"Catch-22" is that no other treatment can be administered until the six-to-eight-week course of mistletoe injections is completed. The doctor's prime targets, naturally, are desperate women who know that their mastectomies did not stop the spread of the cancer. These unfortunate victims do not have six to eight weeks to waste on something that is utterly useless. If they go to the Swiss doctor, it may be too late for proven treatments to do them any good. As far as I have learned, the promoters of laetrile, hydrazine sulfate, and abscissic acid make no such demand, but leave the patient free to go ahead with alternative therapies. Nonetheless, these have been denied FDA authorization for use as cancer treatments, and the NCI trials show that laetrile is still quackery.

"Cures" come and go like long skirts. So-called "vaccines" turn up periodically on unauthorized markets. One, reported in 1968, was a liquid saturated with bacteria, which was to be inhaled by means of an aerosol spray. The unique feature of this treatment, so its promoters said, was that if the patient was too weak to get out of her car, it could be administered at the curb outside the doctor's office. There is a "cure" that stuffs the patient with grapes, and another of red cabbage, either eaten raw or applied as a poultice of some kind. Many similar "miracle" diets are based on the belief that eating an excess of a particular food, vitamin, or mineral will cure cancer.

Then there are the gadgets—panels of knobs, colored lights, and switches, with controls to measure whatever response the patient is supposed to be giving. A wooden box lined with zinc has been touted as a device to renew the body's store of a cosmic energy called orgone, which, the manufacturers claim, is a very beneficial treatment for cancer.

These examples do not come from medieval medical tracts; they are from advertisements in pamphlets and newspapers published in the last half of the twentieth century. There is an underground cancer press that has many subscribers. For when cancer strikes and all hope is gone, intelligent, normally well-balanced people grab at anything. What do they have to lose but money? And someone is always there to take it.

Another kind of quackery must be mentioned, along with the grapes, gadgets, and orgone: the kind perpetrated by the doctor who deceives a patient. Moreover, general practitioners and surgeons who know little or nothing about the management of cancer but who, nonetheless, insist on treating patients with the disease are, in my opinion, just as dangerous as real quacks. Although they are physicians and they "mean well," they, too, cause patients to lose valuable time by giving inadequate or inappropriate treatment.

Most cancer specialists probably agree, although it is unlikely that any would ever say so for the written record. General physicians and surgeons should not be angry or insulted, since no one can fairly expect to be experts in cancer when they have to deal with almost every ailment that exists. Unfortunately, however, they do not know what they do not know.

In the first few months after my mastectomy, I had a personal experience with a woman whose doctor either deceived her, out of misguided kindness, or was unaware of his lack of knowledge. She was a friend of a friend, and not long after I came home from the hospital she called to wish me good luck. She had undergone a mastectomy the previous January and knew what I was going through. "My doctor said he got it all out," she said happily. "He said I didn't need radiation, chemotherapy—anything. All my nodes were clean as pins."

Two or three months later she called again. This time she was hoarse and coughed after every other word. "That son of a bitch!" she cried. "I went in to see him because I had a cold that just wouldn't go away. He did a chest X-ray, and my lungs are loaded with cancer. It must have been there all along—it couldn't have spread that fast. Why didn't he put me on some kind of treatment? Why didn't he tell me it was spreading, instead of saying I was clean as a pin?"

A month later, I heard that the cancer had metastasized to her brain. Less than a year after her mastectomy, she was dead.

Her doctor was a general surgeon, with no expertise in the management of cancer. He knew only how to amputate malignant organs. She did not have preoperative scans of her bones or X-rays of her lungs taken during her postoperative checkups. Until that chest X-ray eight months after the mastectomy, she had nothing but general physical examinations. (Recommended staging and follow-up procedures are described in chapters 8 and 14.)

Perhaps the surgeon did not lie to her. Maybe he really thought she was all clear. Only he and the pathologist, of course, know what was found when her breast and nodes were removed. But *she* knew what was done afterward: nothing. If he did not deceive her, he was at best incompetent to manage a breast-cancer patient. Either way, he deprived her of perhaps a year of treatment as surely as the Swiss doctor takes away six or eight weeks. That year might only have further postponed her death, but even so, the extra time would have been worth it to her.

"Most women can't take the truth" is what one general surgeon gave me as his reason for not telling his patients the whole truth after a mastectomy. "If I find eight or ten positive nodes, they're lost anyhow. Why tell them? Or even their families? There's nothing to be done."

For this Hippocratian healer, and for all others who think as he does, I have one answer: You tell her, so that she can find someone who *does* know what to do about the eight or ten positive nodes, especially in this era of adjuvant therapy. She is *not* "lost anyhow." Unless the cancer is so far advanced that all a woman can look forward to is a great deal of pain, even an extra six months is worth aiming for.

Of course, this inexcusable fatalism of general doctors does not apply only to breast cancer; it is true for all cancers. Oncologists are not so quick to write their patients off. They know of many things that can now be done to prolong life and keep it pain-free.

Fortunately, as I will explain in Chapter 11, few general surgeons insist on following their patients anymore if malignant axillary nodes are found at the time of mastectomy. (The speed with which the news about the effectiveness of adjuvant chemotherapy descended to the physicians and surgeons in Middle America may well be unprecedented in medical history!) So this bit of "quackery" is no longer as common as it once was.

But there are still some well-intentioned doctors out there who believe there is no reason to do anything, because the inevitable outcome is death within five years; these paragraphs are directed to them. Please, do your best to remove all physicians from inclusion in anyone's "quackery" chapter. Tell your patients the truth—they can take it, or their families can—and help them find good cancer specialists to continue their treatment. You will be surprised to see how long we women can live today—even with eight or ten positive nodes.

Everyone, apparently, wants to make money from our free-enterprise medical system; and some doctors, misled by delusions of omniscience, are not excluded.

In the autumn of 1974, when both Betty Ford and Happy Rockefeller were struck by breast cancer, panicky women began stampeding to doctors' offices and hospital radiology departments for breast examinations. Established and reputable X-ray clinics suddenly had waiting lists that were weeks—sometimes months—long. To accommodate those who would not wait, general practitioners and gynecologists around the country began buying thermographs, the only breast-cancer detection device a physician who is not a radiologist was then legally permitted to buy. Several of them established detection clinics, while others used the equipment as a supplement to their regular physical examinations—at an additional cost of $40 to $50.

I will explain thermography in detail in Chapter 7, but I think it is important to say here that the technique has not yet been shown to be as reliable as mammography. In the hands of a trained expert, this device that measures heat retention is a useful aid, especially for monitoring young, high-risk women who should not be mammographed. In 1974, thermography could not be counted on for an accurate diagnosis of either benign or malignant tissue. It simply shows changes of heat patterns in the breast, and—as I said—an experienced person can interpret these changes to show that something may be wrong.

That was true in 1974, and it is still true today.

Now, I still receive letters and telephone calls asking me about breast-screening clinics that have been set up as for-profit businesses. Most of these seem to be located in "Sun Belt" areas where relatively affluent senior citizens have moved for their retirement years. For two or three hundred dollars, women are promised a thorough examination with the latest fool-proof equipment. A Florida "chain" of such firms offers thermography, graphic-stress telethermometry, and ultrasound (also explained in Chapter 7).

While all of these screening modalities are under study and are useful adjuncts to mammography, *none* at this time can be relied on for "a clean bill of health." Most senior citizens are over 50 years old and should be screened by X-ray periodically in addition to having a thorough physical examination. Doctors should be experts and certified by the appropriate Board or College of their specialty, although paramedical personnel (like X-ray technicians) can be well trained to assist them.

A check with the National Cancer Institute's Cancer Information Service (toll-free) 800-638-6694 (except in Maryland: 800-492-6600), the local chapter of the American Cancer Society, or of the state or county Medical Society may show these "clinics" to be selling useless and perhaps dangerous breast-cancer examinations.

I do not want to leave the impression that *all* such screening centers—even if they are for-profit businesses—are frauds, because there are some excellent ones here and there in the United States. But women reading advertisements in newspapers or hearing about them on radio and television should investigate first and get in line later.

As a thermography salesman told me, "Somebody will always come along to try to make a fast buck out of somebody else's troubles."

4

Epidemiology
Who? When? Where?

"It looks as if breast cancer is a cold-weather disease, doesn't it?" the statistician said, pointing toward a world map with the high-incidence countries colored red. "Look at them. Except for Israel, where a large part of the population originated in Europe, breast cancer seems to be confined to the top and bottom of the globe."

I studied the red blotches. "What could cold weather have to do with it?" I asked.

"I'm just commenting on the geography, that's all." He smiled. "As far as we know, weather—cold or hot—doesn't have anything to do with breast cancer. But there is a strong geographical pattern world-wide. You shouldn't ignore the epidemiology of the disease. It could give us valuable clues toward finding a cause."

I stared at the map hanging on his office wall. The United States and the southern half of Canada were a solid red and so was the northern part of Europe, including the British Isles and Scandinavia (except for Finland), from the top half of France across the eastern border of European Russia. In the southern hemisphere, South Africa was red, as were sizable portions of Australia and New Zealand. Iceland was colored in red, and there was a red spot for Israel and a red dot for Bombay, India. There certainly did appear to be a pattern.

"Not only does it seem to be geographical," he continued. "There are other interesting epidemiological aspects as well."

First, he reminded me that the term *"epidemiology"* has nothing to do with whether or not a disease is contagious and thus can cause an epidemic. "Both words, *"epidemic"* and *"epidemiology,"* come from the same Greek root, meaning "staying among

80

the people." But epidemiology is the scientific study of the kinds of people who get a disease, at what ages, and where it is most prevalent. Obviously, mammary carcinoma is primarily a disease of women, but there the obvious ends. There are dozens of epidemiological mysteries—especially the concentration in the upper northern hemisphere.

The statistician went on to say that until recently his young scientific field had been virtually ignored by cancer researchers. "Their ears perked up when we talked about medical factors. But life-style, nutrition, industrialization—nothing doing."

"I've never read anything about those . . ."

"And the incidence of breast cancer keeps nosing up every year," he continued, not even hearing me. "There doesn't seem to be any clear-cut explanation. It may be nothing more than earlier detection and diagnosis. But it could also be a real rise of incidence. We don't know yet."

I called Dr. Sidney Cutler, then the associate chief of the Biometry Branch of the National Cancer Institute, keeper of the records of cancer-incidence rates and those dire statistics known as "end results." (Biometry is the investigation of biological phenomena using mathematics and statistics.)

"In 1974," he said, "cancer of the breast achieved the dubious distinction of having become the number-one cancer in the United States. That is, if intestinal malignancies are separated into colon and rectum, as they should be, it outranked lung cancer of males and females together." Dr. Cutler added that these data had not yet been published, but would be in the next edition of the NCI's epidemiological report. The 1972 edition still showed lung cancer in the top position.

"But be careful to distinguish between incidence and mortality," he warned. "Breast-cancer incidence is higher—more women are getting it. Lung and bronchus still have the greatest mortality, however; fewer people are getting this carcinoma than breast cancer, but fewer survive. That's important to remember. Caught early, mammary carcinoma is more easily cured."

"Of course, it's mostly women," I said, "so half the population is counted out right there."

"About 99 percent female," he agreed. "One out of every hundred mammary carcinomas is found in the breast of a male. When you take that into account, the impact is enormous."

For unknown reasons, Dr. Cutler said, the age of onset appeared to be dropping, and the disease was attacking younger women more than it did in earlier decades. He also suggested that the wide publicity given to early detection, breast self-examination, and the mass screening programs of the NCI and the American Cancer Society contributed to the seeming increased incidence of breast cancer at younger ages.

"More younger women have been made aware of breast-cancer risks and are finding tumors. That could account for a diagnosis at age thirty-five instead of forty-five.

"But early detection would have absolutely nothing to do with the kind of increased incidence we've been seeing within the past few years," he said flatly. "That has been going on too long. If the entire cause of the increase was earlier detection, there woud have been an abrupt hook in the graph, showing a sudden upward swing when the early-detection programs began. Then you would have a plateau beginning at a high level—providing, of course, that the programs created permanent habits. If not, there would be a downward swing when women stopped examining themselves and returned to their former habits."

He predicted that such a hook would appear on graphs for the last three months of 1974, reflecting the thousands of breast cancers discovered after Betty Ford and Happy Rockefeller had their mastectomies.

"But this kind of rise is usually temporary," he added. "It happens every time a famous personality announces that she's had breast-cancer surgery. The steady annual increase in the incidence of mammary carcinoma and the fact that it appears to be attacking younger women must be due to something other than just earlier detection."

At a breast-cancer conference held at the NIH two days after Mrs. Ford's surgery, I overheard a visiting oncologist talking to a colleague at the coffee table.

"I've never seen anything like it," he said. "It's almost an epidemic in Connecticut. What's it like in Cleveland?"

If the doctor from Connecticut had seen Dr. Cutler's graphs and charts, he would have learned that there was not much difference between his state and Ohio. In both, about ninety-nine percent of all cancers were found in women. Around the country, one of every fourteen women (about seven percent) could expect to develop a breast cancer at some time in her life. Grimly, in spite of all the treatment advances and earlier detection, about one-half of these women would eventually die of the disease, even though chemotherapy and improved radiation techniques and equipment were prolonging the years they would be living with cancer.

These kinds of data come from ordinary statistical analyses of incidence and mortality figures collected from hospital records and death certificates. Epidemiology begins where biometry ends, because these scientists take the numbers and try to find certain factors breast-cancer victims (indeed, victims of any disease) have in common. The statisticians are hopeful that this new, dynamic science of epidemiology will yield clues that will result in pinpointing the cause of breast cancer.

Epidemiological research has already shown that certain women have a higher risk of developing breast cancer than others do, and it has already found many clues that will ultimately identify these women so accurately that vigilant monitoring will detect their cancers when they are 100 percent curable.

Learning this about the importance of epidemiology made the red-blotched map far more interesting to me. In a mortality-rate table titled, "Cancer Around the World, 1968-1969," published by the World Health Organization, I discovered that the United States was not first in the breast-cancer column at all, but was twelfth. The Netherlands had the highest mortality rate of the countries listed. Second was Scotland, third was England and Wales combined, then Israel and Northern Ireland. Denmark, Ireland, Iceland, Canada, New Zealand and Switzerland all had higher mortality rates than the United States and all are "cold-weather countries" except for Israel. Even there, most of the women are Caucasians who came from cold-weather countries.

At the other end of the statistical pole, the Dominican Republic had the lowest death rate, according to the table. "But who knows what data are available there?" said the medical librarian who had found the chart for me. "There are a lot of countries where cancer is still unmentionable—even if it is diagnosed."

I noticed that Taiwan and Japan had the second and third lowest reported mortality rates. "How are their data?" I asked.

"Well," the librarian answered, "Japan is mentioned by statisticians quite a lot, so I suppose the figures from there must be fairly reliable. I don't know about Taiwan."

A word must be said about statistical charts, graphs, and tables, and the various ways they are compiled. With respect to incidence data, some countries collect absolute figures—the actual totals of patients during a given year, based on doctors' reports and hospital admissions. In other countries, where years of record-keeping have marked a specific region as being typical of the nation as a whole, biometricians often collect figures from that single region and use them as a model to project the nation-wide average. This is faster, but not as accurate. Still others average the rates of selected areas in different regions.

Most incidence data (and survival-mortality rates, too) are expressed as the number of cases per 100,000 of the total popula-

tion. With breast cancer, many countries more realistically base
the rate only on the female population. However, this usually
includes females below the age of twenty, not just those in the
vulnerable age groups. Since children and teen-agers rarely get
breast cancer, their inclusion in the base has the effect of lowering the incidence rate. Some tables "age-adjust" the data, to take
this distortion into account. Others correct for "death from other
causes."

Some countries collect no raw data at all; some may collect
data but do not report them to the World Health Organization or
any other international agency. Within a country, the quality of
data can vary from region to region, city to city, or even neighborhood to neighborhood within a city. Comparing statistics of one
country with those from another can, therefore, result in considerable confusion. So in these pages, I give comparative figures
only when they all come from the *same* table or graph.

Returning to the 1968-69 WHO table, I studied the numbers for
Japan. More than the Pacific Ocean separated that country's 4.01
breast-cancer deaths per 100,000 from the United State's 22.18
per 100,000. Even a data-collection system that was full of errors
could not alone account for the huge difference.

The librarian was watching me. "I don't think you should be
looking at death rates at all if you want meaningful information,"
she remarked. "Diagnosis, treatment and reporting are so spotty
in some countries that mortality rates aren't necessarily a
reflection of anything. After all, if only two out of 100,000 women
in a place develop breast cancer and both of them die from it, you
have 100 percent mortality, but only a fraction of a percent in
incidence." As a case in point, she found a mention of a small
town in Argentina that had a 50 percent-higher mortality rate one
year than the United States had. "And yet the incidence rate is
much lower in South America than it is here." She smiled. "So,
you see, there's no real connection between incidence and mortality in some countries."

She was right, of course. Not only would her suggestion to look
at incidence rates be more accurate; it would also be more cheerful.

I began with the "who." Who are the women most likely to
develop breast cancer?

The highest-risk category of all is made up of women who, like
me, have already had one cancerous breast removed. We are the
most likely of all to develop another one, in the second breast.
This I had already been told. But nowhere could I find a

comprehensive summing up of other high-risk or low-risk groups. I had to wade through isolated and scattered reports from all over the world to make some sense of all the statistics. It became a fascinating detective story.

An interesting discovery I made at the outset was that, where breast-cancer incidence rates are concerned, epidemiologists and biometricians distinguish between Hispanic women and women having Mediterranean backgrounds, and other white women—though all are Caucasians—because the Latin-Mediterranean incidence rates are considerably lower. Overall, in the United States, white women have a higher incidence than women of other races, and this pattern seems to prevail all over the world.

Several surveys I read stated outright that being black was in itself "protection," but Dr. Marvin Schneiderman, then the associate director of field studies and statistics at the National Cancer Institute, told me this is not so. Several studies had shown no difference in incidence rates between the two races. The puzzle was cleared up by a report that linked affluence and breast cancer.

"As black women climb socioeconomically," it said, "their life styles change and their breast-cancer incidence by income and social status is the same as that of white women in the same group." The survey concluded that there simply are far fewer affluent black women in the United States than affluent white women and this statistic distorts the data.

"It's what we call a statistical artifact," I was told by one statistician. "You can't always go by absolute numbers. There are other factors."

It will be interesting to see if the breast-cancer incidence rates of American black women continue to rise along with a better life style and higher incomes.

An international study done in 1970 compared the breast-cancer incidences of six countries. The United Kingdom and Wales were rated "high," Brazil and Greece "intermediate," Japan and Taiwan "low." Why? No one knows. But, again, the implication is clear: being a non-Latin white raises the risk.

So does being Jewish—sometimes. An American Jewish woman whose parents or grandparents came from Europe is in a higher risk group than the rest of American white women. But if her family is from a North African or Asian Jewish background, her risk of developing breast cancer is lower than the average for all other American women.

Being overweight is another factor that increases the risk of developing a mammary carcinoma, and scientists theorize that there is an "extraglandular" hormonal system in all women's bodies, a system that secretes more estrogens in heavy women. Excess avoirdupois also makes it more difficult to detect a breast cancer that is already present, if the fatty tissue is deposited on a woman's chest as well as on other parts of her body.

Cancer frequently "runs in the family," and whether this meant the disease is actually hereditary, the way brown hair and blue eyes are, is still being debated in 1981. Familial diseases can be caused by factors other than genetics—such as having the same diet or being exposed to the same general environment. However, in the past few years, enough data have been collected to erase any doubts about the role of heredity. A woman whose close relatives—on both her father's, as well as her mother's, side of the family—developed cancer is at higher risk of developing the disease herself.

Even in 1974, most epidemiologists were convinced that breast cancer had a genetic component. Dr. Schneiderman had even anticipated a finding that was not accepted as fact until the end of the decade. He told me he believed the most important factor is the age of the relative at the time she found her cancer and whether or not the disease involved one breast or both.

"If a woman's sister, mother, aunts, or grandmothers were seventy-five or so and had cancer in only one breast," he said, "there would be little risk. But if they were premenopausal and had had cancer in both breasts, the woman would have an exceedingly high risk of developing the disease." This has since been supported by virtually everyone in the field.

Having a history of benign breast disease also increases a woman's risk of developing breast cancer at some time in her life. These include mastitis, abscesses, fibroadenomas, papillomas, chronic cysts, etc. Women must be warned, however, that a biopsy per se does not mean a benign disease was found. They may simply have had insecure, unsure general surgeons who were afraid of possible malpractice suits. They may also have had knife-happy surgeons who believe every lump and bump should be removed, especially if a patient is older than thirty-five. At Roswell Park, I met a woman who had had fourteen biopsies (she could play tic-tac-toe on her breasts)—all with benign diagnoses. After she had finally put herself in Dr. Dao's expert hands, she still grew lumps and thickenings, but he had the expertise to know they did not need to be biopsied.

There is now a furious controversy about benign, but abnormal, growths, an issue that was not even a mild argument in 1974. At that time, all of the scientists I interviewed told me benign masses did not become malignant but should be removed anyhow, because they might "mask" a true cancer. Since then, a classical study done by Dr. Stephen Gallager—a top pathologist at the M. D. Anderson Cancer Center in Houston—has shown evidence that the evolution of cancer may be a "continuum" from benign hyperplasia, dysplasia, metaplasia, etc., until these finally transform into frank invasive carcinomas. This is the theory I refer to frequently when I use the words, "precursor cells."

Whether or not atypical cells are the first step in the transformation process from normal to cancer was never a clinical problem before mammography and other super-sensitive screening devices were invented. If a woman's breast contained such cells, neither she nor her doctor knew about them so long as they remained microscopic. But if they did grow large enough to be felt, the mass had to be removed, studied, and—if it was cancer—surgery was performed. However, now that doctors have the technological know-how for finding clusters of such abnormal, microscopic cells in a breast, this "breakthrough" has caused serious differences of opinion regarding appropriate treatment. There are hundreds of documented cases where older women, autopsied to determine the causes of their deaths, had cancers in their breasts, carcinomas that—for one reason or another—had never grown and were not the reasons they died. Had mammography been available when they were younger, these women would undoubtedly have had mastectomies.

I will discuss precursors and premalignant cells in more detail later, but it is imperative to state here that a history of multiple biopsies *does not* necessarily mean a woman has had confirmed diagnoses of any benign breast disease. A breast may develop cyclical cysts and other abnormalities related to menstruation, and these are *not* pathological processes or "diseases."

A variety of factors involving reproductive life—the years from the onset of menstruation through the menopause—also affect a woman's risk of getting breast cancer. No one knows exactly why, except that the secretion of female hormones—estrogens—must somehow be involved. Women who begin menstruating at an early age (in the United States, before twelve) are more likely to develop breast cancer. Early menarche, the medical term for early menstruation, presupposes a long reproductive life. If a woman has her ovaries removed before she is thirty-five or has a natural menopause at an early age, her chances of developing breast cancer drop considerably. Conversely, women who have a late menopause—after age fifty—have an increased risk of developing breast cancer.

For reasons no one understands completely at this time, a

woman whose first full-term child was born before she was twenty (the age that applies to the United States) has a substantially reduced risk—some statisticians estimate the risk is one-third what it would have been otherwise. At the other end of the age line, a woman who has a first full-term child when she is older than thirty has an elevated risk, and—again, for unknown reasons—her risk is higher than that of a woman who never has any children at all. Again, estrogens are suspected.

The effect of breast-feeding and the possible significance of the number of children a woman has borne—her "parity"—is a subject of debate among breast-cancer experts around the world. There is no question that nulliparous women (those who never have children) are high-risk candidates as are those who wait until they are more than thirty years old. The protection conferred by having a first child at an early age is also widely accepted, and—somehow—female hormones are involved. The dispute that is yet to be resolved centers around whether having many children and breastfeeding them is also protective.

In Moscow, I was given a plausible explanation by Professor O. V. Sviatukhina, a slim, graying woman of perhaps fifty-five, who is both a surgeon and an endocrinologist. She heads the all-female staff of the breast-cancer section at the Institute of Experimental and Clinical Oncology. Professor Sviatukhina believes that a woman is less vulnerable to mammary carcinoma *while she is actually breast-feeding*. Therefore, if she has four or five children and nurses each for two years, she gains eight or ten years of immunity that a non-breast-feeding mother does not have. If Professor Sviatukhina is correct—and other experts abroad agree with her—it is not the number of children but the years of breast-feeding that count.

The value of breast-feeding is probably the most controversial international breast-cancer issue extant. Does nursing a baby protect the mother against the disease? For decades, it was taken for granted that it did, but Dr. Brian MacMahon—a world-famous cancer epidemiologist—conducted a study that convinced him that breast-feeding even a dozen babies ". . . does nothing, one way or the other."

As a result, all breast-cancer experts did a sudden about-face. In his book, *Early Detection,* published in 1974, Dr. Philip Strax, a diagnostician-radiologist at the New York Guttman Institute, agreed with Dr. MacMahon.

"It used to be thought that breast-feeding—especially prolonged breast-feeding—was associated with a lower incidence of breast cancer," he wrote. "The latest data on a world-wide basis refute this concept. Apparently there is no relationship between nursing and breast cancer." Since I had been weaned on the gospel according to La Leche League, this was heresy to me. But science is science, and I moved "protection conferred by lactation" firmly into the myth category.

But when I visited Russia and heard Professor Sviatukhina describe her theory, I asked her what evidence she had found in her laboratories or clinics to support it.

She explained that the hormone prolactin, which triggers milk production, but is always present in a woman's blood in small quantities, contributes to the growth of mammary carcinoma during periods when she is not nursing. For reasons not yet known, prolactin seems to lose its ability to promote breast cancer when a woman is breast-feeding. The professor believed it happens because the brain triggers the production of some kind of inhibiting hormone during this period. The more children a woman has and the longer she breast-feeds them—three years or more is common in the Soviet Union, Professor Sviatukhina said—the longer she has this protection against the adverse effects of prolactin.

And she told me the theory had been proven in her clinics. Russian women who live in cities usually work; therefore, few of them are able to breast-feed. They are also more likely to take oral contraceptives, which could increase their prolactin levels. In rural areas, most women breast-feed and few of them take the Pill—and there is much less mammary carcinoma than in the cities.

When I visited Japan in 1976, I heard the same theory. Dr. Mitzuo Segi, a cancer epidemiologist whose statistical analyses of Japanese data have become classics, believed his country's low breast-cancer incidence rates were associated with a high rate of breast-feeding.

"Bottled milk was always difficult to obtain in Japan," he explained, "and infants were traditionally breast-fed until they reached the age when they could digest solid food or until another baby was born. Now that Japanese women are having fewer children and are adopting Western habits, this may change. But I think breast-feeding has been beneficial."

Dr. Segi pointed out that most Japanese firms have in-house nursery facilities for employees' children, and nursing mothers are encouraged to breast-feed their babies on company time.

Professor Sviatukhina had already begun my conversion on the breast-feeding question, and Dr. Segi completed the process. In spite of data to the contrary from top American physicians, I have taken breast-feeding out of myths and put it back into epidemiology—but with a question mark. Every woman must decide her superstition for herself.

On caution: Some evidence indicates that a woman who has had one cancerous breast removed may transmit suspicious particles via the milk of the other breast. For this reason, most doctors recommend *against* breast-feeding by anyone who has had a mastectomy.

Now, according to all this data, who in the United States is most likely to develop breast cancer? Jewish women of northern European descent who are affluent, overweight, have cancer in their families, have personal histories of confirmed benign breast disease, began menstruating early, and had a first child after they were thirty years old.

And who, so far, is least likely to develop it? Poor black, Oriental, or American Indian women with no history of breast disorders, no cancer in the family, late beginning of menstruation, and motherhood before age twenty. A short reproductive life because of an early menopause—surgical or natural—helps lower the risk.

When is breast cancer most likely to appear?

The disease rarely develops in girls under twenty, and until recently, it was seldom found before thirty. Today more and more women under thirty are becoming victims. For unknown reasons, but probably related to higher levels of circulating estrogens, when it does occur under thirty it is more virulent than is the case with older women.

The incidence peaks between the ages of forty-four and fifty-five. Then an eight-year plateau appears on the graphs—the statistical phenomenon known as "Clemmesen's hook."

The term describes a "bump" in graphs on which age and frequency of occurrence are plotted together. The bump occurs after about the age of forty-five. Until then, the graph shows a steadily climbing line, beginning at about age thirty and continuing until forty-five. Now comes the bump, and the line levels off into the eight-year plateau. Starting in the mid-fifties, the rate again climbs, though not as steeply, until very old age.

Many experts interpret this as statistical proof that breast cancer in young women is a different disease from that in older women. The theory also received support from American investigators in a study published in December 1974. Three Johns Hopkins researchers, Dr. Thomas J. Craig, Dr. George W. Comstock, and a nurse, Patricia B. Geiser (the study was done at the

Johns Hopkins University with funds from the National Cancer Institute), reported a distinct difference in the histories and risk factors of women who developed breast cancer before the age of forty-five and women who developed it later in life. According to their findings, a family history of breast cancer and a later age for the birth of the first child were more often associated with the younger women, while breast-feeding was a factor mainly with the older ones. Since the Johns Hopkins data were published, there have been numerous studies from surveys done worldwide supporting this "two disease" phenomenon.

Many women think the risk of getting breast cancer disappears after age seventy, but this is not true. The absolute number of new cases does drop with age, because fewer women are still alive, but the incidence rate among women over seventy actually increases, if percentages of women are counted. Anyone lucky enough to have reached threescore and ten must not think she is home free. She should pick a set day every month for self-examination and never forget to do it, as well as have an annual physical examination by her doctor.

On the following page is a simple "scorecard" by which a woman can test herself and see roughly where she falls in the risk areas discussed so far.

Anyone scoring 225 or higher should practice monthly breast self-examination (BSE), have a physical examination of the breasts by her doctor every six months, and, perhaps, periodic mammograms. Between 100 and 220, she should examine her breasts monthly and have an expert breast examination twice each year. Over the age of fifty, she should have a periodic mammogram. Below 100, BSE remains a must, along with a physical exam as part of an annual checkup.

Where are the risks highest?

Only within the past few years has much attention been paid to the possible role of the environment in relation to breast cancer. But today, when we have more and more potentially harmful substances all around us, the "where" of breast-cancer incidence has become increasingly significant, and the epidemiologists are beginning to come into their own.

For example, they have found that the region around Birmingham, England, has more cases of breast cancer than the Liverpool area.

Why?

That women living in the European republics of the Soviet Union have more than five times the breast-cancer incidence

SELF-TEST SCORECARD

Age group   Your risk

20-34 10 points	35-49 40 points	50+ 90 points

Race group

Oriental 10 points	Black 20 points	Caucasian 30 points

Family history

None 10 points	Mother, sister, aunt, or grandmother with breast cancer 50 points	Mother and sister with breast cancer 100 points

Your history

No breast cancer 10 points	Previous breast cancer 100 points

Pregnancy

First pregnant before 25 10 points	First pregnant 25 or after 15 points	Never pregnant 20 points

Your total

rates of those in the Asian republics. Yet when Asian women move to the European sections their rates rise to match the existing ones.

Why?

That in Israel, Jewish women from American or European families have at least three times the incidence of breast cancer as do Jewish women whose backgrounds are North African or Asian, while those from Yemen have less than the Africans and Asians.

Why?

That the Parsi women of Bombay have twice the breast-cancer incidence of Hindu, Christian, and Moslem women there.

Why?

What about the United States?

In 1976, a monumental work compiled by Dr. Joseph Fraumeni and his colleagues in the Department of Epidemiology of the NCI was published. Titled the *Atlas of Cancer Mortality by County, 1950-1969,* the book contains maps of the United States showing, in color, the parts of the country where certain cancers were causes of death. According to the breast-cancer map, the urban area of the northeast corridor between Washington and Boston is mottled with red, high-mortality spots. So are the industrialized areas around the Great Lakes, the San Francisco-Oakland region, and Los Angeles. Curiously, there is a white blotch for Penobscot County, Connecticut (populated primarily by Indians, I learned during a visit to the Yale Cancer Center) and a few red counties sprinkle otherwise low-risk states like North Dakota, Minnesota, Wisconsin, and Maine.

Why?

I remembered the warning from the NIH librarian that mortality rates are not as reliable as incidence rates are in trying to determine a disease's etiology (or cause).

"Mortality rates are especially unreliable in mobile societies of the kind we have in the United States," Dr. Dao told me. "It is not only the variability of the quality of care but also the fact that many people are living their retirement years far away from the areas they lived in when they were younger, when their breast cancers probably began to grow."

He looked at the white and pale yellow coloring of the Sun Belt.

"I am willing to bet that when these data are revised to reflect mortality rates through 1980, the warm, southern states will have many red counties as well."

Of course, Dr. Dao is probably right. People were not migrating southward during the twenty years covered by the Atlas the way they are now.

Still, until more and more accurate incidence data are accumulated in state, county, and municipal registries, death certificates are all scientists have to rely on. Besides, all people in the United States do not move away to Florida or Arizona as soon as they are eligible for monthly Social Security checks.

"The map showing liver cancer was the first clue about vinyl chloride," Harvey said, "and I saw a TV documentary about China's program to get rid of stomach and esophagus cancers using these kinds of maps. They're probably going to help find the causes of a lot of different kinds of cancer—even though people are moving around."

Harvey works with statistics, charts, and graphs and understands the potential value of these epidemiological tools. With his help, I studied the World Health Organization's complicated tables to look for clues about breast cancer. The highs were primarily cold-weather countries; the lows were the Dominican Republic (whose data may not be the best), Japan, Taiwan, and the Philippines—all Oriental.* With a mental reservation about the reliability of data, I saw that Mexico, Colombia, and Mauritius, also toward the bottom of the list, had mortality rates so low that even bad reporting could probably not explain the gap between them and the high-risk countries. Not quite so low, but far lower than the United States, were Bulgaria, Chile, Rumania, Venezuela, and Greece. Toward the middle were Finland and Italy.

Finland?

Its relatively low incidence did not fit the northern-hemisphere, cold-weather geographical picture I was trying to paint at all! What was Finland doing so low? I called a cancer epidemiologist.

"Well, you know that heredity plays some role in breast cancer," he began.

I nodded, even though he could not see me. "Yes, I've read about the Parsi women and about families with a lot of—"

"Centuries ago," he interrupted, "Asiatic tribesmen came westward on horseback to escape Genghis Khan. Some of them settled in the Danube basin and became Magyars—now Hungarians. Others kept going northward and became the ancestors of today's Finns and Estonians. I would guess that their Asiatic heritage may have given Finnish women some kind of built-in hereditary protection, which has survived over the centuries of intermarriage and exposure to a different environment. Their incidence rates are higher than Japan's aren't they?"

Hereditary protection?

*Data are not available from most Oriental countries.

My thoughts turned to those Parsi women, who have twice as much breast cancer as the Hindu, Christian, and Moslem women of Bombay. The Parsis, some 100,000 strong, are decended from Zoroastrian refugees who escaped from Persia about 1,300 years ago. They live mainly in Bombay and have kept themselves very much segregated from their neighbors, so that they are perhaps the most inbred people in the world. And their women have so much breast cancer that it accounts for half of *all* Parsi cancers. No wonder breast-cancer researchers are interested in them. The value of having a naturally bred 1,300-year-old population like this cannot be measured. I couldn't help wondering if modern Persian women have high unreported incidences.*

But what is the reason for all the Parsi breast cancer? No one knows, except that it must be something hereditary—a predisposition of some kind these women have to develop the disease.

This is when I stumbled onto another mystery, which made no apparent sense in relation to what I had already learned about breast cancer at that time—differences in diet. Dr. Frits de Waard, a professor at the University of Utrecht in Holland (the country at the top of the mortality list), had spent years studying nutrition and the role it might play in mammary carcinoma. He found a definite correlation between what he calls total-body-volume—a combination of weight and height—and the incidence of the disease. He has shown that large women—those who are unusually tall or fat or both—are at very high risk.

To support his argument, Dr. de Waard cited the differences in the diets of Yemeni women in Israel and of Israeli women who have a more European life style. "Yemeni food was very tasty," he told me, "but I would not like to eat it every day. There is very little meat, mainly vegetables and starches. They use primarily vegetable fats, no butter. In Holland, we are not accustomed to that kind of food."

"Did I understand you correctly?" I asked. "Height is a factor, as well as weight?" Most authorities, I knew, agreed that obesity is a factor in computing risks, but until then I had heard nothing about height.

"Height as well," he insisted. "It is total-body-volume. Height and weight cannot be separated. You know that in your country children of immigrants are usually much bigger than their parents. Not only are the girls taller than their mothers, but also they are

---

*My request to go to Iran to visit the Cancer Institute in Teheran had been approved by the late Shah, before the revolution toppled his government and forced him into exile in 1980.

heavier in general. And they tend to begin their reproductive lives earlier. In the United States, the average age of menarche is twelve or thirteen. But elsewhere, in Finland, for example, it is not at all unusual for it to be sixteen or older."

Dr. deWaard did the pioneering research indicating that every cell in a woman's body makes some minute quantity of estrogen—the "extraglandular system" referred to earlier. The more cells a woman has, the more estrogens she secretes into the bloodstream.

He reminded me of studies of the Japanese in California and Hawaii, where Japanese-American women are being surveyed for just this kind of generation gap. Those who were born in Japan and who have maintained a basically Japanese diet and way of life in the United States have breast-cancer incidences as low as in Japan. However, their daughters, who have adopted American dietary habits, have more breast cancer. Now the granddaughters are reaching the vulnerable age, and they are developing more breast cancers than their mothers did. While some kind of racial genetic protection may exist to keep their rates below our average, the incidence has been increasing with each generation. Japanese women are slender and small, and their low incidence—so long as they eat traditional foods—also supports the deWaard hypothesis.

I learned that a similar survey was done on Jewish women in New York. Being Jewish, and knowing that women with my background have a higher risk than others, I looked into this as soon as I read of it. Between 1949 and 1951, American Cancer Society epidemiologists compared the breast-cancer incidence among immigrant Jews with that of their American-born daughters. The older women had about the same rate as did the control group of non-Jewish New Yorkers. Their daughters' rate was higher. Although diet and nutrition were not specifically mentioned, different environmental factors were pinpointed, and diet is certainly part of the environment.

Herbert Seidman, the Cancer Society expert who ran the survey, said the explanation was really quite simple. "The daughters became more affluent and were able to afford things their mothers could not." He agreed that probably the first things people buy when they have money are richer and more varied foods. "Certainly they began eating better," he said. "But there are other factors. A good many of them went to college, and this meant marrying later and having their first children later. That sort of reproductive change would also be significant, I think."

So Dr. deWaard's theory was convincing. When I was in Moscow, talking with Professor Aleksandr Chaklin, chief of epidemiology at the oncology institute, I brought up the question of diet. He, too, felt Dr. deWaard's conclusions made sense.

Professor V. M. Dilman, an endocrinologist at the Petrov Research Institute of Oncology in Leningrad, was even more emphatic than Professor Chaklin had been. "Fat women have more mammary carcinomas than skinny women," he said. "Of that, there is no question. There is something found in some foods that contributes. There is also a high correlation between women who developed both diabetes and mammary carcinoma in later life—and, as you know, diabetes is a disease connected with foods."

He showed me some of his data. "I feel strongly," he said, in his excellent English, "that a young woman who shows signs that she may have diabetes should be doubly watched for signs of mammary carcinoma as well." He explained that one early diabetic symptom is giving birth to a baby that weighs ten pounds or more. "Rich diet, obesity, and diabetes go together," he said. "And I believe mammary carcinoma goes along also."

My beautiful northern-hemisphere geographic picture was being badly muddled by affluence, nutrition, and now diabetes. Also, several references had been made to city women versus rural women. And the hereditary factors could not be forgotten. What about those countries whose people were descended from Asiatics—Hungary, Finland, and Estonia?

"How are Estonian incidence rates?" I asked Professor Chaklin. "Pretty low, no?"

His eyebrows lifted to his hairline. "Oh, very high! All of the Baltic republics have very high rates of mammary carcinoma. See here." He showed me a chart. "Here we see Turkmen has an incidence rate of 5.4." (He pronounced it as "five and four.") "Now here we have Estonia." He pointed higher on the list. "Estonia has 28.6. In Estonia, there is almost six times the mammary carcinoma as in Turkmen."

"That doesn't make sense, Professor Chaklin," I said, surprised. "Estonians and Finns are first cousins. Even their languages are alike."

"You mean because they are both descended from Asians?"

I nodded. "The Finnish incidence rates are much lower than they are in other northern countries."

Professor Chaklin shrugged. "Estonia is higher than Finland, and, as I told you, the republic of Turkmen is much, much lower. By my data, it seems that Estonia is even higher than Holland." He suggested I go to Tallinn, the capital of Estonia, to talk to Professor Maret Purde, that republic's chief cancer epidemiologist. But it was impossible to hop a plane for a fast interview with her.

I recalled my conversation in Helsinki with Dr. Matti Hakama, one of the chief epidemiologists in Finland. "Finnish women have a lower incidence than other Scandinavian women because our people still are more rural and have a lower standard of living. The diet has far less protein and fats. Our women marry earlier and have their children earlier, and—especially in the rural areas—they have many children." He rejected the Asiatic theory emphatically, and I dropped the subject. "It is simply not true," he said—sharply.

Dr. Hakama went on to say that breast-cancer incidence in Finland had been climbing since the urban population began to grow. "In 1967, there were 550 city women and 354 rural women with the disease. In 1971, the totals were 704 for women living in cities and 452 in the country. I think there is a definite correlation between urbanization and the rising incidence in Finland."

His opinion about city living agreed with what I had been told by Dr. Helen Westerberg, at the Karolinska Institute, in Stockholm. "In Sweden, I suppose the incidence rate is about the same as in the United States," she said. "We have around 3,000 cases annually—somewhat more than Norway, but far fewer than Denmark."

"Why is Finland so much lower?" I asked.

"Well, because Finland is, I think, predominantly a more rural country than Sweden is," she replied. "There is some work showing a correlation between high blood pressure and breast cancer. That would be urbanization as well, don't you think?"

I remembered what Professor Sviatukhina had said about the differences in the city and country women who came to her Moscow clinics, and Professor Chaklin confirmed this with data from the rest of the Soviet Union. "In the cities and in the European republics, there are many more mammary carcinomas," he said. "Estonia is an excellent example." Again he urged me to visit Professor Purde in Tallinn.

"Next trip," I promised, thanking him for his help.

Help? Now I had the added puzzle of what had happened in Estonia to make it so different from Finland.

Back home, I found there was not much information available about breast cancer in Estonia. I wrote Professor Purde, but received no answer for several months. When she replied, she said that her statistics showed Estonia's breast-cancer incidence rates to be *lower* than those of Finland. However, Dr. Schneiderman thought she must have been using different statistical bases for her data, and he referred me to Professor Calum Muir, director of the International Agency for Research in Cancer in Lyon,

France. By telephone, Professor Muir confirmed that, according to his agency's data, Finland's breast-cancer incidence rate was lower than that of any of the Baltic Soviet republics or of the other Scandinavian countries.

But I did not know this until about three months after my return from Europe. Until Professor Purde's reply arrived, I had not been sure I would have her answer in time to include the information in *Breast Cancer*.

What to do?

People who live in Washington (especially reporters) get into the habit of picking up the telephone to ask the federal bureaucracy for information about anything, and this is what I did. I called William E. Colby, a friend who was then the director of the Central Intelligence Agency. Naturally, I assumed the CIA knew all that was going on in the world.

Bill referred me to a long-time Agency physician who preferred to stick to CIA tradition and remain anonymous.

"I'm sorry, Mrs. Kushner," he said, "but we've never had any reason to keep track of breast cancer in any country. However, we do have other recent information about Estonia, and if you have any non-medical questions that we might be able to answer, please put them in writing. We'll do our best."*

I struggled with all the risk factors I had collected. Race? Ethnicity? Being Jewish? (Genetics???) Diet and nutrition? Affluence? Urban versus rural? (Environment???) Oral contraceptives? Breast-feeding? Age at first birth? Onset of menstruation? Menopause?

How could the CIA help me answer the strange and motley assortment of nonpolitical questions?

Finally, I boiled it all down to the following letter:

"Using World War II as a dividing line, is the over-all population [of Estonia] still as ethnically (genetically) related to the Finns? Has there been much migration between Estonia and other European republics of the USSR? What are the possible ethnic breakdowns, if available, between women with Asiatic heritages? Jewish women? Other non-European stock, such as Laplanders or Eskimos? Are more women working in factories than formerly? Do more women live in urbanized areas than on

*When my first book *Breast Cancer* was written in late 1974, my anonymous correspondent requested that I not give the Agency credit for its help in collecting the data about Estonia. After the book's publication, Bill Colby asked me why I had listed "State Department Office of International Demographics" instead of the CIA as the source of these data. After hearing the reasons for my fib, he said, "It's about time the CIA got credit for doing something good." This new book can now give my public thanks to the Central Intelligence Agency for its help.

farms? Are they marrying later—or, more directly, are they giving birth to their first child at a later age? Are they having fewer children? Are they taking oral contraceptives? Are they breast-feeding their infants as they did before?"

In the middle of the composition of the letter I received a report that Seventh-day Adventists (who eat no meat at all) and Mormons (who eat much less meat than the general population) have lower breast-cancer incidence rates than the rest of the United States population. Meat! Dr. Hakama had said that Finns ate little animal protein or fat; Professor Chaklin had said that Estonia was a big cattle-raising country.

"Have there been changes in diet?" my letter continued. "Is more animal fat used in cooking and baking, as opposed to vegetable oils? Is more meat being eaten? What kind? What is butter consumption?"

The letter was sent, but I expected to hear from Dr. Purde in Tallinn first. In the meantime, I studied a risk chart I had put together and tried to guess from it what could have pushed the Estonians' breast-cancer incidence rates higher than those of their cousins in Finland. Estonia, I discovered from our tattered and worn *World Book Encyclopedia*, is a "granary" of northern Europe. Granaries mean cattle and the people were described as having one of the highest per capita consumptions of beef in Europe. It might be a clue. Also, there were strong suggestions that the population of Estonia had changed after World War II, while Finland had remained quite homogeneous.

But who knew? The various military occupations during World War II, the deaths and immigrations and emigrations, might have left Estonia without many ethnic natives. Certainly the environment must have changed considerably since the country became part of the Soviet Union. Collectivization of farms usually means mechanization and fewer people needed in the countryside. If city women there are like the women in Moscow and Leningrad, they were working, not staying at home. This could mean later marriage, later first babies, and little or no breast-feeding. More important, perhaps, it would mean two family incomes: affluence.

Now that my projections were made, based on what I had learned from other high-risk areas, I waited impatiently for a reply from the CIA. Considering that Washington was still going through the post-Watergate upheaval, the answer came surprisingly quickly. I had it in less than three weeks.

In 1970, only 68.2 percent of the population of Estonia was composed of ethnic Estonians. The rest were mainly Russians and Ukrainians. During and after World War II, the native population apparently was reduced. So almost one-third of the people were *not* first cousins to the Finns.

"Prior to World War II," the letter (on plain bond paper: no CIA letterhead) said, "Estonia had been predominantly a rural nation. With war [came] a large-scale industrial build-up and urbanization, primarily in Tallinn and the surrounding areas. More people are living in urban areas now than earlier. There are many more women in factories now than prior to World War II." More women in factories had to mean more women in the cities.

The report went on to say that since Estonians were among the more westernized of the Soviet peoples, the women might be taking oral contraceptives; there was no real knowledge, however, just an assumption. There were also no data about the average age of marriage or the average number of children. But the report did say the birth rate had been dropping and that the average woman in the Soviet Union married between the ages of twenty and twenty-five. As is the case everywhere, rural women were having more children than city women.

"We have no statistics on whether Estonian women breast-feed infants as often as was done prior to World War II," my researcher wrote. But he guessed that, with more women working, there was an over-all decrease in the number of nursing mothers.

"There was a 14-percent increase in meat consumption between 1965 and 1971." My old *World Book Encyclopedia* had already confirmed what Professor Chaklin had said: that Estonia is a top cattle-raising region, known for beef, milk, butter, and other milk products, and that apparently it produces enough for export. If there was enough to sell abroad, I guessed, the local consumption had probably continued to increase between 1971 and 1974.

Everything in the report fit the format.

Meanwhile, I had managed to obtain one report (in Russian) about breast cancer in Estonia, written by the same Professor Purde I was waiting to hear from. Translation showed that the paper concerned the role of several hormones in breast-cancer development. In addition, to my surprise, she gave some evidence that in Estonia there is a high correlation between breast-cancer incidence and a certain kind of goiter (not the one caused by an iodine deficiency) called thyrotoxicosis. Could that be another high-risk factor? Thyroid trouble?

Library research showed that scientists in the United States were also hot on this trail. Dr. Bernard Eskin, in Philadelphia, had been working for years to find a relationship between thyroid disease and breast cancer. His goal: to use possible thyroid problems as early indicators of potential breast-cancer victims just as Professor Dilman wanted to follow diabetics.

Professor Purde made another point that did not fit my format. According to her data, a large number of breast-cancer patients began their reproductive lives *late*—at age seventeen or older. If she had not emphasized the age several times, I would have passed it off as a printer's error. But she did repeat it more than once, and data cannot be changed simply because they fit no epidemiological format.

The Estonian reproductive time-clock seemed to be a few years later than ours. In the United States, girls usually begin to menstruate between the ages of twelve and fourteen, and the average age-at-first-birth was twenty, in 1974. (Since then, college graduates and career women in this country are frequently delaying childbirth until age thirty or even later—a possible contributor to increased breast-cancer incidence rates by the year 2000.) Professor Purde's comparable age in 1974 was twenty-six.

Since her report was primarily about hormonal aspects of breast cancer, environmental factors were not mentioned. But genetics were. In 1,802 families of breast-cancer patients, she reported finding twice the number of cancer victims she had expected from general-population statistics.

What to make of all this? Some of the new factors made sense; others were a puzzle. Elsewhere, I found still more new correlations—I should say "suspected correlations." For example, Dr. Nicholas I. Petrakis, of the University of California, had been comparing breast fluid extracted from Chinese women with fluid from Caucasian women in an attempt to link the low Oriental breast-cancer incidence to the presence or absence of some substance in the body. In the course of the study, he and his colleagues found an association between breast-cancer and ear-wax secretion. Women with small amounts of dry wax, common among Orientals, have a much lower incidence than do those with wet, sticky ear wax, which is more prevalent in Caucasians. No one knows why.

Another correlation, reported in 1968, is that women having a certain kind of salivary-gland carcinoma have eight times the normal breast-cancer incidence. Again, no explanation.

There is even a funny side to breast-cancer epidemiology. A serious scientific study several years ago said that a woman is more likely to develop a first cancer in the breast opposite from her husband's handedness. In the fall of 1974, at the Royal Marsden Cancer Hospital in London, one of the younger oncologists took me aside during a tea break. "Is your President Ford, by any chance, left-handed?" he asked.

"Yes," I told him. I explained that much had been made in the American press about the southpaw President.

"From newspaper pictures, he looks to be left-handed, but that, of course, could be a reversed negative as well."

"I am certain he is left-handed," I insisted. "There was a lot about it the first time he signed a batch of bills."

"That's all very interesting," the doctor commented, telling me about the study.

The risk charts on the following pages may help women find their personal risk-pigeonholes. Imagine having an old-fashioned balance scale and a stack of poker chips. The scale has a high-risk side and a low-risk side. Precise weights—numbers of poker chips—have not yet been worked out for the various high/low risk factors, but some educated guesswork can help determine the number of chips to put on each plate of the scale. Women like me, who have already had one breast cancer, are at highest risk: this is worth about four chips on the high side. Giving birth to a first child before age twenty is worth three or four low chips; over thirty about three or four high chips. A family history—especially in premenopausal, first-degree relatives (mother and/or sister)—requires that four or five high chips be added to the scale. If the relatives' disease involved both breasts, still another high chip must be added.

On the other hand, being poor and black or American Indian reduces the risk of breast cancer, and at least two chips can be placed on the low risk plate of the scale. Oriental women, who live as their ancestors did in Asia, may also add two chips to this plate. Long-term usage of any estrogen-containing substance adds high chips; women who have never used such medications may put one or two low chips on the scale.

Intermediate factors, by the way, are zeros and do not count at all.

To illustrate using the chart: a sixty-two-year-old Japanese woman who had the first of her five children when she was eighteen, who has no history of breast cancer in her family, and who began to menstruate at twelve, has little reason to worry. However, an overweight Jewish woman of thirty-seven who had her first child at thirty-two, has taken oral contraceptives for years, whose mother and older sister had breast cancer, who began to menstruate at ten, and who has had two benign fibroadenomas removed surgically is at high risk. If her sister or

HIGHEST
BREAST-CANCER RISKS FOR U.S. WOMEN

WHO	WHEN	WHERE

1. History of cancer
  Self—breast or other
    cancer
  Sister
  Mother
  Grandmother or aunts,
    fraternal as well as
    maternal
  First cousins
  NOTE: RISK IS HIGHER
    IF RELATIVES' DIS-
    EASE WAS FOUND
    PRE-MENO-
    PAUSALLY IN BOTH
    BREASTS
2. Prior history of confirmed
    benign breast disease
3. Reproductive history
  Early onset of menstrua-
    tion
  Long-term use of estro-
    gens
  First child born after age
    30
  No children
  Late menopause
4. Race and ethnicity
  Jews of European an-
    cestry
  Non-Jews of northern
    European background
    (including Iceland)
  Affluent blacks
5. Diet
  Obesity due to large
    amounts of animal
    proteins and fats,
    including butter, lard,
    cheese, whole milk,
    and milk products.
	Age 40 and up
	(including women
	over 70)
		Urban centers throughout
		U.S.A. Regionally: Mass.,
		Conn., R.I., N.Y., N.J.; parts of
		Penna., Md.; areas adjacent
		to Great Lakes.*
		
		Places having Incidence
		registries:
		San Francisco-Oakland;
		Minneapolis-St. Paul; Detroit;
		Pittsburgh**

*Based on Atlas of Cancer Mortality for U.S. Counties, National Cancer
Institute, 1975
**Based on Third National Cancer Survey, 1969-71 Incidence, National
Cancer Institute, 1974

INTERMEDIATE
BREAST-CANCER RISKS FOR U.S. WOMEN

WHO	WHEN	WHERE

1. Family history of cancer
   No close relatives
2. Prior history of benign
   breast disease
   Presence of some
     masses during men-
     strual periods
3. Reproductive history
   Menstruation at ages
     12-13
   Start of sexual activity
     between ages 20-28
   First child between ages
     23-27
   Menopause in mid-40's
4. Race and ethnicity
   Middle-income blacks
   Latin Americans
   Southern European
     ancestries
5. Diet
   Moderate amounts of
     animal protein and
     fats (e.g., Mormons)
	Ages 25-39	Wash., Oregon, Calif., Idaho,
		Nev., Montana, Colorado,
		Wyoming, N.D., S.D., Neb.,
		Kans., Iowa, Mo., Wisc.,
		Minn., Ill., Ind., Ohio, Mich.,
		Pa., N.H., Vt., Me., Del., Md.
		(excepting very large urban
		centers., e.g., Milwaukee)*
		
		Places having Incidence
		registries:
		Dallas-Fort Worth; Atlanta**

mother were diagnosed when they were pre-menopausal and had both breasts removed, this woman's risk is probably so high many experts would recommend prophylactic mastectomies.

Certainly, she should be sure to examine her breasts regularly and see an expert in breast diseases for periodic examinations. And—even though current NCI recommendations are that she not be screened by mammography until she reached forty years of age most specialists would feel she should at least have a base-line mammogram for future comparison.

While the science of epidemiology is relatively new, it is growing quickly, because the information obtained from surveys and interviews of patients (as well as of healthy people) are proving to be so valuable. Most of the data in this chapter have come from epidemiological studies. Even if breast cancer cannot be prevented, simply knowing who is at high risk will save tens of thousands of women's lives—if they do something to take advantage of all that has been learned.

LOWEST
BREAST-CANCER RISKS FOR U.S. WOMEN

WHO	WHEN	WHERE

1. No family history of cancer
2. No history of prior breast disease
3. Reproductive history
    Late menstruation
    First child born before age 20
    Early beginning of sexual activity
    Early menopause (natural or artificial)
    No use of estrogens
4. Races and ethnicity
    Jews of North African or Asian ancestries
    Non-Jews of Finnish ancestry
    Low-income whites
    Low-income blacks
    American Indians
    Oriental ancestries
5. Diet
    Mainly nonmeat protein and vegetable fats (e.g., Seventh-day Adventists)
	Under age 25	Utah, Ariz., N.M., Texas, Ark., La., Ala., Fla., Ga., N.C., S.C., Va., W.Va.;*
		
		Also: Penobscot Cty., Me.; Tolland Cty., and—for unknown reasons—many isolated, scattered counties in otherwise high and intermediate areas*
		
		Places having incidence registries: Birmingham, Ala.**

Other possible risk factors, effect unknown or subject to debate: Breastfeeding, number of children, above-average height, blood pressure, role of paternal ancestry, diabetes, enlarged thyroid gland, salivary-gland cancer, emotional stress, mental depression, quantity and quality of ear-wax secretion.

5

And Why?

It was a day to be marked in red on my calendar. The bandages were coming off, and I was told I could wear a loose bra and stuff absorbent cotton into the empty cup. I cannot explain why, but it made an enormous psychological difference to look down and see two mounds instead of one.

As if this were not enough, Dr. Dao suggested I get dressed that afternoon and come over to see what his Endocrine Research Laboratory was doing about finding a cure for breast cancer. "I am a biochemist as well as a surgeon, you know," he said. "Being able to do a good mastectomy is only part of dealing with this disease. We must find a cure, so that we won't need mastectomies at all. The really important work is going on in the laboratories. Why don't you come down after lunch? I'll be expecting you."

The invitation was exciting for two reasons. I did want to see what the lab looked like and what was going on. But, more important personally, it showed that Dr. Dao felt I was in the clear and rid of the cancer. He was treating me like a science writer, not a patient.

Elated on all counts, I surveyed my wardrobe: a blue-and-white-striped cord pantsuit and a sleeveless blouse. They were what I had had on my back when I rushed to New York. After lunch, I dressed and scrutinized myself in the mirror. Nobody, but nobody, would be able to guess which one was real and which one was absorbent cotton.

Dr. Dao was wearing the white, stiffly starched laboratory overcoat researchers all over the world wear. It changed his personality completely. No longer was he my surgeon making daily rounds. He had become *Herr Direktor,* chief of the Endocrine Research Laboratory. Even his floppy, brightly dotted bow tie did not detract from the picture of scientific endeavor.

I looked around at the banks of expensive electronic equipment, with names ending in -meter and tongues of computerized print-outs drooping from mouth-like slits, that could measure and analyze a minute fraction of a substance in a droplet of fluid. Although there were also traditional centrifuges, microscopes, and test tubes, the laboratory looked like a Mission Control Center. It was not what I had expected.

Dr. Dao walked over to greet me at the door. "First of all, you can see from the name of the lab that my research is concerned with the hormonal, or endocrine, aspects of breast cancer," he began. "We have known since 1896 that removing a woman's ovaries often caused her breast cancer to improve. But it took years to find out why."

"You mean estrogens?" I broke in.

He nodded, "Yes, estrogens—female hormones. These substances are produced by the ovaries, and removing them from the blood stream has a marked effect on slowing the growth of a breast cancer in many cases."

I was about to break in with another question, but Dr. Dao was not to be interrupted.

"Although the principle had been known since 1896," he repeated, "the reason was not discovered until much later. Removing the ovaries helped, and that was it. So oophorectomy, or ovariectomy—surgical removal of the ovaries—was done routinely after a mastectomy in younger women for decades."

"Did doctors think female hormones caused the breast cancer?" I managed to ask.

"Some did and some didn't," he replied. "But no one could disagree that oophorectomy improved the condition of many breast-cancer patients." Dr. Dao went on with his brief history of the rather confused estrogen picture.

First, while a good many women improved, some did not respond at all after their ovaries were taken out. Their tumors continued to flourish, unaffected. "In these cases," he said, "we had to assume the cancers were different—what we call hormone-independent, not influenced or controlled by estrogen secretion. Another inexplicable factor was the presence of estrogens in a patient's blood stream even after oophorectomy. This means that there must be other glands in the body that either take over estrogen production when the ovaries are removed or produce female hormones along with the ovaries. A third mystery was that many women—especially postmenopausal women—were considerably improved when given the very same estrogens that were causing so much trouble in younger patients."

After more research, Dr. Dao continued, scientists learned that the adrenal glands, near the kidneys, and the anterior pituitary gland, deep inside the brain, are also involved in estrogen production—the pituitary directing the ovarian hormone factories' production. To stop secretion of the female hormones altogether, it was necessary to get rid of all these glands.

"The anterior pituitary also secretes the hormone called prolactin," Dr. Dao went on. "This is the hormone that causes milk production to begin after childbirth, but it is also present in the body at other times, although its function aside from lactation is not clearly understood.

"Why would the body do that to itself?" I asked.

He smiled. "The brain must intend for the body to have a correct balance of all the hormones, but the delicate balance somehow becomes altered. We don't know exactly what 'correct' is. We know only that when an imbalance exists, it creates a nourishing endocrine, or glandular, environment for the growth of breast cancers, as well as carcinomas of other reproductive organs."

"Then what about oral contraceptives? The Pill? They've got estrogens in them. And what about the female hormones given to cattle and sheep so they'll get fat faster? What about—"

"Wait a minute now. You are getting ahead of the story. What I have been talking about are endogenous estrogens—hormones made by the woman's own body, to prepare her for menstruation, ovulation, possible pregnancy, and then lactation. These are all normal secretions, which are controlled by the brain, probably the hypothalamus."

The hypothalamus? That is the part of the brain involved with the emotions. Could cancer be psychosomatic? I tried to ask, but got no chance.

"For a long time, scientists thought it was the pituitary gland that regulated all other glands. It was called 'the conductor of the body's hormonal orchestra.' Now we know it is only the concertmaster, not the boss."

He stopped. Here was my chance. The Pill or the hypothalamus? "What about the oral contraceptives?" I asked quickly. He probably was not much interested in psychological side of cancer, anyhow.

He paused. "We have no proof that such exogenous hormones—those obtained from outside the body—cause breast cancer in humans." He seemed to be choosing his words very carefully. "However, three of them, estrone, estradiol, and diethylstilbestrol—as well as prolactin—do stimulate breast cancers in lower animals."

"What do you mean by stimulate?"

"Exactly what I said. Most estrogens enhance the growth of a mammary carcinoma. For example, in mice who have first been injected with a carcinogen—a substance known to cause cancer—tumors appear much earlier, their rates of growth are much faster, and the tumors are larger if they are also given female hormones, especially prolactin. But prolactin alone does not do this without estrogens. Remember, though, that in these experiments the initial cancers were not *induced* by hormones but by a chemical we are certain is carcinogenic."

"Where does that leave the exogenous estrogens in oral contraceptives?"

"In the suspicious category." Dr. Dao smiled. "Anything that upsets the body's hormonal balance contributes to a favorable environment for cancer growth in the breast. We have evidence of this in several species of animals, but not in humans."

"What about heredity?" I asked, changing the subject. "Cancer seems to run in families, doesn't it?"

"There's no question that there seems to be some kind of inborn predisposition. In our own lab, for example, we use certain strains of mice that have been deliberately bred to develop mammary carcinomas quickly and with very little stimulation. The same principle could apply in human families. It could be a predisposition for the body's endocrine balance to be upset easily."

"Are there strains of mice that never develop breast cancer, no matter what you do?"

He nodded. "However, as these mice get older, they become more vulnerable, too."

I was the only breast-cancer patient in my family on both sides, as far as I knew. Was I starting a new, awful strain? But then, I had been given hundreds of hormone tablets. Could it be that?

"Where does a breast-cancer virus come into the picture?"

"It could be a trigger. Like the chemical we used in those mice to set off cancer growth."

"And X-ray?"

"Not the tiny quantities from dental examinations or tuberculosis checkups. But, in larger quantities, X-ray has been proven to trigger breast cancer. First, however, there must be that nourishing endocrine environment, before a cancer will grow at all. If the environment is hostile, the original microscopic tumor will die and disappear."

"And the hypothalamus helps to create a good environment?"

"Yes."

"Do you think there is a psychological cause of breast cancer then? After all, that's the part of the brain that controls things like sex drive, fear, and anger."

Good grief! Too much sex? Too little sex? Too many arguments?

"Not sex drive." Dr. Dao laughed. "But some investigators have mentioned stress as a factor, and it might be. Plenty of hormones are secreted during stressful times. One hormone could stimulate another. A stress hormone that stimulated estrogen secretion could help to create the nourishing endocrine environment the cancer needs."

Looking for the cause of breast cancer was like wandering in a labyrinth. One path that seemed clear ran into another that was blocked.

"Breast cancer is a multifactorial disease," Dr. Dao concluded. "There just is no one, single cause that works alone."

Later, while trying to digest all I had learned, I realized Dr. Dao had not said anything about why postmenopausal women respond to treatment with estrogens, but younger women have to have their ovaries removed. This mystery was finally cleared up for me months later, in Finland, when I first heard the theory that breast cancers in the two age groups are two completely different diseases.

Dr. Dao had given me some reports published by his laboratory, and, from them, one problem in studying breast cancer in humans was apparent immediately. His mice developed tumors within weeks of being injected, and the entire life span of a mouse is only a few months. In humans, the trigger setting off the first malignant cell could be separated from the appearance of a tumor by more than twenty years. I tried to recall some events of the last twenty years of my life.

I had never taken birth-control pills, but now that I was thinking of the Pill as a female hormone, an estrogen, rather than as a contraceptive, I realized how many times I had been given prescriptions for one estrogen or another: to regulate menstrual periods, to prevent miscarriages, or to "dry up" after weaning my children from the breast. And who knew how much diethylstilbestrol (DES)—the hormone used to fatten livestock—I had eaten in chopped liver and chicken soup? Even without the Pill, I must have taken in plenty of exogenous estrogens.

Dr. Dao had very cautiously shied away from discussing oral contraceptives. However, I was left with the strong impression that he frowned on their widespread, indiscriminate use, and he was not alone among the experts. But there was no proof of any connection between use of the Pill and human breast cancer. Of course, there had not been enough time yet; oral contraceptives had been best sellers for only a few years in 1974.

What Dr. Dao had said about the significance of endocrine environment for breast-cancer growth meant more to me after I learned about the epidemiological aspects of a woman's reproductive life. The start and the finish of reproductive life are especially dependent on the proper balance of female hormones, and now I understood why early or late beginning of menstruation and early menopause affected the risk category.

While the significance of the mother's age when her first child is born remains a mystery, it must have something to do with her hormonal balance.

Understanding that breast cancer can be stimulated by excess hormones also made it easier for me to see why diet might be a major factor. A 1953 experiment restricting the caloric intake of cancer-prone mice, for example, showed that a one-third reduction in calories virtually wiped out their breast cancers. In the German concentration camps during World War II, cessation of a woman's regular menstrual periods was one of the first signs she was suffering from food deprivation, and the same symptom was found in Japanese internment camps. A shortage of food must lead to a shortage of estrogens and thus to an imbalance in the endocrine system regulating the monthly cycle. And there was that link between diet and breast cancer in countries where, like the Netherlands, the consumption of animal fats is very high, while in Japan and other countries that use few animal fats, the breast-cancer incidence rates are very low.

Some scientists have suggested that the cholesterol in the animal fats is somehow converted inside the body into estrogenlike substances, thus upsetting the hormonal balance. Although animal fats were the suspects in one survey, other experts think meat proteins as well as fats are responsible.

Several researchers have pointed out that most of the meat we eat comes either from female animals—hens and ewes, which are loaded with natural estrogens—or from castrated males—steers and capons, whose androgen-producing testicles have been removed. (Lambs, calves, and piglets have not yet developed their hormone-producing equipment.) Since even male animals secrete some estrogens, most people get only female hormones in their meat from these eunuchs. Although no study has been done to ascertain what this means in relation to breast cancer, it has been established that Seventh-day Adventists (who eat no meat at all) and Mormons (moderate meat eaters) have far fewer cases of all kinds of cancer, including breast cancer.

Some such diet factors probably explain why obese women are in the high-risk category. They may also explain why the daughters of low-incidence immigrants to the United States develop more breast cancers than their mothers—too many hamburgers and creamy milk shakes. And the quantity of animal fats or meat in their diets might account for the difference in the incidence rates of Israeli Jewish women with Sephardic and those with European backgrounds.

With regard to the high risk of obesity, Dr. Frits deWaard, the Dutch epidemiologist who evolved the total-body-volume theory, believes each cell in the body is a microscopic factory that produces estrogens independently of the ovaries, the adrenals, or the pituitary. This extraglandular phenomenon, as Dr. deWaard calls it, would give large women extra estrogen-producing equipment and, therefore, more hormones in their bodies.

In recent years countless articles and several books have been written insisting that adding or avoiding certain foods can prevent or even cure all cancers, including mammary carcinoma. In 1978, a Senate subcommittee went so far as to ask Dr. Arthur C. Upton (then the director of the NCI) to present Congress with an "anti-cancer diet."

Public interest in and public pressure for more research in nutrition became intense, and in late 1980, the NCI's new director, Dr. Vincent T. DeVita, created a special program for nutrition research. In addition, a "chemoprevention" section was established to study substances like vitamins C, E, and A as well as certain trace elements that had been given much publicity as cancer-fighters in the general media—selenium being the most prominent.

The preceding Chapter 4 shows the strong case which is building against animal fats of all kinds and perhaps against animal proteins, as well, in terms of their being possible causes of breast cancer. One of the major problems, however, is studying diet in a free society where habits and life styles cannot be regulated or controlled. Let me give one example.

Not long after *Breast Cancer* was published, a Canadian doctor and his wife contacted me for a meeting. It was immediately clear that it was not I they wanted to talk to, it was my daughter Lesley. Their hope was to collect as many high-risk young women as they could and pay them to keep diaries of everything they ate for ten, fifteen, or twenty years.

There were *no* dietary restrictions at all. Lesley would have earned money every week simply to list every piece of cake, stick of chewing gum, every apple, or hamburger she put into her mouth.

"I won't lie to you and tell you I'll do it," she told the doctor and his wife. "I just know that I'd forget to keep it up, and it would be dishonest to lead you into believing I'd do something like that for such a long time. Maybe a month . . ."

Mice, guinea pigs, cats, rabbits, dogs, and even apes can be kept in cages and fed premeasured quantities of desired food: high-calorie, low-calorie; high-carbohydrate, low-carbohydrate; high-fat, low-fat. But humans who are not prisoners (and even prisoners can cheat!) cannot be counted on to follow instructions or to keep reliable records.

A second serious problem scientists encounter in nutritional research is the multitude of processes a food goes through between the time it is planted as a seed and the moment its end product is on the table in front of a person, ready to be eaten. What was grown in the soil before? What chemicals, if any, were added to the seeds to color or preserve them? Were pesticides used? Fertilizers? How was the product packaged? Were additives used? How were the foods cooked? Finally, how do they behave in combination with other foods or with chemicals in a person's body?

Clearly, studying the role of diet in the cause and cure of cancer is much more complicated than it appears to be on the surface.

Yes, there is animal evidence that selenium may attack cancer cells or, prevent the disease from developing by enhancing immunity. The same is true of Vitamin A, in doses too enormous and toxic to be used by humans. Vitamin E is thought to eliminate some of the breast tenderness associated with menstruation, but this may be totally unrelated to cancer. Vitamin C may prevent cancer by strengthening the immune system, but so far, there is no proof that any of these substances can cure the disease. Anyone who relies on any vitamin therapy for an existing malignancy is courting death.

But there is hope. For breast cancer, this hope is that adding or subtracting certain foods or nutrients may affect a woman's cellular biochemistry and prevent an excess of female hormones from making a nourishing home for cancer cells in her breast.

But what triggers that first cell and causes it to transform from normal to malignant?

Scientists have learned there are four basic causes of any cancer: genetic mutations, chemical carcinogens, irradiation, and oncornaviruses (*onco*-is a medical prefix meaning "cancer"; the "rna" is the middle distinguishes this "retrovirus" that may or may not be carcinogenic from the types of oncogenes that do cause cancer all the time). In one way or another, any of the four can do the evil work of wrecking a cell's control over its growth and reproduction.

To find out about genetics, I went to see an epidemiologist at the National Cancer Institute. "Is breast cancer hereditary or isn't it?" I asked. "On the one hand, I have read that Dr. Brian MacMahon thinks genetics plays a minor role in breast cancer, and on the other, there are Jewish women and the Parsi women in India. And what about the Japanese and Yemeni women?" I fished a paper from my briefcase and put it on his desk. "Now I have just found this study, done at the M. D. Anderson Hospital and Tumor Institute, in Houston, saying that women have forty-seven times the risk of getting breast cancer before the age of thirty-nine if both their mother and a sister had it. It doesn't make sense to insist it isn't a genetic disease."

He shook his head and laughed. "I can see why it's so confusing. You get the epidemiologists and the statisticians on one side, and the doctors in the clinics on the other side. They seem to conflict, don't they?"

"They certainly do." I sighed. "I hope you can straighten it out."

"Well, I'll try," he began. "But first, MacMahon used the term 'genetic role,' not hereditary. What do you mean by hereditary?"

"Running in a family," I replied.

"There are many ways a disease can run in a family and yet not be hereditary in the same way as hair and eye color are," he said. "Traits like coloring are passed along physically, by the genes in the sperm and egg of the parents, and these are genetic. But a characteristic can be transmitted to the next generation in other ways."

In 1936, he went on, Dr. Joseph J. Bittner, a scientist at the University of Minnesota, did a series of now classic experiments that proved there is a mammary-tumor virus in mice—the scientific shorthand for it is MuMTV, for murine (mouse) mammary tumor virus—and that the virus can be passed along to their young via their milk. Baby mice fed by mothers with breast cancer subsequently developed breast tumors too. Then Dr. Bittner took a group of baby mice away from their cancerous mothers immediately after birth and had them suckled by healthy mothers. None of these babies developed breast cancers. Nor did the offspring of healthy mice who were fed by their own mothers; but they did if nursed by the cancerous mothers.

"Do you think something like this happens with humans?" I asked.

He shook his head. "Nobody knows. Particles similar to the MuMTV have been found in human milk, and some women swear that their infants refused to take milk from a breast that later became malignant. But the only way to prove anything would be by a Bittner-type experiment, and scientists can't ethically mix and match people the way they can mice."

I persisted. "There must be a reason for the high risk of a woman who has a sister or mother with cancer, compared with the risk of a woman who has no cancer in her family. Not everyone is breast-fed. I'm sure thousands of women with breast cancer were fed by bottle."

"It could be a statistical artifact." He smiled. "Don't forget, 7 percent of all American women get breast cancer. This means there is one chance in fourteen for any woman in the United States to get it. Now, in a family with three sisters, two grandmothers, possibly a few aunts, and lots of female cousins, there's a good chance that some of them will develop breast cancer just because of its national incidence, not because it runs in the family."

Statistical artifact? That is probably what is meant by "doing anything you want with statistics." But here it made no sense. "That wouldn't explain the Finnish, Japanese, Jewish, and Parsi women," I said. "What about the Jewish women from Yemen compared with—"

He laughed. "I'm just putting you on. Of course there must be a genetic factor somewhere. All cancers have a genetic component, to a greater or lesser degree. For example, there's an eye cancer, retinoblastoma, that is caused by a mutant gene. We don't know why the gene changes, but we know what happens afterward if the children's lives are saved by removing their eyes, and they grow to adulthood and marry someone else with the same problem. Half of *their* children will also get retinoblastomas, but half won't. The risks of passing this mutant gene on are so well established that patients are usually advised not to have children."

He also explained how hereditary factors can influence the development of a cancer even if they do not actually cause the disease. For instance, blond, light-skinned people are more vulnerable to skin cancers that come from long exposure to the sun than are dark people, whose skin pigmentation and thickness—both hereditary qualities—protect them from the ultraviolet rays of the sun. "But," he stressed, "both light- and dark-skinned people would have far less skin cancer if all of them stayed out of the sun."

"There are no hard-and-fast rules about genetics and breast cancer," he said. "If all the risk factors were based on heredity, Japanese women, for example, would have a low incidence rate no matter where they lived. But they don't. Low-risk women develop more breast cancer when they move from their native countries to high-risk areas."

A few months later, in Moscow, I asked Professor Sviatukhina what she thought. "The evidence is there for all to see," she said, adding that she had known of too many families spotted with breast cancer from one generation to another to say that heredity is not a factor. But not the only factor.

In other countries I visited, in different accents, the same opinion was given again and again—whatever the cause may be, there is no doubt that breast cancer does run in families. But why? Another mutant gene, like the one that causes retinoblastoma?

In studying the possible role of genetics in diseases, scientists try to find sets of identical twins who grew up in different environments. If the twins have been separated throughout their lifetimes and yet have had illnesses in common, those diseases could be genetic. But apparently no such twins with breast cancer have been found, for I discovered nothing of this nature in the medical literature.

A second-best approach is a computerized study of family incidence now in progress in Iceland. That northern island has a high incidence of breast cancer. It also has a relatively closed society: there has been little migration in or out for decades. Because of this, most Icelandic family trees can be traced back to 1910, many back as far as 1842.

It has not always been so. Professor Calum Muir, of the International Agency for Research in Cancer, in France, told me of a historical study of breast-cancer incidence in Iceland showing that ethnic Icelandic women (not Danish or other European immigrants) once had incidence rates as low as those of Japanese women. Then the population began to change and become more European, and the incidence rates rose and have remained at the same level since. All this, Professor Muir said, seems to be evidence of a strong genetic component introduced by the European immigrants. But as far as the "why" of the high breast-cancer incidence in Iceland is concerned, he too believed that family history is just one factor and not the only answer.

The historical data were entered into the computer for the study beginning with the year 1910, after Iceland had already become Europeanized. Since 1911, the island has had 1,600 cases of breast cancer, and of these, ninety were chosen at random for computerized analysis. Each woman's family was traced back as far as its records went, and the data are in the computer in a "linkage file," so various family relationships can be studied.

The project will take a long time to complete, but preliminary results have been announced by the NCI, financial sponsors of the research. The scientists in charge warn that high family correlations do not necessarily establish a definite genetic cause-and-effect, because the same environment, the same foods, or other characteristics of Icelandic life—such as marrying late and having a first child late—could also be factors. However, the computer can and is calculating relative breast-cancer risks for granddaughters, daughters, sisters, first cousins, and nieces. In addition, the results have already shown with certainty that "running in the family" is *not* confined only to the maternal side but also involves women members on the father's side of a family.

Only two chemicals (estrogens are not considered chemicals) have been proven to cause breast cancer: urethanes (no relative to foam-rubber products) and anthracines. Neither chemical—I have been told—is present in the air or in any food, household product, cosmetic, or medicine. I have been assured that both are laboratory chemicals, not used for any purposes other than scientific experiments in mice.

Some drugs have been implicated in causing breast cancer. One is reserpine, a medication used to reduce blood-pressure levels, that increases the production of prolactin, and thyroid supplements (in connection with the Estonian data). The most recent attack descended on Valium, the top-selling prescription drug in the United States. (There have also been some questions raised about anti-depressants like Elavil and Tofranil.) Dr. David Horrobin, a Canadian physiologist, launched his campaign against Valium early in January 1981 at the annual meeting of the American Association for the Advancement of Science in Toronto. His data (twenty-nine listings long) claim that diazepam (Valium's generic name) is a "promotor," not an initiator, however. Since the drug's manufacturer is Hoffman-LaRoche, there are millions of dollars worth of clout against Dr. Horrobin.

The studies implicating Valium were published in prestigious international peer-reviewed journals (not magazines given away free or published as for-profit newsletters), and the results were impressive enough to convince the FDA that studies should be done under controlled conditions to see if diazepam does cause mammary carcinoma.

At the beginning of the controversy about Valium, there was a tug-of-war about who would pay for the FDA-ordered tests: we poverty-stricken taxpayers or Hoffman-LaRoche, whose stock is worth thousands of dollars per share on the Swiss Stock Exchange.

According to Dr. Richard Adamson, chief of the NCI's Division of Cancer Cause and Prevention, the Valium issue is finally being resolved within ongoing studies by the Boston Drug Surveillance Program and at the Kaiser-Permanente pre-paid health plans. In addition to questions about the use of other medications, breast-cancer patients are being asked about their use of diazepam. As of this writing, there appears to be no relationship between taking the drug and developing breast cancer.

The problem of cancer initiators, promotors, and of co-carcinogens is complicated. But incriminating drugs like reserpine, thyroid, diazepam, and other psychotrophic medications brings another problem to scientists' attention: are the drugs themselves responsible in some way for the growth of a malignancy or are the women who take such substances at high risk because of the disease being treated? Remembering Dr. Dilman's theory about diabetes, Dr. Purde's data about thyroid trouble, and the intricate mechanism involving the brain's hypothalamus makes me wonder whether having certain problems like high blood pressure, diabetes, thyroid trouble, or manic-depression is an indication of being at high risk for developing breast cancer.

"Of course it is possible," Dr. Dao told me. "Until the cause of breast cancer is known, anything is possible. But when you are dealing with diseases that are so common and affect so many women, how can anything be proven? Almost ten percent of American women are going to get breast cancer, millions of others are receiving insulin for diabetes, thyroid medications for underactivity, reserpine to lower blood pressure, diazepam for anything at all. How can any scientific sense be made when so many women are taking pills, perhaps for no good reason?

"No correlations whatsoever can be made under such circumstances."

As always, Dr. Dao unraveled the tangle with plain common sense by reminding me that the only cause of breast cancer that cannot be questioned is low-dose ionizing radiation: X-ray. Although non-ionizing radiation, the ultraviolet rays that come to earth from the sun, have no effect on breast or any other cancers except skin, ionizing radiation is dangerous. Except for a fetus, the female breast is the most vulnerable human tissue in terms of radiosensitivity.

Yet there are no federal controls over the usage of ionizing radiation, and the Bureau of Radiological Health (BRH) has no regulatory authority once equipment has been assembled and installed in a doctor's office or a hospital's X-ray department. Several other government agencies, including the Department of Energy (now incorporating the former Atomic Energy Commission) and the Nuclear Regulatory Commission, have been responsible for setting "acceptable" levels of radiation emission. But, as we all learned during the aftermath of the Three Mile Island catastrophe (an aftermath that may not yet be over), no one really knows what an "acceptable level" is.

Randolph S. Rae, a physicist and a government consultant, explained how maximum acceptable levels are computed.

"We know how much exposure is dangerous," he said. "So we go down and say, 'Well, a thousandth would certainly be safe, and a millionth even safer.' " That, according to Rae, is why no one need worry about "small multiples" of the so-called maximum acceptable levels.

"Usually," he continued, "these levels are even less than what we are exposed to all the time from irradiation in the atmosphere. There is no way—it's absolutely impossible—for anyone to be protected from what is in the air around us all the time."

Scientists do know a great deal about the cancerous effects of irradiation, however. Results of the atomic blasts in Hiroshima and Nagasaki, which are still showing up in Japanese incidence rates, have taught them much. The many experimental explosions that took place above ground, underground, and in the air have also yielded a great deal of information. It is known, for example, that ionizing irradiation is, paradoxically, both a cancer cure and a cancer cause, and for the same reason: it does something to the gene on the DNA molecule that controls the cell's growth and reproduction. In the massive doses given to cancer patients, irradiation destroys a malignant cell by preventing it from reproducing. In lesser doses, irradiation damages the chromosomes of a normal cell, but without killing it. If the damage takes place in the growth-and-reproduction gene, the mutation can create cancerous daughter cells.

While it had been known since Marie Curie's day that ionizing irradiation causes cancer, for many years mammary carcinomas were thought to be an exception. The reason its danger to breasts was not recognized is logical: it takes a long time for a breast tumor to become apparent, and the X-rays that might have caused it are usually long forgotten by the time the tumor is discovered. So, until four years after World War II, X-ray was used to treat anything from bleeding nipples to tuberculosis to eczema. By then, bits and pieces of evidence appeared occasionally in medical literature telling of women who had developed cancer in the affected breast as long as twenty-five years after X-ray therapy for a benign problem. Indiscriminate use of X-ray declined, because doctors believed it aggravated a cancer already in existence. They did not know X-ray could cause one to develop.

Not until six Japanese survivors of Hiroshima and Nagasaki developed breast cancer in 1965, twenty years after the blasts, was the cause-and-effect of X-ray considered proven. Six cases are not many here, but in Japan it is a large number, and the fact that all of the victims had been A-bombed was too much to be a coincidence. As a result, scatter-shot use of X-ray stopped, and it is rarely a cause of primary breast cancers today.

Many physicians are reluctant to expose their patients too frequently to the quantity of irradiation from a mammogram or chest X-ray. But this is one of the times when possible risk must be weighed against possible benefit. (The mammography controversy will be discussed in detail in chapter 7.)

But *take special note:* I am talking about diagnostic X-ray, *not* necessary and prescribed radiation therapy used to treat cancer.

Two avoidable sources of irradiation, aside from sunlight and X-rays, should be mentioned briefly—microwave ovens and color television sets.

"Is there anything to the scares we had about them in *The Zapping of America?*" I asked Dr. Joseph Sharp, formerly a radiation specialist at the Walter Reed Army Institute of Research in Washington.

"As far as we know," he said, "they're as safe as they can be—by current standards, whatever the standards are right now. No one has really gotten any evidence to show that either machine, in good working order, can cause cancer." He smiled. "For that matter, there is no evidence that either machine in bad working order can cause cancer. I would say that the best thing to do, based on the information we have now, is just to turn the contraptions on and keep your distance. We might as well play it safe with the few things we can do something about."

That is a fair summary of irradiation and cancer: play it safe wherever you can.

If extrapolating results from mouse to man is a problem in studying hormones, genetics, chemicals, or radiation as causes of cancer, it is an almost total road block in viral research.

Scientists have known about the MuMTV—the virus that causes breast cancer in mice—for more than four decades, but they have found no way to investigate whether a similar virus causes breast cancer in humans. The reason is obvious: scientists can't duplicate the crucial animal experiments in humans without running the risk of causing cancer in their subjects.

The usual procedure for proving that a particular agent causes an illness is to inject tissue suspected of harboring it into an animal, causing the disease to develop. After that "guinea pig" becomes ill, some of its diseased tissue—in the case of cancer, the tumor—is injected into a second animal. If the same illness appears again, the process is repeated several more times. Then, and only then, can it be stated without any doubt or qualification that this disease was caused by that agent. The procedure is known as Koch's postulates, and it has been successfully applied in finding the causes of a great many diseases. With the common cold and other minor diseases that simply don't "take" in experimental animals, scientists have used paid human guinea pigs or have gotten volunteers for their Koch's procedures. Prisoners have occasionally been recruited, in exchange for early release. But to do this with cancer? Impossible.

"How was it done with polio?" I asked Dr. Ernest Plata, a virologist at the National Cancer Institute. "They certainly didn't go around inoculating human beings with polio to find that virus, did they?"

"This is the cause of a lot of confusion," Dr. Plata said. "The agent we suspect of causing some breast cancers—*some,* not all, by any means—is totally unlike the polio virus or the viruses that cause the cold, measles, mumps, and so on. First of all, no one has been able to transmit this suspected virus from humans to lower animals, as was the case with polio.

"In the second place, it is *not*—repeat, *not*—contagious. With contagious viral diseases, the virus invades a cell and reproduces, using the machinery of the cell to make new viruses. In the end, the cell may be killed and will expel through its membrane dozens of newly made viruses into the surrounding tissue. To study these simpler diseases, all the scientist must do to get a sample of the virus is to break up a piece of diseased tissue and extract it."

Dr. Plata went on with his explanation. "In cancer, the process is different. As soon as the virus invades a cell, its genes—because viruses have them too—hide in some way among the genes of the cell itself. The body of the virus disappears. What is left is an extra, infinitesimal piece of genetic material—a dot."

Dr. Plata added that these small pieces of gene, these dots, had only recently been found in the cancer cells of lower animals. The sophisticated technical know-how was not available earlier, he explained. Again, progress in cancer research was directly related to the higher lens power of the latest microscope and to the development of other technologies.

He gave a thus-far-imaginary scenario of how an HuMTV—human mammary tumor virus—might work. The "thing," or virus, would enter a healthy cell and be incorporated so that nothing remained of it but the dot of gene among the host cell's chromosomes. The dot would somehow change the growth genes of the cell—and, by doing so, create a malignant state. During the S period, when the cell's DNA molecules were twinning, the genes of this malignant state would be duplicated in both sets of new chromosomes. In the succeeding dormant period, the daughter cells would be born transformed into cancer cells.

Dr. Plata said that this viral theory does not conflict with any

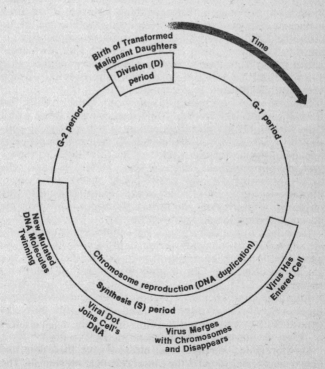

The HuMTV Scenario

known facts about breast cancer. In addition to the transforming mutation, he explained, it is possible that a genetic predisposition makes the body's defense mechanism vulnerable; otherwise, the transformed cells would simply be killed.

A concept, supported by many immunologists, is that every "immunocompetent" body has an elaborate immune surveillance system to kill off invaders when they appear. The system includes the lymph nodes, bone marrow, the thymus gland, and the spleen, as well as individual cells, which are constantly roaming through the lymphatics and bloodstream searching for and destroying foreign invaders.

Studies have shown that patients with malignancies have large numbers of living cancer cells floating around in their bodies, but not establishing new cancer colonies. Dead cancer cells have been found as well. Immunologists who support this surveillance-system concept suggest that only about 1 percent of the stray malignant cells manage to live long enough to become metastases; the dead cells were killed by the various components of the immune system. If this were not so, they argue, few cancer patients with metastatic disease would live very long, because every live cell that was shed into the blood stream or into a lymph vessel would grow into a new tumor.

Sometimes, however, even in immunocompetent bodies, this front-line militia is overcome. Some immunologists blame it on a "sneaking-through" phenomenon, by which malignant cells somehow manage to evade their killers. Of course, if the patient is immunodeficient, for one reason or another, the surveillance system is already weak, and it is much easier for the cancer cells to sneak through. As we know, breast cancer, in sneaking through, usually spreads first to the axillary lymph nodes by way of the lymphatic vessels and then, if the nodes themselves become cancerous, to other parts of the body.

In addition to a genetically deficient immune system, a hospitable endocrine environment—natural or artificial—would aid and abet the viral breast cancer's growth. As Dr. Dao had told me, the cancerous cells could not multiply without lots of nourishing hormones.

Like irradiation, chemical carcinogens, and genetic mutations, the oncornavirus is one more instrument that could foul up a cell's control of its own destiny.

"How can you ever prove this theory if the virus disappears?" I asked Dr. Plata. "Have you been able to take cells from a human breast cancer and grow a tumor in a laboratory animal?"

"In reality, no. With extracts from tumors, no." Dr. Plata

shook his head regretfully. "But we learned a trick from the heart transplants of a while back, when doctors discovered how to prevent the body from rejecting foreign tissues. By knocking out an animal's ability to reject foreign tissue, we can grow human tumor cells in its body. In other words, the animal acts as an incubator."

"Can you grow healthy human breast tissue in a test tube or Petri dish?"

"Only for about twenty or thirty generations," he replied. "That generally means from one month to, at most, three months. Healthy cells eventually stop living and growing *in vitro*—in glass. Only cancer cells keep on growing indefinitely. That is one way we have of knowing when cells have been transformed— when the tissue in the dish never stops growing. We don't even need a microscope."

"Then you have grown human cancer in a dish?"

Dr. Plata nodded. "Human cancer cells are now grown routinely in most laboratories. But, as yet, a confirmed human cancer virus has not been detected or produced in any cultured human tumor." On the other hand, he added that several researchers have obtained suspicious particles "somewhat resembling" viruses from human milk. Attempts are being made, without success so far, to have the particles invade and transform healthy human breast tissue growing *in vitro*. "These human particles have some of the characteristics of the MuMTV—the mouse virus," Dr. Plata said. "Some even look a little like it. But that is as far as we have come."

Before going to see Dr. Plata, I had made up a list of questions to ask him based on the polio-virus kind of invasion. I had planned to ask why scientists were diddling around trying to decide whether a virus did or did not exist. Why not simply assume there was a HuMTV, develop a poliolike vaccine, and forget the whole Koch's-postulates business? Now that I knew the suspected cancer virus is completely different from the polio virus, the fancy argument I had concocted evaporated. I must have looked quite disappointed.

"It's not so very hopeless." Dr. Plata smiled. "There are some really promising human, breast-tumor cell cultures, in several laboratories around the country, that, with a little work, may yield viruses worthy of study."

He told me about the first "particle-producing" culture of cancer cells taken from the chest fluid of a woman with breast cancer. The culture—named MCF-7, for the Michigan Cancer Foundation, where it was first grown—was being intensively studied in several laboratories, including those at the National Cancer Institute in 1974. "There isn't yet a large enough quantity of the particles to do much experimentation—only a few micrograms," Dr. Plata had explained. Now there are enough MCF-7 lines for every laboratory that needs it. In 1974, in anticipation of this, Dr. Plata had fifteen normal and malignant human, breast-cell lines already growing *in vitro* in his laboratory. "If I could infect"—in cancer jargon, to "infect" means to cause an invasion; no contagion involved!—"any of my well-defined cultures of normal breast cells with a purified virus, and if those cells transformed to resemble the cultured breast-tumor cells, there would be little doubt that the MCF-7 was the breast-cancer virus we are looking for," he told me.

"And then what?" I asked hopefully. "Will you be able to develop a vaccine?"

He shook his head. "Oh, perhaps yes, but that is not the immediate answer. Let me explain. Take measles as an example." Doodling on a pad of paper, he pointed out that, before the measles vaccine was developed, the disease was very widespread—much more so than breast cancer is. But, he reminded me, as prevalent as it was, it was not generally a serious or fatal disease.

Breast cancer is another story. "We must look at the fatality rate of the disease before we begin to think of giving every woman a vaccine against it. Even a vaccine that is 99.999999-per cent perfect is potentially too risky. Suppose there is a bad batch. It happened with polio, if you recall. The catastrophic results of having a bad batch of a breast-cancer vaccine are too enormous even to consider."

I leaned back in my chair, discouraged. "Then are you playing scientific games here just to prove that breast cancer is caused by a virus? What's the point? Why spend all this time, talent, effort, and money to find something that won't do any good even if it is found?"

"It would do a lot of good." Dr. Plata smiled. "If we find a virus, we will be able to look for a part of it—an antigen on its surface, a completely harmless substance—that we can use for a vaccination. If necessary, once that antigen is recognized, it could then be synthesized. By copying it chemically," Dr. Plata continued, "we would totally avoid the possibility of virus contamination. The antigen—the small part of the virus—would trigger the body into producing antibodies against just that antigen. Then, by attacking the antigen wherever in the body it would be found, the antibodies would kill the entire virus or the tumor cell of which that antigen formed a part."

"Is that what's meant by immunotherapy?" I asked.

"Yes," he replied. "This would be especially effective if a particular breast cancer were found to be caused by an exogenous—external—oncornavirus."

"What other kind of virus is there?" I asked. "Don't all viruses come into the body from outside?"

Dr. Plata shook his head. "That is true for most viruses. But unfortunately, in cancer, according to new evidence and the oncogene theory of Dr. Robert Huebner and Dr. George Todaro of NCI, at least some oncornaviruses may be an integral part of the animal host to begin with. There may well be an oncogene built into every cell." He told me of experiments by many investigators showing that these oncogenic viruses can be "demonstrated"—shown to be present—in nearly all animal species tested so far by activating healthy, normal cells with certain sophisticated chemical and irradiation procedures.

"In almost every case," Dr. Plata said, "the oncornavirus 'pops out' of the cell when these are done."

"What does that mean?" I asked.

"It may mean that every cell in the body has an endogenous, or internal, gene that could trigger a cancer if all the other circumstances were suitable for its growth."

"Are you telling me that everyone has a genetic predisposition to get cancer?"

He nodded.

When I described this interview in *Breast Cancer,* I had added a grim footnote that three other laboratories in the United States and another in Germany had replicated the Heubner and Todaro study supporting the theory of "an inborn, suicidal oncogene!" In 1974, before so much was known about cancer, it was awful and awesome to hear that animals (including humankind) might carry a "built-in cyanide pellet" that will kill them by cancer if something else doesn't kill them first.

Or, as Dr. Plata put it, "If the theory turns out to be reality, it may be one way by which most animals are preprogramed to die."

In 1974, his words were terrifying to hear. But somehow, I don't feel that way now. So much has been learned about the fantastic machine we call a human being, that the notion that nature has created us with a "preprogramed" way to keep the world's population under control seems to be something that we should expect.

6

The Problem of the Pill

I was talking to Frank Korun, a public-information officer for the Food and Drug Administration, about the rumored relationship between the Pill and our rising breast-cancer rates.

He recited the standard litany: "At this time, there is no proof that oral contraceptives cause breast cancer." Then he added, "When Betty Ford and Happy Rockefeller both got it, the first thing that popped into somebody's mind here in FDA was 'I wonder if they were taking OCs.'"

OCs, I quickly learned, is medical jargon for the Pill. "Why would anyone at FDA say that if there wasn't some risk you know about?"

"Don't misunderstand me," he snapped. "We have no evidence at all of a cancer risk with OCs. It was just something someone said."

When I was in the fifth grade, forty-two years ago, The Johns Hopkins Hospital and the Baltimore and Maryland departments of health decided to screen elementary-school children for hearing defects. I was found to have a deficiency in my right ear. The hospital and the two government departments generously decided to do something about the hard-of-hearing children, which included me. Every Thursday, a bus took me to Hopkins for an afternoon of radium treatments. I was the envy of all my "hearing" friends.

"I forgot all about the radium," I told an otorhinolaryngologist (ear, nose, and throat specialist) twenty-five years later. "Then a friend of mine told me her daughter had a thickened eardrum like mine. So I suggested radium treatments. 'Good Lord!' she yelled to me. 'Thousands of people who got radium treatments are getting cancer of the thyroid and larynx.' That's why I'm here to see you," I explained to the doctor. "Is my throat okay?"

He examined me carefully. "Everything seems to be all right." He smiled. "I doubt that, after twenty-five years, anything would happen now. But let's keep checking. You may be walking around with a time bomb inside you."

For the next five years he examined me frequently. Finally, thirty-five years post-radium, he cut me down to annual checkups. "I think you can breathe a bit easier now," he assured me in 1970.

But who really knows?

Now here was Frank Korun insisting that oral contraceptives—after being on the market for less than fifteen years—had no cancer risk.

"You mean there is no risk that you know of *so far*. Isn't that more accurate?" I questioned.

"There is absolutely no proof."

I told him about my radium treatments. "That was thirty-five years ago, and I'm still being watched. It took twenty-five years for most of those radium cancers to show up."

He was silent for a moment. "There is no proof OCs cause cancer," he repeated. "The FDA is monitoring all the time."

That was at the end of 1974, before Drs. Huebner and Todaro announced their oncogene theory. If they are right, if everyone is born with that built-in "cyanide pellet"—and it looks as if they may be—what a nourishing endocrine environment the estrogens in the Pill must create.

The tour through Dr. Dao's lab had made me suspect the Pill immediately. How could it not be dangerous?

"So is smoking," one of the doctors at Roswell Park said. "But people don't read that 'Warning: The Surgeon General Has Determined That Cigarette Smoking Is Dangerous to Your Health' on every pack. As far as the Pill is concerned, there are a lot of women who would rather risk cancer than a pregnancy."

"But do they know there's a risk? Is there a surgeon general's warning on the Pill package?"

"I'm sure there is," he insisted. "The risk is too obvious. The government must have made the drug companies put a warning on."

"Don't be so sure. The government can be very strange," I told him.

"Well, get some and see. There must be contraindications

where cancer is concerned. There is a Food and Drug Administration, you know."

I followed his advice. No, there was no warning of possible cancer risk on the label attached to the package, which is known, in FDA jargon, as the "patient package insert" or "PPI." It carried the manufacturer's instructions for use of the product, prefaced by this warning, printed in boldface type:

ORAL CONTRACEPTIVES (Birth Control Pills)
Do Not Take This Drug Without Your
Doctor's Continued Supervision

The oral contraceptives are powerful and effective drugs which can cause side effects in some users and should not be used at all by some women. The most serious known side effect is abnormal blood clotting which can be fatal.

Safe use of this drug requires a careful discussion with your doctor. To assist him in providing you with the necessary information, [the manufacturer's name is inserted here] has prepared a booklet written in a style understandable to you as the drug user. This provides information on the effectiveness and known hazards of the drug including warnings, side effects and who should not use it. Your doctor will give you this booklet if you ask for it and he can answer any questions you may have about the use of this drug.

Notify your doctor if you notice any unusual physical disturbance or discomfort.

Caution: Oral contraceptives are of no value in the prevention or treatment of venereal disease.

I asked a pharmacist for the booklet mentioned in the label, but he had none. They were only available from obstetricians and gynecologists, or from drug-company "detail men." Other physicians did not receive copies. Finally my husband's secretary got one for me from her obstetrician.

"You aren't given one of these automatically," she explained. "My doctor only gives it to patients who ask for it." She had been taking OCs for several years, and the booklet she had, *What You Should Know About the Pill,* contained the name of the brand she was using. However, I found out that all Pill manufacturers were required to use the same text, filling in the blanks with their tradenamed product. Alice had not read the booklet before. As soon as she finished the last page, she decided to stop using OCs.

"Oral contraceptives, like all potent drugs," it said blithely, "have some side effects. Fortunately, serious side effects are relatively rare."

Among the nonserious side effects it mentioned were: tenderness of the breasts, nausea and vomiting, gain or loss of weight, spotty darkening of the skin, vaginal bleeding, elevated levels of sugar or fat in the blood, nervousness, dizziness, some loss of scalp hair, increase in body hair, an increase or decrease in sex drive, and appetite changes. Also, a nursing mother was warned that she may find a decrease in her supply of milk.

There were also light references to migraine headaches, mental depression, fibroids of the uterus, heart or kidney disease, asthma, high blood pressure, diabetes, and epilepsy. These were all listed under "Special Needs."

The *serious* side effects? Statistical evidence about thrombophlebitis—a potentially fatal circulatory disorder—had forced drug firms to give women some information about a risk of blood-clotting problems resulting from use of the Pill. One of about every 2,000 women on OCs, the booklet said, is hospitalized every year because of blood-clotting trouble; also, one in 66,000 pill-taking women under thirty-five dies each year from thromboembolic disorders. But only *one in 500,000 women not taking OCs dies* annually from clotting disorders.

Although cancer was omitted from the patient package insert, it *was* mentioned in this booklet. "There is no proof at the present time that oral contraceptives can cause cancer in humans," it said. "However, the possibility that they may continues to be studied, based on observations that large doses of female sex hormones have produced cancer in some experimental animals."

And, buried deep in "Special Needs": "There are some women . . . who should not use oral contraceptives. These include women who have cancer of the breast or womb." This booklet did not say that the Pill is contraindicated where there is a family history of cancer, although I was told by Dr. Louis Hellman, chairman of the FDA advisory committee that approved the Pill for sale in November 1959, that his copy of the *Physicians' Desk Reference*—a drug guide for doctors—did have the warning. The 1975 edition did not, however.

Dr. Hellman, then the deputy secretary for population of the Department of Health, Education, and Welfare, (now the Department of Health and Human Services—HHS) was not aware that breast-cancer incidence rates had been climbing steadily upward. He also did not know that the package insert carried no warning aimed at women who had had cancer, in spite of having helped write the first label.

"The original insert specifically mentioned cancer . . . as a contraindication," he told me. "Certainly whatever is in the booklet and the physicians' instructions about cancer should also be on the patients' label."

Oral contraceptives and an asthma medication were then the *only* drugs on the market in the United States that carried a warning label about contraindications addressed to patients. Although there were (and still are) many medications that should not be taken by certain people, only their doctors had this knowledge.

A former obstetrician-gynecologist and a professor of both, Dr. Hellman had testified before former Senator Gaylord Nelson's Select Subcommittee on Monopoly in January 1970—shortly after the Pill's tenth birthday. He had told the senators then that he was "uneasy" about possible carcinogenic effects on the breast, that the fear "is always at the back of my mind." But, he said, there was no evidence that a cause-and-effect relationship existed, and so he had advised the FDA to approve the Pill for marketing. Women were to be warned, however, about the possibility that estrogens should be avoided if they or close relatives had cancer.

He stressed to me that correlation must not be confused with cause and effect. "Just because the breast-cancer rate is going up at the same time as use of OCs is going up, that doesn't necessarily mean the drug is causing the increased incidence."

Another witness at the 1970 Senate hearings was Dr. Roy Hertz, then an associate medical director of the Rockefeller University. He had also been a member of the FDA committee that evaluated the Pill. During his career, Dr. Hertz had been a professor of obstetrics and gynecology and had taken part in research programs at the National Institutes of Health. At the time of my telephone interview, in late 1974, he was a research professor in obstetrical pharmacology at the George Washington University Medical School in Washington. He is now retired.

He told me he stood by his 1970 testimony. "I don't think that between then and now we have obtained the definitive information we need to know whether the estrogens in the Pill are carcinogenic or not. The same possibility of risk is still there."

In 1970, he had testified that "it was clear from the outset such an innovation, like all new medications, [carries] with it certain inherent risks." Increased cancer of the breast and uterus, Dr. Hertz had said, were his prime concerns. Asked by one senator if he thought estrogens were the whole cause of breast cancer, he replied, "I think they are to breast cancer what fertilizer is to the crop. They are not the seed."

Dr. Hertz had helped to write the physicians' instructions, which warn that women who have had cancer should not be given OCs. He had assumed the patient package insert repeated the warning.

The 1970 Nelson hearings brought together an impressive array of medical experts on all the diseases that might be affected by the Pill, not just cancer experts. As far as mammary carcinoma was concerned, the consensus was that it was too soon to know. Even one of the FDA's own witnesses, Dr. Robert Kistner, of the Harvard Medical School (also, at the time, a grantee and part-time consultant to Searle Pharmaceuticals), admitted that ten years were not enough time to judge.

Dr. Hugh Davis, a Johns Hopkins professor of obstetrics and gynecology, was vehement in his objections. "Shall we have millions of women on the Pill for twenty years and then discover it was all a great mistake? Breast cancers have been induced on at least five different species of animals by treatment with the same synthetic hormones being marketed in the oral contraceptives."

Dr. Marvin Legator, then the chief of the Cell Biology Branch of the FDA's Division of Pharmacology, a defender of the Pill, nonetheless agreed that its effects had to be carefully watched. "The earliest period for detecting an increase in genital or mammary tumors . . . would be the mid-'70s," he told the subcommittee.

It was the mid-'70s and there had been a definite increase in mammary-tumor incidence rates. Yet oral contraceptives carried no warning of cancer on the patient's label.

Paradoxiclly, in 1959—the year before OCs went on the market—the Food and Drug Administration banned the use of diethylstilbestrol (DES) in poultry feed, because tests had proved this synthetic female hormone caused breast cancer in mice. Edible tissues of poultry which got the feed, the FDA ruled, retained traces of DES that were too high to be safe, under the food section of the 1938 law that authorized the supervisory agency's creation. DES was also banned in feed for cattle and sheep in August 1972. However, in January 1973, the District of Columbia Court of Appeals reversed the latter ruling on a legal technicality.

Edward Nida, an information officer of FDA, explained why estrogens were FDA-OK for women but prohibited for chickens. "Oral contraceptives are voluntary and available only by prescription," he said. "Drugs put into animal feed are what we call 'surreptitious,' and consumers may not be aware they're getting them."

Nida, like Korun, repeated the line about there being no proof that estrogens caused cancer in humans. "The pharmaceutical firms are required by law to report any adverse effects immediately," he declared. "If they don't, somebody goes to jail. We don't play around with them."

The FDA was depending on the proverbial fox to guard our chicken coop.

"We have medical officers who follow all drugs," Nida added. "We also have literature searches and automated medical libraries." He said the FDA continues monitoring all drugs even after approval is granted.

The questionable efficiency of the FDA's estrogen monitors was demonstrated on October 9, 1974, when the approval of an injectible contraceptive—Depo-Provera—was delayed just three days before it was to go on drugstore shelves. The delay was at the direct order of Secretary Caspar W. Weinberger, the former head of the Department of Health, Education, and Welfare, of which FDA is a member agency.

Congressman L. H. Fountain of North Carolina had told Weinberger that his Intergovernmental Relations subcommittee—the House's biting watchdog over the FDA—had evidence showing Depo-Provera to be the possible cause of cervical cancer in twenty-two of 1,000 women involved in clinical trials of the drug. In the course of his eleven-page, single-spaced letter, Congressman Fountain said the relevant data had already been published by the National Cancer Institute in 1971.

There were other examples of the FDA's failure to exert tight surveillance over the Pill. For example, its Metabolic and Endocrine Section did not know that breast-cancer incidence had increased since OCs were approved, as Frank Korun admitted. "But let's thank God it's easily cured," he said.

Korun did not know that the "cure" is to have the breast amputated and then to be given a fifty-fifty chance of living longer than ten years.

Korun said he knew of no work in progress to study a possible relationship between the Pill and breast cancer. Again the FDA's monitoring system had failed. Several investigations were under way.

Two contracts to study the problem were being funded by the Center of Population Research (CPR) of the National Institute of Child Health and Human Development. Dr. Philip A. Corfman—whose name was mentioned by several FDA officials as that agency's unofficial monitor of OCs—is the director of the center. The chief of CPRs Contraceptive Evaluation Branch, Dr. Heinz Berendes, was tracking the results. He told me one investigation involved 200 women in Connecticut and the other about 450 women in California. Both were "retrospective studies": women with recent diagnoses of breast cancer were compared with a closely matched control group.

"We ask the cancer patients, 'Did you take the Pill?' " Dr. Berendes explained. "Then we analyze to see if there is an association." After two years, he said, no cause-and-effect relationship had been found. However, he admitted that 650 is a small sample and "it is too soon to know with certainty."

I did not try to track down the Connecticut scientists. However, I did call Dr. Ralph Paffenbarger in Berkeley, California and was referred to Dr. Elfriede Fasal, who directed the California investigation Dr. Berendes had cited.

"I did not say there was no relationship," she told me. "I simply gave some preliminary findings at a national public-health meeting. At that time, I merely gave these findings with no conclusions, except that some of the comparative data were not statistically significant. The actual report has not even been published yet." (This was in April 1975.)

As an example of the study's statistical insignificance vis-à-vis breast cancer, Dr. Fasal told me she found that all the women over the age of thirty took the Pill less frequently than did those under thirty—regardless of their illness. (The control group, by the way, was composed of hospitalized patients who had medical or surgical problems other than breast disease, *not* healthy women chosen at random.) The thirty-to-thirty-nine age group averaged 65.6 percent Pill users; the forty-to-forty-nine group, 38.6 percent. She said the differences in usage between breast-cancer patients and others in the older age groups were not "statistically significant"—only a few percentage points.

However, Dr. Fasal said that of the fifteen women between the ages of fifteen and twenty-nine who had breast cancer, *100 percent* were on the Pill at the time their tumors were found. Only 81 percent of the younger women in the control group, on the other hand, used OCs. This difference, according to Dr. Fasal, is also not statistically significant, because the sample was so small. But, since breast-cancer risks are normally low in this age bracket, she thought the 100-percent use of the Pill by the young cancer patients "warranted further investigation."

I found no mention anywhere of this aspect of the Berkeley study, and when I called Dr. Corfman for more information, he told me he was not aware of the data. He had not heard the oral report given by Dr. Fasal and was waiting for the final results to be published in an NIH journal. Dr. Berendes was not available.

Then I called Dr. Herschel Jick at Boston University. His Boston Collaborative Drug Surveillance Program had been so widely referred to that I was certain he must have found something important. Also, it involved 25,000 women—an enormous sample.

"We were not primarily concerned with breast cancer," he told me, "but with all diseases—short- and long-term—that could be related to oral contraceptives." He said that only twenty-three of the 25,000 women studied had breast cancer, and the major pharmaceutical suspect was reserpine, not the Pill. However, he agreed that reserpine along with estrogens could have a relationship to breast cancer, because reserpine increases prolactin secretion and because prolactin must have estrogens to interact with in order to be carcinogenic. Logically, more estrogens in the blood, from oral contraceptives, would give the higher prolactin levels a more favorable environment to do their cancerous work. This, Dr. Jick told me in a telephone interview in April 1975, was the suspected link between breast cancer and the various Rauwolfia drugs—reserpine is just one.

As far as I could see, the widely touted Boston Collaborative and Berkeley studies incriminated oral contraceptives even more deeply than I had suspected.

"I just don't understand how anyone could interpret their results as proving no relationship between breast cancer and the Pill," I told Harvey during dinner that night.

"In my business, we're working with statistics all the time." He laughed. "You can always find some number to support what you want to prove."

One problem seems to be that all the Pill studies had been retrospective. As Dr. Berendes said, women with breast cancer were asked if they had ever taken the Pill, and if they had not they were listed in the "no-oral-contraceptive" column of the chart.

When I entered Roswell Park, I was also asked if I had ever taken oral contraceptives. I said I had not. "But," I told the young physician who interviewed me, "I've taken lots of estrogens."

Without even trying to add the gallons of chicken soup (DES-impregnated until 1959) and the DES-impregnated chopped liver I had eaten in my life, I told him about the hormones prescribed for me as a teen-ager to regulate my menstrual periods and to clear up my skin. I added that I had been given estrogens to prevent miscarriages and to "dry up my milk" after breast-feeding.

"Estrogens are estrogens," he said tersely.

"Prospective studies" are analyses of people followed "ahead of time." To study OCs in such controlled surveys, a random group would be chosen and studied for years—some taking the Pill, others not—to see what diseases they developed in later years. Estrogens taken for any other reason would also be included. A prospective study, everyone agrees, is a far more reliable technique, but it takes a long time to get adequate data.

So, as of early 1975, all the evidence against the Pill as a carcino*trophic* factor in breast cancer—cancer-nourishing, not cancer-causing—was based on retrospective studies, simply because it had not been around long enough.

Another statistical problem was that postmenopausal women with breast cancer were combined in the same data base with younger victims, diluting the impact of the actual number having the disease. Since so much evidence indicated that there are two different age-related kinds of breast cancer, it would have been more accurate to study the effects of Pill use only on younger women.

In contrast to the Food and Drug Administration's policy, Dr. Corfman did not depend on drug firms to report adverse effects of the Pill.

"I don't think the industry has hardly any good data." He laughed. "That's the reason we're doing the studies here." He also placed little reliance on National Cancer Institute research, but for different reasons. "We keep in touch," he said, "but we don't find we get much from their work. The only way to study pills is to study pills and not try to piggyback on bigger studies."

Because of the lack of close communication with NCI, neither Dr. Corfman nor Dr. Berendes were aware that 1974's breast-cancer incidence rate was much higher than it was in 1960. Even without knowing this, however, Dr. Berendes admitted he would be "reluctant" to have his wife take OCs for ten years or longer.

After I told him what the 1974 incidence rates were, Dr. Berendes recalled that during the 1970 Senate hearings there had been unanimous agreement that, unlike cervical cancers (also linked with OCs), breast tumors could take as long as twenty years to develop. The witnesses—including Dr. Corfman—had testified on the need for periodic reevaluations of oral contraceptives. "We knew there would have to be continuing surveillance . . . at least for maybe ten years," Dr. Berendes said. "We simply don't know how long someone would have to be exposed . . . and what the interval would have to be."

In a report published in the medical journal *Contraception*, in late 1974, Dr. Corfman wrote a résumé of the currently available methods of birth control. Using as evidence the Berkeley and Boston studies, as well as work done in Britain, he said, "At least to date, there is no relationship between the use of OC's and breast cancer."

However, the editor of the journal followed Dr. Corfman's report with this statement: "I find myself again in the position of calling for moderation and against over-enthusiasm in accepting and interpreting data in regard to oral contraception. . . . Subjecting well young women over long periods of time to potent drugs with widespread generalized reactions is certainly not good medicine."

Now we are told that all of us have an oncogene—a hidden trigger in every cell in our bodies—which might cause cancer under the right circumstances. What are the consequences of disturbing the delicate hormonal balance of a young woman by adding unnecessary estrogens?

Married women, who usually get their prescriptions for the Pill from family doctors or obstetrician-gynecologists, are usually under their continuing care. Presumably, these physicians know their patients' family backgrounds and personal medical histories. But what about the thousands of teen-agers and young women who get their pills through friends or from various birth-control clinics, most after one-shot visits and with no continuing care? No one is keeping a watchful eye over them.

In Europe, no one I interviewed hesitated to say that oral contraceptives are carcinogenic. This seems to be the "catch-22" of OCs—the three-letter syllable *gen,* Greek for "produced by." Indeed, there is still no proof that the Pill produces breast cancer in humans. There is, however, a great deal of proof that, whatever the seed might be, the estrogens in these drugs are fertilizers that stimulate and speed the growth of mammary carcinomas. Research literature shows evidence that, while OCs may not be carcino*gen*ic in humans, they are certainly carcino*trophic*—cancer-nourishing.

With regard to animal studies, the FDA's spokesman, Frank Korun, told me the law specifies "toxicity" in three species of animals as being enough to rule a drug unsafe for human use. Five species of animals have developed mammary carcinomas after being given the same hormones that are in the Pill. Here is some of the additional evidence.

- Scientists needing cancerous tumors for experimentation routinely grow them quickly by giving estrogens to specially bred vulnerable strains of mice.
- Two compounds, Ethynerone and Neonovum (trade names for estrogenic OCs), were not even submitted for

FDA approval, because they had caused breast cancers in dogs and monkeys over a seven-year period.

- Clinical data show that both the withdrawal and the administration of estrogens affect the rate of growth of existing breast cancers in women.
- Premenopausal women with the disease whose ovaries—a natural source of estrogens—are removed usually improve.
- Women who have had their ovaries removed surgically or who have complete hysterectomies before the age of forty have a lower risk of developing breast cancer; the same is true of women with natural early menopause.
- Most breast cancers that develop in pregnant women are particularly virulent and fast-growing; the accepted reason for this phenomenon is the high estrogen level in the blood during pregnancy.
- From the late 1940s through the 1960s, millions of American women were given diethylstilbestrol routinely to prevent miscarriages early in pregnancy. Many so-called "DES daughters" developed rare forms of vaginal and cervical cancers. An NCI committee, created to study this problem in 1979, found that the mothers were developing "an excess" of breast cancer. This term means the incidence is higher than should normally be expected in that number of women.
- Giving estrogen to men with prostatic cancer has led to the development of cancer of the breast—a rare disease in males.
- Breast-cancer specialists know that some tumors are hormone-dependent and some hormone-independent, and that knowing the type helps determine the best postoperative treatment.

What did the Food and Drug Administration do about warning women of the risks of the Pill? The same thing it did about reinstituting the 1973 ban on feeding DES to cattle and sheep. Nothing.

Ed Nida told me the FDA admitted there were many unanswered questions about cancer and the Pill. "No drug, including aspirin," he insisted, "is absolutely safe. What we look at is the benefit-risk of a drug. Do the benefits of preventing pregnancy outweigh the risks of having a baby?" He said, however, that the Supreme Court decision of January 22, 1973, liberalizing abortion laws had virtually eliminated one of those risks—the danger of botched abortions. In using the mortality rates of childbirth as a risk factor, the FDA seemed to be equating pregnancy with a serious disease. To be pregnant was a pathological illness, where the benefit of a potentially dangerous drug that can prevent or cure (like chloromycetin, which can also cause the destruction of white blood cells vital in fighting disease) is weighed against the risk of possible death. But the dangers of giving chloromycetin are usually spelled out clearly to the patient or the patient's family.

Nida contended that the FDA was doing all it could about the Pill, under the circumstances. "When you have drug companies chewing on us for not approving drugs and creating a drug lag, and the Ralph Naders and the rest of the world chewing on us for putting risky things on the market, questions are not easily answered."

The late Gilbert S. Goldhammer, then a consultant to Congressman Fountain's oversight subcommittee, said that one of the FDA's major problems in dealing with the Pill is simply that the agency is too "business oriented," and OCs are big moneymakers. "There's no real chicanery," he told me. "No bribery or things like that. It's just that the people at the top of FDA are not really scientists. They are medical people, but they're more management types. They have a business outlook on salvaging a product and making it work out." He chuckled. "And if they're wined and dined by the pharmaceutical people, that makes them all pals. You can't turn around and hurt pals."

Goldhammer added that Richard Nixon's longtime friendship with the founder of the giant Warner-Lambert firm, Elmer H. Bobst, undoubtedly had had an effect on the FDA's attitude toward all drug companies. "Bobst is godfather to one of the Nixon girls," he laughed, "and close to Nixon. By taking over Parke-Davis, he got one of the OCs—Norlestrin. Now, you know that kind of relationship had to affect the bosses at FDA. Nixon never needed much encouragement to be on the side of any business, and everybody knew what direction to go in." In early 1975, most of the top FDA officials were still Nixon appointees.

Goldhammer said that the Fountain subcommittee had held hearings on DES in animal feed, but, except for the Depo-Provera matter, it had not devoted much time to oral contraceptives. "I certainly think that all cancer risks should be put where the woman can see them," he said. "That means on the patient-package-insert label."

Paradoxically, in early March 1975, the FDA withheld authorization of an estrogen compound containing large quantitites of DES that had been developed as a "morning-after" contraceptive, citing fears that it could cause cancer. Why bar a morning-after drug but not the standard OC? Who knows? The ways of FDA are strange and uninterpretable. Less than a month later, the potent compound was approved, because, according to Nida, doctors were simply prescribing multiple doses of ordinary DES to be taken for five consecutive days after the "accident."

"We are just recognizing current medical practice," he explained. "This way, the morning-after DES will have a warning on it that it is for emergency use only—rape or incest—and can be taken only once in a lifetime."

Approve a drug so dangerous it can be taken only once in a lifetime? As I said, who can understand the FDA?

Why was DES not permitted in chicken feed when it was all right in the feed of steers, sheep, and other animals?

Why were cyclamates banned as carcinogens on the basis of far less evidence?

It didn't look like the cancer risk would be added. Spokesman Frank Korun told me in late 1974 that the patient package insert was then in the process of being reviewed, "but there are no great alarming facts that are going to be included. There are no plans to mention anything about cancer on the label," he said at the time.

There is still no proof positive that estrogens cause breast cancer in women. Probably there never will be; the hormones are carcino*trophic*—fertilizers, not seeds. And even if they were the cause, a woman who would rather risk cancer than risk becoming pregnant should have the right—in the spirit of the basic individual freedom invoked by cigarette smokers—to make that choice.

I was not suggesting that oral contraceptives be summarily wiped from the shelves, as the "carcinogenic" cyclamates were. But I felt Pill users should be warned, as smokers are. I saw no excuse for keeping the possible consequences from them—especially those in the high-risk breast-cancer categories.

In January 1975, five years had passed since the Pill was last discussed in open hearings on Capitol Hill. Five years and about half a million breast cancers later, it was time for another congressional look. There was none.

Benjamin Gordon and Dr. Frederick Glaser, former Senator Gaylord Nelson's top aides on drug matters, told me that no new hearings had been scheduled because there was evidence OCs were not related to breast cancer and might even be protective.

What evidence?

The Boston Collaborative and Berkeley studies?

"We've also been told that breast-cancer incidence has not been soaring upward, as we and you thought," Gordon said.

"I can't believe that at all," I said. "One of the top statisticians at NCI told me just a couple of months ago that it's been going up about 1 percent every year since 1960."

"Well," he said, "that's all I can tell you. That's what they say."

I called Dr. Sidney Cutler, the NCI biometrician I had been quoting. He was on leave, but Susan Devesa, I was told, would have such incidence information. Immediately, she assured me that I had not been misquoting Dr. Cutler or giving out misinformation. NCI's statistical method had simply been changed.

"What he told you was based on information from Connecticut," she explained, "and we are not using that as our base now." Ms. Devesa went on to say that Connecticut—where the breast-cancer incidence had been going steadily upward, from 65 cases per 100,000 women in 1960 to 74 per 100,000 in 1969—had been the data base because it had a reliable state tumor registry that had been in existence for many years. However, NCI had come to feel that Connecticut was not truly representative of the country as a whole. For example, few blacks, Orientals, Latin Americans, or American Indians were included.

Therefore, in the mid-1960's, money was granted to seven cities and metropolitan areas to establish tumor registries—Birmingham, San Francisco-Oakland, Atlanta, Dallas-Fort Worth, Detroit, Minneapolis-St. Paul, and Pittsburgh—as well as to two entire states, Iowa and Colorado. The registries began collecting and analyzing incidence data in 1969, and their figures for the years 1969-1971 were published as the Third National Cancer Survey. Since most of the areas had no earlier statistics, there were no precedents against which to measure changes.

"But San Francisco has had a registry since 1960," Ms. Devesa told me, "and the breast-cancer incidence in that area has been rising. The age-adjusted rates for 1969-1971 were 84.1 per 100,000—even higher than Connecticut's." Sure enough, telephoned data from Alameda County (Oakland) showed a rate of 66.1 per 100,000 women—including Orientals, who have little breast cancer—for the 1960-1962 period, with a subsequent steady upward climb to 84.1 (which also includes San Francisco) for 1969-1971. I studied the table of statistics to which Ms. Devesa referred me. Birmingham had only 58.8 per 100,000 for 1969-1971. But a phone call to its registry gave no further information; there were no earlier incidence data.

"Maybe I can find out how many women are taking the Pill in the two areas," I suggested to Harvey during my daily dinnertime report. "The difference of incidence around Oakland is enormous. I bet it's even 'statistically significant'."

After hours on the telephone, I discovered it is impossible to learn any details about sales of oral contraceptives. The American Pharmaceutical Association, the Center for Health Statistics, Planned Parenthood, the Population Institute, and even Ralph Nader were no help. Finally I again turned to Benjamin Gordon.

"That breakdown is kept by a marketing research firm named IMS, in Pennsylvania," he told me. "I've never been able to get the information out of them." Sure enough, the appropriate persons at IMS said that information was "privileged."

The Census Bureau told me that women in the San Francisco-Oakland area are generally more affluent, well educated, and sophisticated—all factors that might contribute to an increased use of OCs—but these same factors could contribute to the rising breast-cancer incidence without the Pill, as well.

"Another piece in the jigsaw puzzle," I lamented.

But I did learn a great deal about statistics and their significance—and insignificance—to cancer while I was studying oral contraceptives. For example, I could not find a single scientist involved in breast-cancer research who believes OCs are safe where this disease is concerned. Everyone I queried was positive that adding large quantities of female hormones to a woman's body—especially a young woman's—is dangerous, regardless of the lack of statistical evidence.

The arguments supporting the Pill were coming from doctors in clinical practice and from those scientists who played various numbers games. These are the people who constantly say, "That is not proof," "There is no evidence," and even "OCs are protective." Laboratory scientists like Dr. Dao pay little attention to numbers. When mice consistently develop mammary carcinomas after treatment with estrogens, this is enough proof for them that the female hormones are not safe. Dr. Dao had often told me, "I don't need large samples. For me, ten out of ten are enough to prove anything."

But even the numbers players agreed that a cancer warning should be on the patient package insert.

"Certainly," statistician-biometrician Susan Devesa said, "if the contraindication is in the physicians' instructions and in the booklet or other literature, it should be on the label the patient sees."

So why wasn't it? The reason can be found in the *Federal Register,* Volume 35, Number 113, dated June 11, 1970.

Organized medicine, speaking through the American Medical Association, the Association of American Physicians and Surgeons, the American College of Obstetrics and Gynecology, the American Society of Internal Medicine, the AMA Interspecialty Committee, the South Georgia Medical Society, the California Medical Association, the Rhode Island Medical Society, the Texas Medical Association, and the Medical Society of Delaware, generally opposed [a label with assurances and warnings] on the grounds that (1) it would interfere with the physician-patient relationship . . . (2) that it would confuse and alarm the patient . . . (3) that the package insert cannot provide all the needed information . . . (4) that the physician is the proper person to provide the kind of information to his own patient . . . on a need-to-know basis; and (5) that the regulations should not control what information the prescriber gives to the patient.

Some physicians also felt that label warnings were an "unnecessary government intrusion into medical practice," and they said "the doctor's judgment as to what the patient should be told should prevail."

The Food and Drug Aministration, created to protect and defend the people of the United States against impure, unsafe, and ineffective drugs, had bowed to pressure from pharmaceutical companies and "organized medicine."

"Why should we taxpayers be stuck with FDA salaries?" I complained to Harvey. "The FDA is looking after the drug companies and the doctors—not us."

Then I found an article written by former Senator Vance Hartke of Indiana headlined "FDA Is a Sham That Looks After Its Cronies Instead of the Public." "An inescapable conclusion," he wrote, "is that industry will pay many FDA members' salaries when they leave government. The implication is obvious: Don't bite the hand that will be feeding you."

After weeks of reading, telephoning, and interviewing to find out why we were not being warned about the dangers of the Pill, one short article gave me the answer—"economic incentive."

EPILOGUE

My book *Breast Cancer* was published in September 1975, and I was smugly confident the data in Chapter 6 would at least trigger new Congressional hearings, but my book had the effect of a feather in a hurricane. The matter had to be brought to the attention of the public or of people who had the power to do something. Since I had been a reporter for many years, my first thought was to go to the press. Morton Mintz, then the Washington Post's expert in FDA affairs, wrote some articles and tried his best to reopen the controversy, but his stories were drowned in Watergate coverage. They did not succeed in getting a single congressman or senator to call for new hearings.

In the meantime, we had moved, and I learned that Gaylord Nelson was a new neighbor. After Xeroxing the preceding pages (as they had originally appeared in *Breast Cancer*), I put them into his mailbox. Within a week, a letter came from him telling me his Senatorial duties in 1975 no longer gave him jurisdiction over drug matters.

I contacted the FDA's Committee on Obstetrics and Gynecology and asked to be put on their mailing list so I would be notified of future hearings on oral contraceptives. I wanted to put the data into the official record as "citizen testimony." Since the FDA's Rockville, Maryland headquarters are not far from my home, I went to hearing after hearing and was even given time to testify before the Committee on one occasion. My testimony had no effect.

Giving up on the Executive Branch of Government, I decided to go to the Legislative. Although Senator Nelson could do nothing (he could have responded to a Wisconsin constituent), I thought the Maryland representatives would be required to act. Senator Charles Mathias bombarded the FDA with letters and sent me copies of all the correspondence. He, a U.S. Senator, was getting the same runaround I had gotten as a citizen.

"There's something wrong with the system," I wailed to Harvey, after counting the inch-thick pile of letters that had been going to and fro Capitol Hill and Rockville. "Mathias is getting the same stuff I got. What's the point of being in the 'most exclusive club in the world' if you can't do better than a reporter?"

"Maybe you ought to try the courts," he grinned. "You've struck out with the Executive and Legislative. Why not try the Judiciary?"

He was only joking.

But why not? I remembered reading something about an injunction being requested against the Department of Agriculture by a Nader group to stop meatpackers from using ground-up bones in processed meat without saying so on the label. After Harvey left, my fingers began walking through the yellow pages to find a woman lawyer to file suit on a free (*pro bono*) basis. None of the female attorneys I called said no, but all of them were too busy with other matters. I tried some feminist organizations, and everyone told me such a matter would have to be voted upon by a

Board of Directors or even by the entire membership. It could take years.

In late 1975, Martin Baron—a personal-injury lawyer in Queens, New York—contacted me to help in a malpractice case (detailed in Chapter 7) involving delayed diagnosis of breast cancer. Although he had contributed generously to the Breast Cancer Advisory Center and owed me no favors, I decided to ask him for one anyhow.

"When can you get up here?"

"Whenever you say?"

"Tomorrow?"

"If you have time . . ."

"I'll make the time," Marty said. "This is more important than any of my other cases. Let me know when you'll be getting in, and I'll pick you up."

It suddenly occurred to me that I had not mentioned anything about wanting a *pro bono* lawyer.

"I've got no money to pay you."

"So who asked you for money?" he laughed. "I'll see you tomorrow."

After being turned down by every woman attorney I had spoken with as well as by Sidney Wolfe of Ralph Nader's Health Research Group and miscellaneous women's-lib organizations, I couldn't believe my ears. A private, for-profit, male lawyer was the only person willing to help.

On September 26, 1976, a suit was filed against Dr. Alexander Schmidt, then Commissioner of the FDA, and Caspar Weinberger, the former Secretary of the Department of Health, Education and Welfare. The legal snarls took Marty back to his Tort books to find precedents (including a case involving a steel company), because he had to prove that a private citizen had the right to sue an executive agency. To this day, I don't know all of the precedents and arguments Marty had to file in writing or make orally before someone or another. I do, however, know that the compelling and convincing legalism had something to do with a Commerce Department ruling and was unrelated to FDA regulations.

At that time, over-the-counter medications were required to have every conceivable contraindication, side-effect, and hazard visible on their labels. But labels on prescription drugs were required by law only to bear its pharmacy number, the patient's name, the physician's name, the date, and directions for usage. Marty miraculously found the Commerce Department regulation saying that a prescription drug giving users any additional information about the medication—such as a warning about a single side-effect—had to give *all* known information. Otherwise, the label was "misbranding and misleading," and the drug could not be traded in interstate commerce. Since the Pill had been carrying the Congressionally mandated warning about clotting disorders, the regulation required that all of the information in the booklet had to be put on the patient-package-insert as well.

Even with this ammunition, however, it took from September 1976 to February 3, 1978 before the final verdict was handed down. (By that time, the defendants were Secretary of HEW Joseph Califano and FDA Commissioner Dr. Donald Kennedy.) Judge Thomas Platt of Manhattan's Federal Court ruled that a label warning women who had breast cancer not to take oral contraceptives be printed on the patient's label of all brands on the market. I had asked for a warning aimed at women who had a family history as well, but this part of my request was not granted. At that time, there were not enough data to support this. Still, I savored the victory.

Drug manufacturers were given a few months to comply. It had taken almost a year and a half of legal maneuvering, and the work involved must have cost Marty about $10,000. The secretarial and photocopying costs alone must have come to four figures! Yet he charged me nothing. All he earned for his efforts was a lucite paperweight with a month's supply of pills embedded inside and a framed, laminated copy of the new patient-package-insert. More than a year later, when I had become active in the National Women's Health Network, Judy Norsigian wrote him a letter of thanks on behalf of all women.

Women also owe a debt to Dr. Donald Kennedy.

Furious and frustrated about the refusal of the House of Representatives to do as the Senate did to eliminate diethylstilbestrol in cattlefood, Dr. Donald Kennedy announced an FDA ban on this use of DES on June 29, 1979—a ban that went into effect the following November. I have been told (but Ed Nida—still in his public-information job at the FDA—could not confirm it) that this was his last official act before resigning as the Commissioner of the agency. Like Dr. Schmidt, he returned to a low-paying job in academia and did not—as former Senator Hartke predicted—move into the plush executive suite of a pharmaceutical firm.

During his tenure, the FDA also disapproved (again!) the use of DES as a morning-after or "postcoital" contraceptive. However, since the hormone is still available from any drugstore, all a physician has to do to make it a postcoital contraceptive is to write a prescription for the approved dosage but instruct women to take the pills twice a day for five days.

Except for treating advanced breast and prostate cancers,

there is—I have been told—no reason for prescribing diethylstil-bestrol at all. Many cancer experts I have interviewed believe the time has come to make DES a substance that is available only from oncologists—just as marijuana (or THC) tablets are.

The OC situation is now more complicated and confused than ever. Although enough proof about the dangers of sequential contraceptives (hormones taken separately, one after another, rather than in combination) caused these to be banned, the controversy about ordinary OCs has raged on. A study done by scientists at Yale, published in 1979, showed that some benign breast problems are prevented or alleviated when oral contraceptives are prescribed. Since this is supported by numerous studies done by scientists all over the world, the data cannot be rejected. The "Catch-22," obviously, is that women can't know what kind of benign masses they have in their breasts. Are they the kind that OCs will help? Are they made up of harmless cells that will be transformed to cancer by the Pill? Or are the cells true precursors of cancer that the estrogens will mature so they are transformed years before they would have otherwise become cancerous? There is simply no way to know.

In the fall of 1980, it was widely reported in newspapers and magazines that the health hazards of the Pill were "negligible." The report was based on a twelve-year, $8.5 million study of more than 16,000 women in California. Dubbed the "Walnut Creek Report," its authors, Drs. Savitri Ramcharan and Frederick Pellegrin, called a prepublication press conference to tell the world that they found no elevated risks from pill use in "young, healthy women."

Scientists at the NIH questioned the announcement prior to the report's publication in a journal. There were other problems as well.

"What's young?" Dr. Corfman, whose Center funded the study, asked. "And what do the words "young," "adult," and "white" mean? It's so fraught with conditions and value judgments that I find it's not a useful public health statement."

Of course, Dr Corfman's point is well made. Is a Mexican woman with a deep tan "white?" Who is to say that a woman of sixty isn't young? I know hundreds of women who have had breast cancer but who say they are "healthy"—in terms of other health problems.

When Dr. Ramcharan was asked to explain the Walnut Creek results to the television audience watching Good Morning America on February 17, 1981, she narrowed the population down to nonsmoking women, younger than thirty. The women surveyed were all members of a Kaiser Permanenté medical plan, and critics of the Walnut Creek results added that these women were also probably middle class and prosperous enough to pay the premiums.

When objective reviewers analyzed the study, they decided the science itself was not valid. At the beginning, in 1968, one-third of the 16,638 participants had never taken the Pill, one-third of the women were taking OCs at the time, and one-third had taken oral contraceptives in past years but had stopped. By the time the study ended, only about 2,000 women were still using this method of birth control. So, even though the total number of women surveyed was more than adequate for the results to be statistically significant, the total number who continued to take OCs was not.

The final blow to the reliability and validity of the Walnut Creek data, however, was the stunning news that financial support had been given to Drs. Ramcharan and Pellegrin by six pharmaceutical firms. Not only did the researchers receive almost $150,000 to do a part of the study the NIH did not fund, but Searle, Meade-Johnson, Syntex, Ortho, Wyeth, and Parke-Davis paid the bills to publicize the results in the United States and Canada. Although no one has said that the firms' financial contributions influenced the data, such a conflict of interest is bound to make them suspect.

In spite of all that has been written about the dangers of oral contraceptives, about 150 million women throughout the world are still using them. However, the number of women in the United States using the Pill has dropped from a high in the mid-1970s of almost 10 million to a current estimate (precise sales figures are still privileged!) of about 6 to 7 million users.

The DES mothers are still being followed by the NCI, and the official statement is that diethylstilbestrol has not yet been proven to be the cause of the "excess" breast-cancer incidence found when their daughters were studied. Dr. Robert Hoover, the chief of Environmental Carcinogenesis at the NCI, however, has little doubt that a cause-and-effect relationship does exist. Many scientists also think postmenopausal estrogens (Premarin is the #1 seller) are dangerous as far as breast cancer is concerned (there is no doubt about its role in triggering uterine cancer), but this is difficult to study. By definition, women do not begin using this substance until they are middle-aged, and—since breast cancer can take twenty or more years to reach the size of a pea—the majority would die of some other disease long before an estrogen-induced carcinoma would be found.

Earlier, I used the word *"carcinotrophic"* to describe a substance's ability to nourish a cancer without necessarily being the cause (now sometimes called the "initiator"). Since I coined that word, cancer biologists have found that there are also "promotors" and "co-carcinogens," as well as "initiators." What these words mean is that there are certain environmental factors (including foods and their additives, certain chemicals, drugs, etc.) that, by themselves, do not cause cancer. However, when such a factor is combined in some way with another, the two together cause healthy, normal cells to be transformed into malignant ones. One example of this kind of co-carcinogenicity has already been mentioned in this chapter: prolactin is carcinogenic only in the "presence of estrogens." It does not cause cancer when it is used alone. With this new information, scientists are making an educated guess that the estrogens in the Pill may be harmless to women who carry no other cancer-promotors or co-carcinogens in their cells. On the other hand, estrogens may interact with different individual factors in a woman's body to cause a breast cancer to develop.

Of course, the most obvious of these are dormant cancer cells which might never grow to become life-threatening without large quantities of estrogens. And the women most likely to have such dormant breast-cancer cells are those who have family histories of the disease. A preliminary study linking oral contraceptives with breast cancer in such women was reported in April 1981 at a meeting in Atlanta of the Federation of American Societies for Experimental Biology. Dr. Maurice M. Black, one of the world's most distinguished pathologists, urged caution, because the data must be duplicated by others to be confirmed.

"But in the meantime," Dr. Black said, "I think the data are strong enough to warn women who had either a grandmother or aunt with breast cancer not to take the Pill."

Dr. Black was one of the experts who signed an affidavit supporting my 1976 suit asking that women with family histories of breast cancer be warned specifically. While this is implied in the patient package insert, it is not said loud and clear in bold-faced type.

Dr. Black is still fighting for a change of label. Let us all hope he wins.

7

Early Detection

One morning in 1975, I waited anxiously by the phone for news about a friend who was scheduled for a biopsy that morning. Although she had found the tumor five months earlier, it was "being watched."

After my mastectomy, it seemed as if every one of my female friends and relatives made a mad dash to her doctor for a breast checkup. In July 1974 there were no long lines or waiting lists, and all of them were examined quickly. Jerry was the only one to have a "suspicious" growth—and she had found it herself.

"It's in the left breast," she told me, after seeing her gynecologist. "He ordered a mammogram, and it was benign. So he said to forget about it for the time being. he just wants to keep an eye on it."

"How big is it?"

"About the size of a pea."

"Does it slide around and move, or does it seem to be stuck in one place?"

"It doesn't move a bit," she answered. "As a matter of fact, that's why he wanted a mammogram. He tried his best to move it, but it wouldn't budge, no matter how hard he squeezed and pushed—"

"Squeezed and pushed?" I cried. "What did you let him do that for? You've read the instructions for self-examination. You're supposed to press and massage it with your fingers together, not—"

"I wasn't going to tell him what to do," she interrupted angrily. "He's a gynecologist, after all. He knows what he's doing."

I said nothing. What was there to say? My nephew had just

passed his Obstetrics-Gynecology Boards examination with flying colors; his "cram book" had a total of two paragraphs about examining breasts.

"The mammogram did say it was benign, anyhow," Jerry continued. "Pushing and squeezing wouldn't bother it."

"Maybe you should get another opinion," I suggested. "Even a benign mass should come out."

"As soon as I get enough sick leave, I will," she promised. "I'll wait till next year. The doctor said there was no rush."

To make a five-month story very short, Jerry's "benign" lump grew considerably after the examination. Now she abandoned her gynecologist and visited an oncological surgeon. He did not like the way the mass felt and scheduled a biopsy.

Having breast cancer is bad enough. To know the cancer grew because of the arrogance, ignorance, or inexperience of a doctor must be unbearable. In the many lists of danger signals and instructions we are given, no one warns us about this obstacle to early detection of breast cancer: the inexperienced or incompetent physician who is confident a lump "is nothing."

Although patients are not told about them, the medical profession is very aware of such doctors. "Keeping an eye on it" is such a common habit it even has a name—"professional laxity." Physicians' delay and procrastination are so widespread and the consequences are so grave that *doctors themselves* have done surveys to discover the reasons. The results show that most general practitioners do not know enough about breast cancer to do a proper examination. Unless a woman has a lump or other specific symptom, they do little more than give a perfunctory tap. And if there is a lump, they too often poke and push it, unaware that harsh handling of a cancerous tumor could be dangerous.

After breast cancer reached the front pages in the fall of 1974, more doctors began to order mammograms, but a negative diagnosis usually reassured them into "keeping an eye on it." Yet in the months of "watching it," a small, early cancer can turn into a large, late one that could be lethal. Too few ordinary doctors have heard of doubling time.

Jerry's sister finally called. "They're cutting off her left breast right now," she sobbed. "It is cancer."

In each country I visited in Europe—England, Scotland, Sweden, Finland—and the Soviet Union, the practice is that all suspected cancer patients be referred to a cancer specialist, clinic, or hospital immediately. "As soon as a woman shows up at a clinic with a suspicious symptom," I was told everywhere, "she is sent to oncology."

But not in the United States.

Even though there have been several headline-making malpractice suits for "delayed diagnosis," waiting-and-watching is still going on. In late 1975, when Martin L. Baron contacted me, he was representing a thirty-seven-year-old woman, Marcia Halpern, a mother of four young children. The late Mrs. Halpern had called her obstetrician-gynecologist, a Dr. Henry Gozan, when she suddenly discovered that one breast was larger than the other. Over the telephone, Dr. Gozan prescribed a diuretic, explaining that the one-sized enlargement was due to premenstrual fluid retention.

The water-reducing medication did no good, but when Mrs. Halpern reported its failure, Dr. Gozan increased the dosage. To make a long and tragic story short, it was cancer. When she finally frantically called to tell him the breast had become hard, had shrunk, and its nipple had pulled inward, he told her to rush to a radiologist for a mammogram. By that time, she had several malignant axillary nodes, and subsequently developed a tumor in the second breast. In spite of the fact that the cancer was already evident in her lungs, a second Halsted radical mastectomy was performed. (The importance of presurgical staging is stressed in Chapter 8.)

Baron had read my book and wanted me to help him prepare the case. A prominent New York breast-cancer expert was called in by Gozan's lawyer to say that Mrs. Halpern's cancer was so virulent and aggressive that she was doomed the moment she found the first symptom, no matter what Gozan might have done. However, this surgeon did not defend the negligence in any way; he said only that nothing Gozan could have done would have made any difference.

Gozan lost the case, and the Halperns were awarded $175,000. The relatively small sum was due to the expert's convincing argument that Gozan's negligence had not contributed to the inevitable outcome. Though this may have been true, it does not justify the doctor's negligence. (In spite of having lost the case, by the way, Dr. Gozan did not lose his license to be an obstetrician-gynecologist and was not even given a slap on the fingers by the local medical society.)

So the Halperns won—if anyone can consider it a victory. Somehow, Mrs. Halpern made it through the trial in spite of her pain and the agony and anguish of her cross-examination by the defense attorney. I shall never forget one particular exchange.

"If you saw that Dr. Gozan's medicine wasn't helping," the defense attorney barked, "why didn't you go to another doctor for a second opinion?"

"I trusted him and he told me what I wanted to hear—that it

was nothing serious," she whispered. Then she began to cry. "After all, he delivered all of my babies. How could I not trust my doctor?"

Somehow, Marcia Halpern managed to live until the verdict was handed down on January 17, 1976, but that night, she went back to the hospital, never to leave it alive.

Since then, I have been told, every malpractice suit involving "delayed diagnosis" for breast cancer in New York state has been settled out of court. But there have been other states where a doctor's negligence was taken to judge and jury. In 1980, after the benefits of chemotherapy were established and accepted, a Navy wife won $900,000 from the Department of Defense, because military physicians had ignored her breast symptoms until the cancer had spread.

In February 1981, a similar case was being tried in a Boston court. Mrs. Gena Glicklich found a breast lump in August 1978 and sued three physicians for negligence in misdiagnosing the breast cancer which then metastasized to her brain. This case was not so clear-cut, because the doctors claimed she refused to follow their recommendations to have mammography and a biopsy. According to newspaper reports, however, there was no evidence that any of her three doctors put these recommendations in her record, so it was her word against theirs. For extra protection, her doctors used the brain metastasis to convince the jury that her outcome would have been the same even if she had been diagnosed earlier.

Keeping sloppy medical records is, in itself, medical malpractice, and the argument about "inevitable outcome" is not as solid as it was in January 1976. Data from cancer experts all over the world support the view that if adjuvant therapy of some kind had been given to Mrs. Glicklich in 1978, it would probably have at least slowed or even prevented the metastasis. In February 1981, Mrs. Glicklich and her son were awarded $400,000.

The result of this kind of publicity puts doctors on the defensive, and women are being referred for unnecessary mammograms and biopsies, because once a woman is sent to specialists for further diagnostic tests, the original physician is no longer liable for anything that might happen in the future. This may be causing a trend toward too many biopsies, but—except for the anxiety and cost involved—it is better than ignoring a possible breast cancer.

For women, it would seem to make sense to go to a specialist at the beginning; to go to a person with the training and experience to recognize a symptom and know with more certainty whether or not a mammogram and/or biopsy is needed. But there are 50 million women in the United States older than thirty-five, and there are not enough breast experts in the country to take care of all of them.

It would help a great deal if the 22,000 obstetrician-gynecologists in the country would learn more about breast problems, but they do not seem interested. In 1977, the Gynecological Society for the Study of Breast Disease (GSBD) was founded by a group of OB/GYNs precisely for this reason. About 150 doctors attended the premier meeting in Washington, D.C., and the keynote speaker was Dr. Louis Keith, Professor of Obstetrics and Gynecology at the Northwestern University School of Medicine in Chicago.

"Since 90% of all women who see any doctor at all go first to their OB/GYN," he lectured, "it is up to us to know enough to help them properly."

The following year, GSBD's meeting in Toronto attracted only about 130 OB/GYNs, and finally, GSBD disbanded altogether. It was reborn as the Society for the Study of Breast Disease with a membership that included family practitioners, radiologists, and surgeons. There were not enough OB/GYNs interested in keeping GSBD alive.

What Dr. Keith said is absolutely true. Ninety percent of all women in the United States who see any doctor at all use their OB/GYNs as their primary physicians. Yet relatively few of the 22,000 members of the American College of Obstetrics and Gynecology seem to want to go to the trouble of learning more about women's most dreaded disease. Until they change, there will continue to be delayed diagnoses or too many mammograms and biopsies.

It looks as if we women have to depend on ourselves if we want to be sure we get every chance to survive. Vaccines are still hopes for the future; fighting heredity and trying to avoid suspected carcinogens in foods or the environment are impossible. Except for staying away from estrogens (discussed in Chapters 4 and 6) and having babies when we are teen-agers, there is *nothing* we can do to prevent a breast cancer from developing.

But we can do a great deal to keep the disease from growing and spreading through our bodies. A woman may save her own life by finding a tumor early and being assertive that her doctor do something besides "wait and see." This is possible if she faithfully practices breast self-examination—BSE. It is safe; it can be done as often as she likes, and she needs no appointment. About 95 percent of all early breast cancers are discovered by the patients themselves or by their husbands and lovers, *not* by their doctors.

Then why do so few women examine their breasts regularly? Both the NCI and the ACS spend millions of dollars to educate women about BSE. I have a mountain of studies, attitudinal surveys, polls, and miscellaneous materials about motivating women to do it regularly. Even business has gotten into the act. There are simulated torsos (the most popular is "Betsy") and breasts that have built-in lumps and bumps to help women learn how to examine themselves and to show them what they should be looking for.

With so much money, time, and energy directed toward BSE, it would seem that if all women would practice BSE regularly, breast cancer could be virtually abolished.

Studies done for and by the NCI and ACS about women's attitudes toward BSE conclude that women do not do it because they are not confident in their ability to know what they are feeling. As I explained earlier, women's breasts are often filled with odds and ends of strange growths, and BSE zealots think all that is needed is a perfect teaching mechanism that will give women the missing confidence.

There are at least thirty different scientific studies exploring the best way to persuade women to do the self-examination!

My personal theory about the problem is slightly different, however. Having worked in the field of behavioral modification for a long time, I believe asking a woman to practice BSE is asking her to do something that is time-consuming, often frightening, and perhaps even considered sinful. If she should need further examination, such as a referral for mammography BSE would then also be linked in her mind with money, anxiety, time, and perhaps some risk. Finally, BSE may be the first step in a series that will inevitably take her to the operating room where she will lose her breast. So, from a behavioral point of view, BSE may be synonymous with mastectomy in many women's minds.

In other words, I believe most women do not practice BSE because they do not want to find what they are supposed to be looking for. But there is a behavioral way to break this chain of conditioned reflexes: reward a woman who does BSE faithfully instead of punishing her. Tell her that BSE does *not* have to result in the loss of a breast.

Not too long ago, suggesting that a mastectomy may not always be necessary would have been blasphemous, but in today's medical/surgical climate it is not. When I describe my behavioral theory now, the response I get is often thoughtful consideration instead of angry rejections.

For example, in July 1980, I attended an international cancer conference in London and spoke with Dr. Tony Miller, a director of Canada's NCI. He told me the CNCI was about to launch a breast-screening program in Toronto.

"First, of course, we will devote a great deal of effort to teaching the women how to do BSE properly," Tony explained, in his crisp clipped Canadian style. "In addition, they will be screened periodically by mammography which, by the way, will expose them to the lowest quantity of radiation possible."

"How many women are you aiming for?" I asked.

"We're hoping to accrue 50,000 volunteers."

"Suppose you do get 50,000 women to examine themselves regularly, and one of them finds a tiny dingbat the size of an apple seed?" I asked. "What treatment will she get?"

Tony looked bewildered. "We will *only* be using your two-stage procedure.

"That's not what I'm driving at," I continued. "If she finds a cancer that's only a quarter of an inch in diameter, what will happen next?"

"Oh, you mean if it's a minimal cancer. If it's that small, of course, certainly nothing would be done until several different and independent pathologists reviewed it and agreed. . ."

I interrupted him. "Let's say all of the pathologists' opinions are unanimous: it is a real invasive cancer. How will the woman be treated afterward?"

Tony immediately understood what I had been leading up to. "I suppose she would have to have a mastectomy," he said softly. "The routine practice of the hospital participating in the program is to do a mastectomy, regardless of the size of the tumor."

He brightened up. "But they do only the modified type."

I shook my head. "Why should a woman go to all that trouble to find an apple seed if she's going to lose her breast?" I asked. "After all, that's the same treatment she'd get if she waited a while and came in with a tumor the size of the whole apple. In the meantime, she'd have both breasts for a year to two or maybe longer."

"But an apple seed is virtually 100 percent curable!" Tony insisted.

Again I shook my head. "That may be 100 percent true, Tony," I said. But, unless a woman has had a lot of friends or relatives die of breast cancer, she usually doesn't think an apple seed could ever be a tombstone.

"Unless your women in Canada are a lot different from us down here," I continued, "I think they'll stay away from your screening program in droves. It's not the radiation women are worried about now, it's the fear that they'll lose their breasts for a tiny apple seed."

Tony did not disagree with me.

"I've got an idea that might work," I offered. "Suppose you tell all the participants in advance that if they practice BSE regularly and do find something smaller than a half-centimeter, they'll have only a lumpectomy."

Briefly, I explained my Pavlovian-Skinnerian theory about rewards and punishments, and he nodded.

"It does seem to make good sense when you explain it that way. But I'm an epidemiologist and not a surgeon. I rather doubt that my surgical colleagues would see it in that peculiar light."

The conversation had taken place around a coffee table, and it was time to go. "I still think it would work," I teased, as we stood up. "I bet you $100 right now that it would."

Tony grinned. "As it is, it is highly unlikely that our surgeons would consider offering that guarantee to the women."

"Then send the women with tiny lumps over to Princess Margaret Hospital in Toronto," I laughed. "They would let them keep their breasts there."

Indeed, Princess Margaret Hospital in Toronto is the place where Dr. Vera Peters did her pioneering work comparing minimal surgery plus irradiation with the Halsted radical mastectomy. Now, after following the patients almost forty years, the hundreds of women in that comparative study lived and died at normal mortality rates, no matter what had been done at the beginning.

At that same London meeting, we also heard seven-year data given by Dr. Umberto Veronesi of Milan, with statistics supporting the same kind of minimal surgery for minimal cancer.* As I will document in Chapter 10, there are now data from all over the world showing that the results are identical at five and ten years even if the breast cancer was *not* "minimal."

I have included these paragraphs about minimal treatment for minimal breast cancers in this chapter on early detection to stress that there are excellent reasons for women to do BSE: they can now expect a reward for finding a small tumor. We now have enough surgeons in the United States who will do breast-saving procedures, if the tumors are smaller than one centimeter (about half an inch) at their greatest diameter.

So on with BSE:

The basic technique is probably familiar by now to every

*Front page "news" on July 2, 1981.

woman who can read. Here are the instructions as given in an American Cancer Society pamphlet, available free from local ACS offices or by writing: 777 Third Avenue, New York 10019. The NCI also has excellent material that can be obtained by calling (toll-free) 800-638-6694.

This examination should be done every month. In premenopausal women, the breasts are most normal and free of cyclical bulges about ten days after menstruation begins, and that is when BSE should be done. Women who have already gone through the menopause might choose some date they will not forget and use it as the day for an examination every month. At first, the BSE may take several minutes, but after two or three times it will take no time at all.

As all the standard instructions state, the first step in BSE is done lying down, each arm alternately resting under the head while that breast is palpated with a gentle rotating motion, never a squeezing or pushing one.

A woman with large or pendulous breasts will need to alter this technique slightly. The side of the breast must be steadily held, either with the hand or by resting it against something solid. Otherwise it would be like examining a plastic bag full of gelatin and a marble (the tumor, if one is present). Unless the bag is held firmly or placed against something solid, palpation will simply keep pushing the marble out of the way making it impossible to find.

The axillas must also be palpated for growths, and this examination is also best done while lying down with the arm behind the head.

For more sensitivity, the BSE should be done when the body is slippery from soap or oil. Or the hands can be coated lightly with powder. Even invisible bumps and dips feel like mountains and craters under slick fingertips. For some reason, instruction guides often fail to mention this important part of the examination.

Lumps and thickenings are the most frequent first symptoms of breast cancer, but anything new or unusual should be noted. If this part of the self-check does reveal a lump or thickening, the woman should call her doctor for an appointment immediately. In the meantime, she should ask herself these questions:

Does it hurt? If it does, this is a good omen. Early cancer, unfortunately, seldom hurts.

Does it seem to float freely inside? This is also a good sign. Most cancers are not movable, but are fixed. Nor are they usually symmetrical; they can be irregular and fibrous.

Is she often "lumpy" and "cystic"? Has her doctor said she is

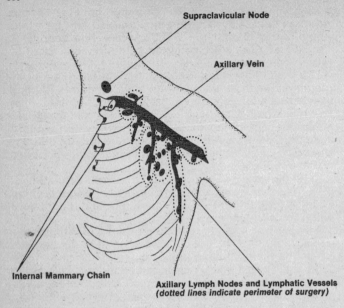

Approximate Location of the Nodes

prone to have chronic mastitis? If so, the lump is more likely to be benign. But the doctor must make the final diagnosis, not the woman.

Most instructions for BSE, excellent as they are, omit the less common symptoms of breast cancer, simply for lack of space in a small leaflet. Also, many symptoms are so infrequent that they are listed nowhere but in medical textbooks. To look for these, I recommend a second part of the self-check, which is done standing before a mirror.

First, the breasts should be scrutinized for any asymmetry. It is normal for one breast to be somewhat larger or to vary slightly in shape. But if such a change is recent it should be reported, even if there is no other symptom. Now for the skin: Is there a difference in the appearance of the skin of each breast? Any flaking or scaling? A variation in texture anywhere, giving an "orange skin" or "pigskin" appearance? Then the nipples: Are they cracked? Is any fluid coming from them?

Breast Self-examination (BSE)

1 1. Lie down. Put one hand behind your head. With the other hand, fingers flattened, gently feel your breast. Press ever so lightly. *Now examine the other breast.*

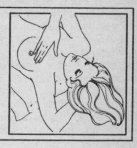

2 2. This illustration shows you how to check each breast. Begin where you see the *A* and follow the arrows, feeling gently for a lump or thickening. *Remember to feel all parts of each breast.*

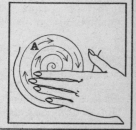

3 3. Now repeat the same procedure sitting up, with the hand still behind your head.

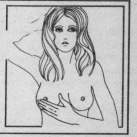

Reprinted by permission of the American Cancer Society

The next step is to perform some gymnastics and contortions. Do the nipples react differently to the same movements? Does one seem to be forced into a different tilt? Any puckering or dimpling of the skin anywhere? Strange bumps or creases in the armpits? Has there been any change? Answers of yes to any of these questions call for a visit to the doctor.

Remember that signs of the two very rare carcinomas described earlier—the inflammatory and the generalized (the one with only pain as a symptom)—must be watched for too. It is improbable that a hot, red, swollen, and sore breast would go unnoticed, but an odd, persistent ache or pain might. Doctors are likely to shrug off pain as nothing but cyclical tenderness, but if a woman knows the pain is not associated with her menstrual period, she should insist on more investigation. Generalized cancer often cannot be discovered by a manual breast examination alone.

Here then—in addition to the lump or thickening—is a list of less common warning signals:

1. Asymmetry in either appearance or movement of the breast.
2. Scaling skin around the nipple, changes in skin texture, cracked nipples, or any secretion from the nipples.
3. Puckering or dimpling of the breast skin.
4. Hot, swollen, and sore breast.
5. An unusual ache or pain that is persistent and not associated with cyclical changes and tenderness.
6. Any change that is unilateral—one-sided.

In his book *Early Detection,* Dr. Philip Strax, a veteran breast-cancer diagnostician, makes the excellent suggestion that every woman have one professional breast examination, including a mammogram and perhaps a thermogram, whether she needs it or not, in order to have a normal "map" for future comparison.

Before going on, I want to stress how the hands should be held during BSE, because it is so important that this be done properly. Use the flat of the hand, keeping the fingertips lightly together. The palpation should be gentle pressure and massage in a circular motion. Do *not* squeeze, push, pump, or pull.

And no doctor should squeeze, push, pump, or pull, either. If he or she does not know how to examine the breasts properly, the patient should put her clothes back on and find one who does.

I have been asked how the average woman can tell whether the doctor is doing a correct examination. My answer is based on Dr. Strax's suggestion: go at least one time to a breast-cancer specialist—even if it means a trip to another city or state—and be examined by an expert. To judge by my experience, any woman who pays close attention to what is done will easily be able to recognize a "correct" breast examination afterward. The difference is so dramatic it could never be missed.

Let's suppose a friend finds a tiny bump that was not there during BSE a month ago, or something else strange or unusual is present. She should never be shy about reporting anything, even a "nonsymptom" like a bruise that refuses to fade. What if her doctor does think she is a hypochondriac? If she wants to be examined and is willing to pay for it, why should he or she object? It's her life, after all.

In choosing a doctor, incidentally, no woman should ever forget: the best BSE does no good if the doctor is one of those who wants to "keep an eye on it." Unless he or she is an expert whose hands have palpated hundred of breast masses, both benign and malignant, no faith can be put in fingers alone. Diagnosis by manual palpation has been proven wrong almost half the time: in hospital surveys comparing doctors' preoperative diagnoses with the postoperative pathology reports, manual examinations were inaccurate 45 percent of the time.

Nonetheless, having an examination by a doctor is the first step after finding a symptom.

Panicked, our friend has telephoned for an immediate appointment. "Don't delay!" instructions insist. Unfortunately she is just another patient wanting an appointment. There is no chance of her being examined for two weeks. Just as the tip of the tongue always finds the gap left by a lost filling, her fingers will automatically wander to the spot. She must do her best to avoid this reflex. When bathing or showering, only gentle patting and pressing are allowed—no squeezing.

Finally the day of her appointment arrives, and she is in the examining room. (This doctor knows how to do a breast check, and she does not have to put her clothes on and storm out.) He finds the growth, but cannot tell what it is.

"Maybe it's a water-filled cyst," he mumbles, turning out the room light and flashing a powerful beam to see if the growth is hollow (this is the procedure called transillumination now newly renamed "diaphanography"). "No." He shakes his head. "It's solid as a rock." Using a hypodermic needle, he tries to aspirate it, in the hope that something will come out that can be analyzed.

"Nope," he repeats. "You'll have to have a mammogram." He writes the request on a prescription blank and gives her the name of the radiology clinic he deals with. "Maybe something will show up on the X-ray," he says.

Mammography has been around since 1913, but not until 1960, when Dr. Robert Egan, a Houston radiologist, demonstrated its value, was its effectiveness in diagnosing early cancers widely accepted. Since then—in less than twenty years—mammography has become routine and its younger sister, Xerography (a process that uses X-ray to penetrate the breast tissue, but reproduce the image on paper instead of film), has replaced conventional film mammography in many institutions and clinics. Xerography, however, has some disadvantages as well as advantages: more of the fine details of a breast's contents can be imaged, but more radiation is required to accomplish this. The development of low-dose film has reduced the need to use large quantities of ionizing radiation, and, while the manufacturers of Xerographs have also managed to lower their radiation requirement, Xerography still exposes women to somewhat higher doses than does mammography.

As far as the superiority of one over the other for diagnosis, both were evaluated by the NCI in the Breast Cancer Detection Demonstration Projects (BCDDPs). After five years, the results showed that the accuracy and reliability of both techniques depend on which method the interpreting radiologist had been trained in or had most experience with.

Oldtimers who had been weaned on film do not do as well with Xerox paper; on the other hand, younger physicians who had never looked at a negative image of a breast cannot make heads nor tails of a conventional film mammogram. So while women should know that Xerography exposes them to somewhat higher levels of radiation, they should *not* refuse this kind of procedure if it is the radiologist's preference. The danger of having a misdiagnosis by far outweighs any small risk from the difference in radiation dosage.

Being mammographed with or without the Xero-, is essentially the same. The woman strips to the waist and is usually seated while a radiological technician squeezes her breasts (one at a time) with some kind of a compression device. (There are different kinds.) Each flattened breast is X-rayed from various angles. If film-screen was used, the films are developed as ordinary X-rays are; Xerograms slide from a machine just as familiar photocopies do. Both are interpreted for diagnosis by doctors trained in radiology—*not* by the technicians. She or he can tell the woman nothing, so there is no point in asking for her/his opinion.

It would not be appropriate for me to omit reference to the "mammography controversy." Here I'll summarize this inflammatory issue as fairly as I can.

In 1963, the Health Insurance Plan of Greater New York (HIP), with the help of the NCI, began a controlled, clinical trial to see if annual mammography plus a physical examination would affect its female members' survival rate, as far as breast cancer was concerned. Two groups of 31,000 women each, between the ages of 40 and 64 were randomly chosen from HIP membership. Women in the group to be X-rayed received a baseline mammogram and a physical examination, and for the next three years breast X-rays supplemented their HIP physical examination. The other 31,000 women got only the routine HIP exams.

The first five year results were published in April 1969. There had been forty deaths from breast cancer in the group that had been mammographed; sixty-three women in the group not mammographed had died of the disease. The difference, however, was seen only in women who were older than fifty. There were no survival differences in women X-rayed when they were 40 to 49 years old. A follow-up report published in 1971 reinforced these first results.

The reason for the significantly better survival rates of the women who had been mammographed was attributed to the fact that 75 percent of them had no axillary-node invasion, while those who had not been X-rayed were found to have positive nodes about 50 per cent of the time. As I explained in Chapter 2, the presence or absence of cancer in the axillary lymph nodes helps determine the prognosis.

Even with the benefit of hindsight, it is impossible for me to understand how the potential danger of exposing the healthy breasts of women to periodic doses of unregulated ionizing radiation was ignored. After all, by 1963 data from the atomic-bomb raids over Japan had already proved the harm X-ray could do to people. But somehow, the Japanese data were neglected.

In February 1972, the success of the HIP study triggered the ACS Board into voting for a major breast-cancer screening program in twelve centers around the country. Government money was then made available to enlarge the program to include twenty-seven centers. The plan of what was to be the Breast Cancer Detection Demonstration Projects (BCDDPs) was to screen 10,000 women, aged 35 to 70, in each center for five years. They would not only be X-rayed (by both film-screen and Xerography) but also thermographed (explained later). In addition, all the participants were to have thorough manual breast examinations and were taught how to do BSE. Then they were to be followed for another five years with manual exams only.

Unlike the HIP study, the BCDDPs did not randomly select the women: they mammographed each of those who voluntarily applied. The reason for this is that the program had no research goal. It was a "Demonstration Project" designed to answer the question, "Will 270,000 women voluntarily agree to be screened for breast cancer?" Before Mrs. Ford and Mrs. Rockefeller had their well-publicized mastectomies, both the ACS and the NCI were not at all sure women would participate in the free program. In other words, the BCDDPs were to be a measure of women's attitudes about looking for hidden breast cancer.

Again, for unknown reasons, the potential risks of ionizing radiation were not considered to be important. I have been told that Dr. Frank J. Rauscher, Jr., then director of the NCI, received a critical letter about this matter from Dr. Saul Harris, Director of the New York Health Department's Office of Radiation Control. In 1977, when the controversy was at its height, I asked Dr. Rauscher if this was true, and he told me he had gotten such a letter and had then checked with appropriate NCI scientists who gave him an all-clear.

Later I learned that no one at the Bureau of Radiological Health, the Bureau of Standards, the National Academy of Sciences, or other agencies with radiation physicists on their staffs, was consulted by either the NCI or the ACS. According to all of the people I interviewed, had these scientists been asked, the BCDDPs and the equipment used in them would *not* have been given an "all-clear."

The joint ACS-NCI screening program began in 1973 and, according to *Science Magazine,* "It sailed along according to plan, by all evidence and appearance a success. Women, responding to announcements in local newspapers and the like, flocked to the screening centers as they opened. Then, after Mrs. Ford and Mrs. Rockefeller had breast cancer surgery, the centers were veritably inundated with women who wanted to have a mammogram. In some places, the waiting list was months long."

By the time the projects closed their doors to new participants in 1976, 280,281 women were enrolled.

In January 1976, Dr. John C. Bailar III, an epidemiologist who was then the editor of the *Journal of the National Cancer Institute,* published a paper in the *Annals of Internal Medicine* and argued that—for women under fifty—the risks from the radiation exposure outweighed their risks of having early breast cancer. He argued that younger women, who had no symptoms of breast cancer and who were not at a high risk because of a strong family history, should not be screened by X-ray.

Once Dr. Bailar started rocking the boat, various federal, state, and local agencies began to measure the amount of radiation being emitted by the equipment in the BCDDPs, as well as in private offices, clinics, and hospitals. The results? Some non-BCDDP mammography machines leaked radiation, were not modified to X-ray only the breasts and used industrial film that exposed women (and men who got other X-rays on the same equipment) to extraordinarily high levels of ionizing radiation. Random spot checks showed that even some of the "special purpose" equipment used in the BCDDPs emitted more radiation than anyone considered safe.

Since the breast is more vulnerable to the effects of ionizing radiation than any other human (except for fetal) tissue, politicians perked up their ears. There were about 280,000 women involved—an awful lot of votes.

Scientists also became interested in the Projects. A flurry of exploration revealed that a group of Nova Scotian women who had been treated for tuberculosis and who were monitored by frequent fluoroscopies later developed high incidences of breast cancer. Women who had received X-ray treatments for mastitis also had more breast cancer than would ordinarily be expected. The BEIR Commission that follows the survivors of the atomic raids in Japan had already shown that there were more cases of breast cancer among these normally low-risk women than there should have been.

Chronicling the details of those two years is difficult for me to do, because as a "patient advocate," I was asked to testify against the BCDDPs before Congress and other interested groups. I spoke and wrote about them and wrote and spoke *against* them—even though I believe good mammography and good mammographers can save women's breasts by detecting cancer when it is microscopic and needs no mastectomy to be cured.

But the BCDDPs are an example of a well-intentioned program that was not well-planned and caused a great deal of harm to a valuable diagnostic tool. So I will only report here that hardly a week went by without some mention of the Projects in the lay and professional media. There were hearings in both the House and Senate: scare stories predicting that the BCDDPs would cause more cancers than would be found seemed to pop up everywhere. Participation in the screening program dropped suddenly and dramatically. Even women with overt symptoms refused to be mammographed, because they were convinced the examination would cause a breast cancer to develop.

Finally, in September 1977, Dr. Donald S. Fredrickson, the former director of the National Institutes of Health, convened the first Consensus Development Conference to bring the matter before a "jury" of lay and professional people not personally involved in mammography.

Like the BCDDPs themselves, even this meeting was hexed. The organizers had apparently not checked with a calender when they picked the dates—September 14 and 15. The first day was the Jewish holiday, Rosh Hashanah, and, as a result, many people did not come on the 14th. Because of so many absences, the Office of Cancer Communictions (OCC) put a notice in the press kits prepared for reporters telling them the information was not to be released until the following day. This is highly unusual for medical events. Suspecting something Machiavellian in that post-Watergate era, everyone fine-tooth-combed the report to see what was so "hot" that it had to be withheld for twenty-four hours.

Unfortunately, there were "hot" data in that report. Of the 1,810 women who had been treated in some way for breast cancer as a result of the screening program, review of the cases showed that 66 of them were not cancer at all. The expert pathologists assigned to prepare the report had gone over 506 slides and disagreed with the original diagnoses made by pathologists in the women's hospitals. News of the "66 benigns" made headlines all over the country, but by the time the re-review of the slides was finished (almost a year later), no one was interested anymore. The damage had been done.

It turned out that two of the 66 benigns were computer errors, and most of the women (37) had had a waiting period between the biopsy and whatever treatment was given afterwards. Certainly, having a two-stage procedure is not proof-positive that a women knows she had only suspicious cells, but it is proof-positive that nothing was done while she was unconscious on an operating-room table.

However these findings were not known on September 15, 1977. The panel of jurors recommended that the guidelines governing participation in the screening programs be changed to include more selected categories of women: all women over the age of 50 should continue being screened; only women between the ages of 40 to 49 who had a first-degree family history of breast cancer; and those aged 35 to 39, only if the woman had already had breast cancer herself.

An ethics subcommittee also urged the NCI to tell all of the women their confirmed diagnoses "forthwith," but this could not be done for legal reasons. Unlike the HIP study, which was a part of a pre-paid medical plan, the BCDDPs were free-standing detection centers funded jointly by the ACS and the NCI. If a woman's mammogram showed something suspicious, notification of this went to her personal physician, and the NCI was out of the picture immediately. Since the woman's private doctor took her to a private hospital that had a private pathologist, the Federal government could not intervene later by telling her anything. To do so would be governmental invasion of the doctor-patient relationship. The only way a woman could (and still can) get her diagnosis is to file a Freedom of Information request.

A book could be written about the petty politics and ridiculous rivalries that emerged from the fiasco, but I will cite only one example. Dr. Bailar, who so vehemently spoke out against the risks of radiation exposure, bore the brunt of heated and vicious verbal attacks.

Women all over the world are indebted to him for disobeying one of the cardinal rules of bureaucracy: "Don't mess around in anyone else's turf." Because of him, low-dose X-ray film was perfected, more special-purpose mammography equipment using film-screen was acquired by radiologists, and more care is taken by everyone involved. Today, it is common to be able to get good, well-calibrated, low-dose mammography equipment that exposes a woman to—at most—one half "rad"* per view. This means no more than two rads should be needed for four X-rays of both breasts.

Even if only one woman lost her breast unnecessarily, the BCDDPs were regrettable, but the most serious outcome of the ill-fated program was (and still is) the refusal of women to be mammographed. Even women in the groups who should be screened, according to NCI's guidelines, are not permitting X-ray examinations. Certainly, women like me—who have already lost one breast to cancer—should welcome the magical machine's ability to see anything that might be growing in the remaining breast.

In addition, all women older than fifty should be screened periodically (although there is disagreement about how often "periodically" is in individual cases), and daughters and sisters of women who have had breast cancer should be checked by mam-

*Radiation absorbed dose; usually an estimate of how much X-ray reaches the mid-point of an organ.

mography after they reach the age of forty. Many experts also think women whose breasts are constantly cystic and lumpy should have a baseline mammogram for future comparison when they are forty—even if there is no family history. Unfortunately, it may take a long time for women to regain the confidence lost because of the excesses of exposure and surgery that resulted from the BCDDPs.

On the other hand, a lot of good also resulted from the Projects. As I said, the most immediate benefit was the development of low-dose film, a product that permits excellent images with minimal radiation exposure.

Women needing mammography should ask if the equipment is being monitored by the Mammography Quality Assurance Program of the Bureau of Radiological Health and how many estimated rads she would be getting. If the total is more than 2.0 rads for two views of each breasts, she should try to find another mammographer. The best place to look is a teaching hospital, because—like any other large organization selling a service—teaching hospitals usually have a high and fast turnover of patients. This means fresh film, fresh chemicals, up-to-date equipment, and better-trained and qualified personnel.

Unfortunately there is almost no regulation over medical radiology in the United States, and—like everything else seems to be—it is *caveat emptor* (buyer beware).

To return to the hypothetical patient I left long ago, her doctor may also suggest she have a thermogram, as well as a mammogram, to get a baseline picture of the heat patterns of her breasts.

Like so many medical advances, thermography came from war. Scientists knew some materials hold more heat than others, and, using this principle, weapons designers invented rockets that were able to home in on enemy targets by following any heat emanating from them. "Smart bombs" used in the Vietnam War, for example, tracked their quarries by trailing their heat radiation. Medical scientists, knowing that malignant tissue and normal tissue also have different heat-retention qualities, then adapted this principle for cancer detection.

Just as the sun's warmth radiates to us on earth, heat in the body is also radiated. A thermograph is a device that visualizes these temperature differences in color* as a thermogram, and experts can interpret the displayed differences on a TV-like

---

*At the beginning, thermograms were black and white, and the "grays" had to be interpreted. Color has enhanced their accuracy.

screen to detect changes that may have occurred between thermograms. An ordinary Polariod photograph can be taken for a permanent record.

For a thermogram of the breast, the only "discomfort" involves being nude from the waist up in a cooled room for about fifteen minutes (before the thermogram is taken), so any "hot spot" in the breast will be apparent. Even slight friction can raise the skin's temperature, and women are usually asked to keep their arms away from their bodies while waiting.

By 1977, thermography had been tried in the BCDDPs for four years or longer. Because its accuracy rate was so poor (about 40 percent reliable), the technique was dropped from the program except in those institutions where scientists were especially interested in learning more about thermography.

The reason for the great interest in perfecting thermography is that, unlike mammography, it involves no ionizing radiation at all and can, therefore, be used as often as necessary, even in children. I have a personal interest in thermography, because its diagnosis in my case was more accurate than the mammogram's.

A footnote to my personal thermographic history is needed here. In Chapter 1, I mentioned that my thermogram was more reliable than the mammogram by diagnosing my lump as being "suspicious." However, I also pointed out that I did not receive the report until six weeks after my mastectomy. At a Washington party I went to in April 1981, I met Dr. Margaret Abernathy, the thermography expert at the Georgetown University Hospital where my heat photograph had been taken. After we were introduced, I told her how accurate her diagnosis had been and said that I had so written in *Breast Cancer.*

"I know," she responded coldly, "and I don't think it was quite fair. You said you were not told for six weeks. I remember clearly calling your physician that very evening to give him the report, because I was so concerned."

I was speechless.

"I'm sorry," I finally blurted out, "but I wasn't told for six weeks."

A lovely, elegant woman, Dr. Abernathy was legitimately angry that I had virtually libeled her and her Thermography Department.

"We may have problems at Georgetown," she said, "but no diagnosis has ever taken six weeks. And in your case, I specifically remember telephoning your doctor at home that same night."

The following Monday, I called Dr. Heckman and asked him what had happened.

"I don't remember it, it was so long ago," he told me. "Let me look in your chart. I write everything down."

A few hours later, he returned my call.

"I've got it right here, in black and white," Dr. Heckman told me. "She did call, and I made a note of it, but I didn't tell you because you had already decided to have a biopsy. There wasn't any reason to get you more upset than you already were."

Had I refused to have the lump removed because the mammography report had been optimistic, he said, he would have told me Dr. Abernathy had been so alarmed she called him at home that same night.

I hope this account can be considered an apologetic retraction to her and to thermography. Lesley, I must add, is being followed by this technique to detect any changes, since she is too young to even get near an X-ray machine.

Even more than mammography, thermography requires a great degree of training and experience on the part of the "reader." X-rays have been around since 1913, and there are few practicing physicians who have not, at some time in their careers, peered at negatives of stomachs, intestines, and brains. Thermography, on the other hand, is relatively new, and there are few well-trained, qualified thermographers in the United States. Unless women have access to one, having a thermogram is probably a waste of time and money. Some names and addresses may be obtained from Dr. Istvan Nyirjesy, current president of the American Thermographic Society, at 5272 River Road, Bethesda, MD, (301) 654-0445.

Ultrasonography, a technique older than thermography is now making a comeback after several years of being out of fashion. Also a by-product of war and weapons research, ultrasound is based on knowledge that different materials transmit different sound (as well as heat) waves, and these can be converted electronically to pictures. A familiar example of this is military sonar used to detect submarines.

Sonograms of the breast have not been successful or reliable in the United States, but my visit to Japan showed that "echograms" are considered to be at least 95 percent accurate—a statistic yet to be achieved in this country. At Tokyo's supermodern Metropolitan Hospital, I talked to a young surgeon who trained at Roswell Park under Dr. Dao.

"Ultrasound works here?" I asked incredulously. "It hasn't been at all useful in our country."

He shrugged. "I know, and I cannot understand it," he said. "Here in Japan, we rely on echograms with almost complete certainty. But when I tried to use my same equipment on the women in Buffalo, I had worthless results."

"What can the reason be?"

"It might be nothing more than the fact that my patients in Buffalo were heavier and had more adipose tissue in their breasts. Perhaps this, somehow, affected radiation of the internal soundwaves to the outside." This was the only reason he could think of to account for the differences in ultrasonography's reliability in the two countries.

Ultrasound equipment being advertised now seems to be more convenient, as far as the patient is concerned. For example, I was told that two of the early problems women had with ultrasound examinations were its awkwardness and inconvenience. They had to be suspended in water in a way that permitted their breasts to be totally immersed. One contraption I saw was a harness that had the woman dangling nude in a tank! According to a recent advertisement for a new type of equipment called "life imaging," this is no longer the case. The brochure shows a woman lying on a special table, partially nude, on her belly. Her breasts are dipping into a tank of water anatomically placed at the table's upper end. "Life imaging" seems to be proof that this aesthetic disadvantage of ultrasound, at least, is being resolved.

I have always rated poor grades as a physicist and could never understand the equations of turning a breast-tissue echo, through water, into a photograph. The best explanation I can give here (without copying *verbatim* from a technical textbook) is to say that there is some kind of computerized "interface" between the breasts suspended in water and the screen the ultrasonographer later interprets. (Like thermography, these may either be black-and-white or color.) The scientific basis for ultrasound's ability, as far as I can describe it, is that an acoustic beam is projected into the breasts, and varying echoes result—based on the type of tissue the beam encounters. After being processed by sophisticated electronic equipment, these echoes ultimately are focused on a TV-like screen, either as an entire organ or as cross-sections showing the contents of the breasts in great detail. Like thermograms, ultrasonograms may be photographed from the screen image.

And, also like thermograms, their reliability in terms of accurate diagnoses depends almost entirely on the training, qualifications, and personal experience of the person reading the screen and/or photograph.

Another problem, I have been told, is a technical one. An ultrasound specialist at the National Heart and Lung Institute said that while ultrasonography is O.K. for diagnosing hollow organs like the bladder and kidney or for locating the position of an infant in the uterus, the beat of the heart and the bellowing of the lungs make echoes that may mask the sounds of the breasts.

"There's just too much racket in the chest to get a good picture of the insides of the breasts," he explained.

However, he believes that advances in noise-abatement (probably paid for by the Environmental Protection Agency) may help dim the background sounds of the upper torso.

For the life of me, I cannot understand why nipple-fluid analysis for the early detection of breast cancer has not become more common, because the technology has been around for years. It is quick, easy, inexpensive, and as reliable as any other modality besides mammography. In 1975, I described it in *Breast Cancer*.

"One detection technique that will probably never be widely used is Dr. Nicholas I. Petrakis' method of analyzing breast fluid. Few women are aware that a constant supply of fluid is manufactured in the breast; it rarely drips out of the nipples, because their openings become plugged, and usually is reabsorbed unnoticed. This nonmilk is made by the acini, the tiny milk-producing glands in the lobules. To remove it from the breasts, scientists aspirate the liquid by suction or, sometimes, by putting fine pipettes into the nipple openings. According to the doctor reporting the research, 'It is uncomfortable.' "

Breast-fluid analysis is not considered a diagnostic tool now, although it may be someday. The technique is being used experimentally in San Francisco to see what differences there are in the fluid composition of Caucasian and Chinese women. There is a difference, by the way, the scientists say. Chinese women have much less breast fluid than do Caucasians, and it contains fewer "atypical cells." Should the latter turn out to be precursors of cancer, breast-fluid analysis might well become a valuable early-detection technique."

Unfortunately, my prediction about its never being widely used has turned out to be true, even though Dr. George Sartorius later invented an ingenious pump for removing the fluid with far less discomfort. At the Peralta Hospital in San Francisco, there is an early-detection clinic that is somehow kept going by Dr. Adeline Hackett to analyze women's aspirated nipple fluid to find cancer long before there are enough cells to be considered even a "minimal" tumor. Yet women are not flocking to Dr. Hackett's doors for the test.

Of course, like all early-detection modalities in use today, including breast X-rays, nipple-fluid analyses have their share of false negatives and false positives. However, the technique has been successful enough in finding evidence of early breast cancer to warrant more popularity. And, as I wrote earlier, the identification of certain precursor cells via these analyses should make the fluid interesting to scientists searching for the elusive "markers" to which I have referred.

But perhaps it is not the fault of women at all, but of doctors, because generally women do as their physicians tell them. Nipple-fluid aspiration has not become popular among members of the medical profession just as needle biopsies of lumps (to be discussed later) has not.

Yet, of all the early-detection procedures known today, nipple-fluid analysis comes closest to being the simple diagnostic tool for breast cancer that the "Pap" test is for cervical cancer.

Sophisticated devices for detecting breast cancer early seem to come and go with the seasons. One that relies on telltale heat patterns—Graphic Stress Telethermometry or GST—had a flurry of fame and publicity in the late 1970s, but it has since faded from the limelight. It involved placing a heat sensor on a woman's forehead and comparing its temperature with that of her nipple and breasts. Afterward, her hands are dipped in ice water for fifteen seconds, and a second set of readings is made in the same way. While no one believes GST can diagnose a cancer, its advocates think GST could be an ideal technique for following high-risk women, especially those too young to be mammographed.

There are several scientists trying to use Computed Tomography (CTM) with some success. These three-dimensional X-rays have reportedly found some deep-seated cancers not visualized by mammography, and although the device does rely on ionizing radiation, the dosage is smaller than that of conventional mammography.

I also have some reports of "aerial photo-mapping" for breast cancer, the use of microwave radiation, injections of radioactive iodine, and electromagnetism—all for the same purpose: early detection. So far, none seems to be reliable enough to consider any clinical trials.

A "new" technique, known as diaphanography, was announced just as I began this chapter on early detection. It seems to be a more sophisticated and, perhaps, more reliable version of an old-fashioned tool I described earlier: transillumination. Used with great success in Scandinavia, diaphanography was brought to the United States by Dr. Ernest N. Carlsen, who hopes to train gynecologists in its use.

Another non-invasive technique, NMR, recently hit the front pages of medical journals, though not newspapers and general magazines. Because I have not been able to find anyone to explain its intricacies, I must quote the explanation of nuclear magnetic resonance *verbatim* from an NIH report of February 1981:

"Known as nuclear magnetic resonance (NMR) spectroscopy, the technique measures the effect of radio waves on the behavior of atoms placed in a magnetic field. Each element exhibits a unique response, which allows chemists to identify compounds and study molecular structure."

In this NIH report, there is no mention of NMR's usefulness for detecting any kind of cancer.

However, in a 1971 paper in *Science Magazine,* Dr. Raymond Damadian, Professor of Medicine and Biophysics at the Downstate Medical Center of the State of New York (SUNY), described NMR's ability to discriminate between benign and malignant tissue. Although he did not specify breast tumors, a hint of the potential was there.

Since I could make neither heads nor tails of the paper, I called Dr. Damadian at his Long Island office for a less technical, more simple explanation. He pointed out that using conventional X-rays may often make it impossible to differentiate between various types of soft-tissue lesions, including cancer. Such malignancies would, naturally, not be discovered by mammography, if they are in the breast. On the other hand, NMR techniques involve the use of "external probes" that read the chemistry of the tissue entirely by wireless electronics. The detector, known as a Fonar spectrometer, is able to pick up radio signals that are broadcast by atoms deep inside the cells of cancerous tissue.

"In other words," Dr. Damadian told me, "NMR is a technique for doing chemistry entirely by wireless electronics."

"Does NMR technology require an "interpreter" with special training and experience to read the diagnoses?" I asked.

"No," he said. "NMR uses quantitative numerical values that can readily be understood by anyone after only a short training period."

"Can NMR scan a breast and find out if the mass inside is the only one or whether there are others? What about scanning the axillary lymph nodes to see if there's cancer."

Dr. Damadian paused. "This, of course, is our hope—that we will be able to help surgeons make clinical decisions about how much must be cut in order to remove all the cancer in a breast. So far, we've had some very exciting and promising results."

In one case, he told me, a mammogram had diagnosed a

woman's tumor as being "95 percent malignant," but the NMR reading was one of normal tissue. And it was normal. According to a surgical biopsy performed at a top hospital by a breast expert, the X-ray had been a "false positive."

The second case involved the diagnosis of a large malignant tumor on the wall of a woman's chest—a tumor that had not been apparent on the mammogram.

"Of course," Dr. Damadian cautioned, "these data are most encouraging, but it's too soon to be able to say anything except that we are 'optimistic' about NMR's use for the early detection of breast cancer. The most enthusiastic comment to make is that 'the results so far are promising'."

If all goes according to current plans, NMR's cost should be equal to that of a four-view set of mammograms. This is still not the cheap, easy and quick PAP test we women want and need. But if NMR should be able to predict which women have other foci and which have positive axillary nodes, the non-invasive technique will be worth countless millions of dollars—not only to breast-cancer patients, but to all people who develop cancers. Fonar and NMR may be the most exciting early-detection technique on the horizon.

No chapter on early detection is complete without a discussion of the brassieres that have been invented to detect changes of breasts' heat patterns. In 1974 several were being tested. Since then, Fabergé has bought a patent to develop another one, but all rely on thermographic bases: heat sensors are embedded into the bra to detect retention by potentially diseased tissue. According to the promotional information, the brassieres need to be worn only a few minutes a day for accurate results. So far as I know, none of those results has been published.

Still another gadget, the "Mammoscan," is coming from Israel. But except for BSE, which may or may not be an excellent early-detection technique, all the techniques I have described in this chapter rely on expensive gadgetry. No matter how good and/or safe they may be, they are, by definition, devices that are practical for, at most, ten percent of the women in this country. In other countries, the number of women who can afford them is even smaller.

Screening examination—i.e., one where no obvious symptoms are present—are not covered by most medical insurance plans, including Medicare.

So even though the NCI urges all women over the age of fifty to be screened periodically, the cost is prohibitive for women whose Social Security checks barely cover the minimum essentials of survival. Many physicians do pretend they have found a symptom, but this can happen just so many times before they are caught by sharp-eyed Medicare staffers.

Younger women have the same insurance restrictions, and they have the added worry about babysitters or need to take time off from work. In the Washington, D.C. area, a clinical examination, four mammographic views, and lost time (not to mention a parking fee) can mount to more than $150. For an annual routine expense, this is, clearly, for only a chosen few of the 50 million women at risk.

A former president of the United States is famous for having said, "What this country needs is a good 5¢ cigar." What we women of the world need is an accurate, safe, and *cheap* breast-cancer test.

We also need tests that are 100-percent accurate for detecting recurrences when they are early enough to be destroyed by chemo-, radio- or endocrine therapy of one kind or another. At this time, doctors have the technical know-how to find some occult metastases, especially in the bone, if only they would use them.

Shortly after Christmas 1974, on a Washington TV talk show, I saw an interview with Ann London Scott, a once dynamic feminist leader and one of the founders of NOW—the National Organization for Women. Ms. Scott, only forty-five, had advanced metastatic disease and did not expect to live much longer. Her cancer had begun little more than a year earlier as a breast tumor.

"Are you bitter about the prospect of dying?" the interviewer asked sympathetically.

The fiery organizer, her eyes flashing, stared into the camera. She was emaciated and clearly very ill, but her spirit was far from beaten. "Not about dying itself," she hissed, "but because it might have been postponed if I had had follow-up care. I thought the mastectomy would be the end of it, that I had to wear a stupid prosthesis and that was all. Finished."

Ms. Scott's luxurious black hair glowed with highlights under the television lights, and her fierce, expressive eyes blazed with anger. The rest of her slumped weakly in her chair.

"What I'm bitter about is the total lack of anything after the surgery—the X-rays, scans, and tests that could have spotted the cancer when it first began to spread. I never had any of them. If I had been put on chemotherapy immediately, it might have been stopped." She continued, her fury carrying across the air-waves onto my screen. "Okay, so I did all the right things. I found the lump and had the mastectomy. That was all I was told *I* had to do.

For the rest, a woman depends on her doctor, and there is a lot of work that still needs to be done about that."

It was obvious that Ann Scott wanted to be around to do it. Unfortunately, she died not long afterward, on February 17, 1975.

There is no shortage of publicity about early detection of a first cancer. When the first and second ladies had their mastectomies, it was hard to find a newspaper or magazine, a radio or television program that had missed giving instructions in BSE and the seven danger signals of cancer. For the general education of women, this is a marvelous contribution. But women like me, who have already had one cancer, have a very high risk of developing another one, and *nowhere* have I seen an article printed or a discussion aired on how to detect early signs of a recurrence or a metastasis.

In the reams of expensive brochures, pamphlets, leaflets, and booklets published by the American Cancer Society, there is not a single line addressed to patients to warn them about a second cancer. Ann Scott was right. All a woman hears about are BSE, biopsy, and the different kinds of surgeries, as if these were the end of breast-cancer troubles. In fact, primary treatment of any kind is only the beginning of a lifetime of watching, examination, and testing—if the patient is lucky enough to have a doctor who knows what should be done.

An American Cancer Society spokesman told me the ACS has many and frequent meetings and conferences to "educate the profession." It is assumed, he said, that "once the cancer is discovered, the patients are under the care of physicians, and we direct our follow-up information to them." Having attended many a medical conference and meeting, I know how many doctors consider them nothing but tax-deductible vacations for brushing up on their golf, tennis, or fly casting. Science reporters covering such conventions usually return home knowing more about the subject of the meeting than the doctors do.

Until recently, the National Cancer Institute also gave no information to women about the early-warning signals of a recurrence. However, in July 1980, Dr. D. Jane Taylor, the director of the Coordinating Office of the Breast Cancer Task Force decided the NCI should do something about filling this void.

"It wasn't much of an issue before," she told me. "First of all, even if there was some way to find microscopic metastases—a 100-percent accurate way—there wasn't much anyone could do about them. It seemed to be better not to make women anxious about something that couldn't be treated."

Dr. Taylor, a thirty-year veteran of the war against cancer, explained that the scientific research establishing the theory that treating any cancer when its "tumor burden" is small is relatively recent.

"With what we knew before the mid- to late-1960s," she said, "there didn't seem to be any benefit in beginning treatment until a woman developed clinical symptoms of metastatic disease. So why alarm her and have her worrying all the time?"

With the knowledge now firmly accepted, new technologies available for finding microscopic spots of cancer in other organs at least some of the time, and the use of powerful anticancer agents, the Breast Cancer Task Force decided the time had come to tell women what to watch for and report to their doctors.

As a result, Dr. Taylor and J. Paul Van Nevel, the associate director of the Office of Cancer Communications, asked me to write a leaflet, "If you've had breast cancer . . . ," and this has been included in Chapter 14—After Treatment: Physical.

Like adjuvant therapy given prophylactically to women at high risk of developing a recurrence because they have malignant lymph nodes, treatment of microscopic metastatic disease is only a few years old. It is too soon to know if its use will have any effect on ultimate survival rates. But I know hundreds of women who had never developed any obvious symptom of metastasis when eagle-eyed oncologists spotted microscopic "hot spots" on scans and began treating them immediately. Common sense tells me that these women will live longer, even if the "statistically significant" ten-year data are not available yet.

8

The Real Controversies: Separate Biopsies, Staging, Aspiration, and the Estrogen-Receptor Assay

When *Breast Cancer* was published in 1975, it had a chapter called "The Real Controversy." It began: "Everyone by now, must know that a breast-cancer controversy is raging in the land. Are too many mastectomies being performed? Too many radical mastectomies? Why are most surgeons in the United States still doing the disfiguring and disabling Halsted radical when the modified radical is just as good?

"This is the blazing controversy we have been hearing so much about. But I think the real breast-cancer scandal has nothing to do with the kind of mastectomy at all . . .

"The single underlying basis for these practices is the penchant in the United States for performing the biopsy on the operating table and combining it with an immediate mastectomy if the frozen-section pathological diagnosis is cancer. Aside from the psychological trauma to the patient of going into the operating room without knowing whether she will awaken with one breast or two, there are good medical reasons for separating the two procedures."

In late 1974, I was most concerned about the barbaric custom—virtually universal in the United States—of doing a diagnostic biopsy and a mastectomy (if necessary) in a single procedure. As I mentioned in Chapter 1, I had called nineteen surgeons before I could find one who would deviate from this ridiculous procedure. And I still think he agreed only to humor a silly, scared woman. After all, my mammogram had said the lump was benign.

Instituting the "two-stage procedure" then became a personal crusade—almost a vendetta, because there is no valid medical reason for combining diagnosis and treatment. The practice is nothing more than a bad habit surgeons acquired as a result of two politico-economic changes that occurred in the United States after World War II. The first was the passage of the Hill-Burton Act in 1946, legislation giving local communities federal grants-in-aid to build hospitals all over the country. In earlier decades, there were few towns that had hospitals staffed and equipped to do mastectomies, and a woman's breast lump was routinely removed in a doctor's office. Afterward, it was sent off to the closest big city where a pathologist made the diagnosis. Then, and only then, if the mass was malignant, the woman cleaned her cupboards and closets, stocked the pantry, arranged for her children, and packed a suitcase for a trip to Big City.

(This is an historical tidbit I like to tell whenever I hear the myth that a breast cancer will "spread like wildfire" if the breast is not removed immediately.)

The second change involved insurance coverage. When prepaid medical plans first began to be popular, most insurance companies refused to cover any surgery unless it was done in a hospital instead of in a doctor's office. So a breast biopsy became an in-patient rather than an out-patient procedure in order to save women money. Naturally, if the operating room was already reserved, the patient draped and unconscious, and doctors and nurses were standing by, why not do it all at once? It was just plain common sense.

What about the woman's state of mind?

The probability is high that she will be sure the mass is benign until the second the anesthesia puts her to sleep. Few women accept a pre-biopsy diagnosis of cancer, emotionally—even if the doctor says he is "99 and 44/100 percent sure."

Why do women have so little faith in their doctor's pre-operative opinion?

The main reason is simply human nature: all people, not only women, deny the truth and do not accept bad news as final until there is proof beyond any reasonable doubt. (I can personally attest to this: four pathologists examined the slides from my tumor before their diagnosis of "infiltrating intraductal adenocarcinoma" sank into my numb brain.)

But there is another reason.

We know much more about breast cancer now, because so many articles, books, and television programs have educated us. For example, we know that no matter how sure a doctor may be that a diagnosis will be cancer, he cannot really be certain until a pathologist examines the mass and declares it benign or malignant. And later, no matter how positive the pathologist may be about the quick, frozen-section examination of a sliver of tissue, women know that he/she cannot really know until the longer, more reliable "permanent section" is studied. The media have told us that this requires the tissue to be stained and embedded in paraffin, and we have learned that the permanent section may indicate that the cell is not malignant after all.

True, this happens rarely with common "garden variety" breast cancers, but there are also uncommon, non-garden-variety benign masses (e.g., something called sclerosing adenosis) that can easily be mistaken for cancer. There are also those microscopic clusters of cells too small to be diagnosed as anything other than "atypia." We women have been told again and again that diagnosing these miniscule droplets of tissue is an "interpretive art" and not an exact science. Such errors are even more likely now that ultrasensitive devices can find "tumors" so small they can only be seen under a microscope or with special X-ray equipment called specimen radiography. The result has been a united front among women against the biopsy-mastectomy as a single procedure.

In 1974, my personal reason for insisting on a separation had nothing to do with scientific data, however, but on a 25-year-old memory of a shaggy-dog joke Johns Hopkins Medical School students used to laugh about when I worked there. A young man, the tale went, arrived at the student health clinic complaining of pain in his penis, and a biopsy under general anesthesia was recommended. When the surgeon visited him in his room a few days afterward, he looked grim.

"Son," he said, "I've got some good news and some bad news. Which do you want to hear first?"

The student looked down at the bandaged stump between his thighs.

"The bad news first, I guess."

"I had to cut your penis off," the surgeon said. "I did a penectomy."

The student flinched and cried, "My God! What can the good news be?"

The surgeon put his hand on the student's shoulder and smiled happily. "It was benign on permanent-section study. The frozen-section was a false-positive."

Of course, this was only a joke, but it stayed with me for more than twenty-five years, locked in a corner of my fond recollections of Johns Hopkins. When I found out I needed a breast biopsy, the story leaped from 1947 to 1974 within microseconds.

There would be no false positives based on a quick frozen-section for me!

As a matter of fact, I had no scientific data to support a two-stage procedure until late 1975 when I interviewed Dr. Maureen Roberts at the Royal Infirmary in Edinburgh. We sat in her office discussing the differences in the way breast cancer was treated in Scotland and in the United States.

"What do you do here?" I had asked her.

"When a woman presents us with a suspicious symptom in the clinic," she explained, "we of course do mammograms or xero-mammograms immediately. If these are inconclusive, we biopsy the mass."

"In the operating room?" I interrupted.

"Oh, that is only a last resort," she said. "Surgery for a biopsy is usually not necessary, because there are several other ways of finding out, in the clinic. First we try a fine-needle biopsy."*

That was what my first surgeon did when he tried to aspirate my tumor with a hypodermic needle.

"That's what was done with me," I told her, "but nothing came out."

"Of course, that does sometimes happen if the tumor is very solid. However, if it is filled with fluid that can be aspirated, the cyst simply collapses. Then we analyze the fluid, to be certain it was benign and not malignant,"

"But what would you do if nothing came out? Wouldn't you have to do a surgical biopsy then?"

"Not straightaway," she said quickly, surprised. "We then use what we call a Tru-cut needle. It's a bit larger, and needs just a dab of anesthetic on the breast, but it invariably gets some tissue out, without requiring surgery. We rarely have to use surgical biopsies for the preliminary diagnosis here at the Royal Infirmary."

In *Breast Cancer,* I wrote that I remembered hearing a doctor at the National Cancer Institute say something about clinical trials of wide-bore needles for non-surgical biopsies, but the program was still in the talking stage. In Edinburgh, it was already routine. (The Royal Infirmary was only the second stop of my European tour. I learned afterward that, under one name or another, wide-bore-needle biopsies were also routine in Sweden, Finland, and the Soviet Union.)

"If neither of the needles extracts enough tissue for a definite

---

*In cities in the United States, where good cell pathology (cytology) is available, fine needle aspiration biopsy is becoming more routine. Where such aspiration and cytology are done, if cancer is present, it may show up 85 percent of the time without the need for a surgical biopsy at all.

diagnosis to be made," Doctor Roberts continued, "then and only then will we excise the mass. As I said before, this is rarely necessary, but sometimes—yes, it must be done. If the lesion is not too large or deeply embedded, this procedure, also, might be done on an outpatient basis, without hospital admission.

"But there would be no frozen-section histological—pathological—examination," she explained. "The growth would be studied in paraffin, a permanent section. While waiting for the diagnosis, the patient is at home."

"Do you remove the lump if the needle biopsy says it is benign?"

"As a rule, yes. If the patient has objections, no. However, we do instruct her to come to the clinic frequently to be watched."

"And if the pathological examination shows it's malignant?" I asked.

She looked surprised. "Why then the patient must be staged, of course."

At the time, all I concentrated my thoughts on was the routine separation of the biopsy from further treatment and not on presurgical staging. Therefore, the two-stage procedure was what I urged in my book and in almost all of my subsequent articles and lectures. Instead of fighting back with the antiquated and disproved argument that the cancer would spread immediately if there was a delay, surgeons found another specious "medical" reason for doing the one-stage procedure: that considerable anesthetic trauma would result from putting patients to sleep twice. However, this argument boomeranged. Instead of supporting continuation of immediate mastectomy, it began a trend of doing biopsies under a local anesthetic on out-patient bases—thanks to medical insurance companies who saw this change as a way to cut hospital costs.

It was not difficult for me to accumulate more solid reasons to support the separation between diagnosis and treatment.

For example, biopsies are usually performed under light anesthesia, an injection of a narcotic drug, which does not involve a pre-operative chest X-ray. All good hospitals require that patients who are to be given inhalation anesthesia, gases, be X-rayed first to be sure their lungs are free of infection and disease, but this is not always done before a breast biopsy. If the frozen-section diagnosis is "benign," it makes no difference. But the injected narcotic is not a deep enough anesthetic for doing a mastectomy, and gases of some kind must be added. Although these should never be used unless the lungs have been examined and pronounced clear, there is no time for chest X-rays when a mastectomy of any kind is done immediately after the biopsy. I know of one young woman who died during a mastectomy, done under endotracheal anesthesia, because no X-rays had been taken of her lungs. She had undetected "walking pneumonia."

In addition to these known and accepted contraindications for the one-stage procedure, evidence began to come from immunology studies. These showed that if the mastectomy is postponed for a few weeks after an excisional biopsy (removal of the entire tumor), the patient's defense system seems to gain strength to attack and destroy residual cancer cells left behind in the area of the tumor. While this hypothesis has still not been proven definitively yet, there are some clinical data to support it. Certainly there is no reverse evidence: there are no data showing that those of us who waited a week or two between our biopsies and further treatment have had bad effects.

What began as my personal "crusade" in 1974 was quickly picked up by women's groups, by many surgeons, most health maintenance organizations (HMOs), insurance companies and, finally by the U.S. government. The Department of Health, Education and Welfare (HEW, now HHS: Health and Human Services) began to urge all Americans to get a second opinion before having surgery of any kind, including breast biopsies. Obviously, it is impossible for a woman to get a second opinion if she is asleep on an operating-room table.

The final result was astonishing.

On May 22, 1979, the Massachusetts legislature passed a law requiring that all women be told every treatment option and alternative, if they should have breast cancer. Since then, this law has been passed in California and is in the legislatures of several other states. Implicit in such legislation is separating the diagnosis from further treatment: no one can expect doctors to explain all options and alternatives to every woman who finds a breast lump.

By early 1979, the political stage was set for a national recommendation. Two years earlier, Dr. Donald S. Frederickson, then the director of the National Institute of Health in Bethesda, Maryland, had established a "science court" to be a regular part of technology-transfer—getting the latest advances in all fields from the NIH to the public where they can be used. Called Consensus Development Conferences (CDCs), the first science court was held in September 1977 and concerned the BCDDPs, mammography, and breast-cancer screening. The Conference's recommendations, detailed in Chapter 7, were quickly accepted. Their success in resolving the confusion and controversy about breast X-rays convinced the powers-that-be that Consensus Development Conferences were ideal for getting a broad range of views regarding what new products, programs, and procedures were ready to be used on the community level. Since that first CDC, there had been seventeen by mid-1979, and—even though the recommendations do not have the force of law—the prestige of the international panelists helped them become quickly accepted.

Of course, not all of the CDCs involve cancer. There are eleven institutes at the NIH, and each has issues that need airing and discussion in such Conferences.

One day in 1979 I was surprised to be called by Dr. Seymour Perry, then deputy director of the NIH. He asked me to be a panelist at the Conference planned for "The Treatment of Primary Breast Cancer: Management of Local Disease," to be held in June. It is now routine for most governmental agencies to have lay consumers on miscellaneous committees, boards, commissions, and panels, but, as a rule, most members are professionals. Consumers' voices are usually muted and muffled when final recommendations were issued.

For this panel, Dr. Perry told me, I would be the only non-physician, but I would have an equal vote with the seven doctors invited to participate.

According to the notice sent out to publicize the Conference, its purpose was "to address the following question: Are there clinical alternatives to radical mastectomy which minimize patient morbidity and do not decrease a patient's survival potential?"

A paragraph followed indicating that results of the radical mastectomy would be compared with those of a "total mastectomy with axillary dissection."

I was flabbergasted! Fewer than five years earlier, I had almost been lynched in Atlanta for preaching my heretical gospel to a B'nai B'rith women's group, and in 1979, I was invited to sit on an NIH advisory panel.

"Am I reading this properly," I asked Dr. Perry by telephone, "or is it some kind of a mix-up?"

"Of course it's not a mix-up, Rose," he told me. "We want to have all views represented, and this can't happen unless there's a patient advocate on it too."

"But look who is on the panel," I cried. "I'm not at all sure. . ."

Dr. Perry interrupted me, laughing. "Don't tell me you're afraid."

Then his voice became serious. "This will be a chance for you to say what you've been saying for more than four years, but this time you'll be talking from the National Institutes of Health. If you're too scared to do it, I'm sure I can get someone else."

Embarrassed by my cowardice, I quickly agreed to be the lone consumer on the panel.

Preparatory material came to me from Dr. Perry. The term, "radical mastectomy," was obviously a euphemism for the dreaded Halsted-radical mastectomy, but I knew nothing about "a total mastectomy which removes axillary nodes, but preserves the pectoralis muscles." A visit to Dr. Jane Henney explained that breast-cancer experts wanted to replace the meaningless term "modified radical mastectomy" with more precise language.

"A modified radical is simply any mastectomy that's at all different from the Halsted," she said. "It has no exact surgical definition. Some surgeons take all of the axillary nodes, some take one, some six, some ten or more. There are surgeons who leave both pectoral muscles, and others remove only one. Technically, all of these procedures are 'modified' in the sense that they're different from the Halsted, but there's no way to know exactly what was done."

She said that using the words "total mastectomy with an axillary dissection" would describe only one operation: removal of the breast and of all the underarm lymph nodes.

"The confusion about the precise extent of the surgery done would end."

"But, these words sound worse," I said. "Women are already used to modified radicals. The new jargon sounds like a lot more cutting—especially that word 'dissection'."

Dr. Henney agreed. "But we've got to start somewhere, and this Consensus Development Conference is the best place we can think of. Surgical names have been changed in the past, and people have gradually gotten used to them—even if they do seem harsher when the change is made.

"It's something whose time is long overdue, Rose," she said. "As long as surgeons can say they did a 'modified mastectomy,' there's no way to really get a handle on the comparative recurrence and survival rates."

Of course, she was right. One man's "modified" was often another's "extended simple," and I had seen too many sunken chests where one of the muscles was obviously gone after such operations, even though the women had been told they had modified radical mastectomies. There was a real need to end the babel of terminologies. As Dr. Henney said, this Conference was an excellent place to start the change.

The Consensus Development Conference was to begin at 8:30 A.M. on June 5, 1979 in the Masur Auditorium of the NIH. I read the names and titles of the other members of the panel. Dr. John Moxley, the moderator, was a pediatric oncologist, so I assumed he had no vested interest in the treatment of breast cancer. Dr. John R. Durant of Alabama was an unknown name to me; Dr. Bernard Fisher of Pittsburgh had not done a Halsted since NSABP trials, done in the early 1970s, showed this extensive operation was no better than the total (or simple) procedure. Dr. Samuel Hellman was a radiation therapist whose specialty, for years, had been using X-ray instead of mastectomy for primary breast cancer; Dr. Bernard Pierquin of France, was also a radiotherapist. It was unlikely that he would support the Halsted. Dr. Jerome Urban, I knew, was a radical surgeon but the last member of the panel, Dr. Umberto Veronesi, was an Italian surgeon who was comparing different kinds of mastectomies with partial surgery followed by irradiation of the breast.

After studying the composition of the panel, I was sure there would not be much of a fight about continuing the Halsted. What was I to say?

Before the Conference, all panelists had been asked to send a summary of our formal presentations, and I sent mine, as requested. It was no different from what I had been saying and writing about the Halsted for almost five years. When I mailed the summary to NIH, I also mailed a copy to Dr. Dao. He must have called the second he finished reading it.

"You have no business talking about whether or not a woman needs a certain kind of breast operation," he said angrily. "You may know more about breast cancer than most women do, but you cannot speak as if you are standing over an operating-room table with a scalpel in your hand!"

I was shaken by his anger, to put it mildly. "I didn't write anything there I haven't written or said before . . . "

"You may be perfectly right, Rose. I have not had to do an extensive mastectomy for more than fifteen years, but—as a non-physician—you have absolutely no right to stand before a forum of scientists, physicians, and surgeons and tell them what *you* think they should or should not do when a woman's life may be at stake. You do not have the training or the experience to give you such a right."

"But Dr. Perry asked me to be on the panel specifically to give a patient's point of view."

"Yes," he snapped. "*Your* point of view as a *patient*. There is no way that you can have any credibility standing up and giving your point of view about what might be necessary for women whose cancers may be more advanced than yours was."

I was bewildered.

"I always thought you agreed . . . ," I began.

"Of course, you know I do," Dr. Dao said. Then his voice softened, and its shrill edge disappeared. "Besides, there is no sense whatsoever in your standing up to repeat what everyone else on that panel will probably say. It would be pointless.

"But," he continued, "there is a way for you to make a real contribution that will probably not even be thought of by anyone else on the panel."

"What?"

"You must write a new summary to replace the one I have just read. But in this one, you—as a patient—should urge that there be a separation between the diagnostic biopsy and whatever definitive treatment the surgeon might decide is necessary. This is something you can do to prevent the kind of, as you have put it so well, 'railroading' a woman is subjected to from the time a symptom is discovered until she awakens in a hospital room with one or both breasts lost. This is what you should fight for."

Dr. Dao was right, of course. As a non-physician, no matter how much I might have learned about breast cancer, I had never made the first pointed slash into a woman's chest. How could I vote on the surgical procedure that should be used? Besides, why spend time on this when the majority of the panel was obviously going to do it without me? Asking for a recommendation for the two-stage procedure was the logical proposal to come from a patient. Then I suddenly had another idea.

"What about asking for presurgical staging?"

He laughed. "Give you an inch and you want a mile. You can ask for it, but I doubt the panelists will agree to that. Right now, the tests are still not good enough."

"But scans are getting better and better all of the time," I insisted, "and you know that you wouldn't do a mastectomy on a woman if there was any hint in her chest X-ray that she might already have a metastasis in her lungs."

"Well, of course, you know I examine everything I can before I remove a woman's breast, no matter how small a lesion might be," he agreed. "But don't forget, Roswell Park is a research institution and not a private community hospital. For research purposes, the yield of an expensive examination is not as important as it is when the patient has to pay the bill."

"No woman would worry about some money if she knew a test could mean avoiding an unnecessary mastectomy," I said. "If the cancer is already in another organ, it doesn't make sense to remove the breast. You've told me that yourself."

There was silence at the end of the telephone. "Rewrite your oral presentation and include whatever you think is important to a patient. But keep your fingers and words out of the surgical argument itself."

It almost sounded like a warning.

Because of the vagaries of the U.S. Postal Service, Dr. Dao had received his copy in Buffalo, N.Y. before the original arrived in Bethesda, Maryland—five minutes from my mailbox. So it was easy to retrieve before anyone there read it. Because of the research I had done in writing my book, I had no trouble with the argument against combining the diagnostic biopsy with treatment. However, at the end of 1974, I had little information and few data, except for my conversation with Dr. Roberts in Edinburgh, to support presurgical staging.

"Staging" is the word generally used to cover the many examinations—X-rays, scans, and blood and urine tests—done after cancer is diagnosed in any organ but *before* any extensive treatment is considered. In the case of breast cancer the purpose of staging is clear enough: the only hope of cure by any kind of local treatment, whether it is surgery or radiation, is to stop the disease before it spreads beyond the regional lymph nodes into other organs of the body. If metastasis is already present, there is no reason to do more than to remove "the primary tumor burden." In breast-cancer treatment, most of the time, this may mean only the biopsy and nothing more.

Staging for breast (or any) cancer has always been difficult, because occult metastases that may be growing in other organs are so difficult to find, even with advanced technologies. At this time, examining lymph nodes after their removal is the most reliable staging procedure available for predicting possible metastasis, but this is considered to be a primitive way to find out if the disease has spread. Something better is needed.

Scientists had been searching for years to find a more reliable method than counting malignant nodes, but the techniques available in 1974 were poor. Dr. Dao was right about their low yield: according to everyone I interviewed (anything in print was already obsolete!), radioactive scans of a woman's skeleton were, in the best institutions by the best nuclear-medicine experts, at most only 22 percent accurate. Chest X-rays could show pulmonary metastases, but liver and brain scans rarely showed anything unless the disease was so advanced that clinical symptoms were already present. If the cancer had metastasized to the intestinal tract, uterus, or ovaries, there was no way to detect the spread without major surgery.

Still, I was haunted by Dr. Robert's description of the way breast cancer was managed in the Royal Infirmary. In *Breast Cancer* I had described our conversation, because she told me she had been so puzzled by the way both Betty Ford and Happy Rockefeller had been treated.

"In all of those newspapers and magazine stories about Mrs. Ford and Mrs. Rockefeller, it seems as if the mastectomies were done so very quickly," she said. Her voice had a faint Scottish burr. "When could they have had time to do all the preoperative work-ups properly, if the mastectomy followed the diagnosis so quickly?"

"That's the way it's usually done in the United States," I told her. "What do you do in Scotland?"

Dr. Roberts explained all of the testing done after a diagnosis of cancer was confirmed by the various kinds of biopsies.

"Before anything at all is done about removing a breast here at the Royal Infirmary, we first scan the brain, bones, liver, and lungs, to see whether the disease has spread beyond the breast. If it already has, there's really no reason to do a mastectomy at all, is there?"

When I later reported my interview with Dr. Roberts to Dr. Dao, I asked what he thought about staging. He told me the prevalent surgical opinion: that the low yield did not justify the expense in the vast majority of cases.

"Furthermore," he added, "the public-education programs in this country have made women so aware of the early symptoms of breast cancer that there are not as many patients being admitted to hospitals with advanced disease. That is not true in most other countries."

He credited public education, early detection and screening programs for the fact that, in the United States, breast cancers are now being found in earlier, more curable stages.

He was probably right. Only one or two of the patients I had spoken with in Edinburgh had tumors smaller than walnuts, and this might well have been the reason for the routine staging done at the Royal Infirmary. It also explained why, in many instances, only the primary tumor in the breast was removed and other therapies were begun immediately. The breast itself was not amputated.

"No major surgical procedure is ever justified if there is already evidence of metastases to other organs," Dr. Roberts had told me crisply.

"Then you never have women who don't know in advance that they will have a mastectomy?" I asked.

"No, never," she said, "By the time the woman has come to the day of her operation, we know quite a bit about her. We have scanned her body and know the extent of the disease in terms of the rest of her organs, and we know the diagnosis absolutely. Of course, we have also done the other preoperative examinations—electrocardiograms, blood studies, urinalyses, and so on. The only thing we do not know with certainty is the status of her nodes. We cannot know about that until the mastectomy itself."

Could the different practices have been due to the fact that women in Scotland wait too long before going to a doctor? It certainly made sense. So I had not stressed the lack of routine staging in this country, because its omission was not a "raging controversy" in 1974. The major issue was the routine one-stage procedure.

What had been true in 1974, however, was not true in 1979. Time had brought about many changes. The field of nuclear medicine had exploded with more sensitive and sophisticated radioactive isotopes and scanners, and there were a variety of blood and urinary analyses—carcinoembryonic antigen (CEA), alkaline phosphatase, and human choriogonadotrophin (HCG)—that had shown their value in detecting occult metastases. All this technological know-how, undoubtedly, had increased the "yield" from presurgical staging examinations.

After learning about the progress made in detecting occult metastases since 1974, I decided to incorporate the data for the June 5 Conference and to link a recommendation for routine presurgical staging with my argument for the two-stage procedure.

About six weeks before Dr. Perry called me, I had received a manuscript from one of the authors of a hospital survey done by the American College of Surgeons (ACOS). After scanning it briefly, I had put it aside, because, at the time, it seemed unrelated to anything I was doing. But when I began to write the revised statement, a corner of my mind remembered there was something about premastectomy staging, and I dug it out of my files.

The survey had been done in two phases. The first, "Short Term Patient Care Evaluation Study for Carcinoma of the Female Breast" was published on October 12, 1978, and it described the treatment given to 14,634 women with primary breast cancer in the United States. The second part, titled "Final Report" was issued on February 21, 1979. It reported on the treatment of 23,777 women. Fourteen different kinds of breast cancers and their therapies were listed; and almost all of them got the same treatment: some kind of mastectomy.

There was also a table showing the stage of disease at the time of treatment.

What a find!

Using the ACOS's own data, I had proof that, of this cross-section of cases treated in 1977, 1,626 women already had distant metastases at the time of diagnosis. Yet 48.6 percent of them had some kind of mastectomy—far too much cutting than was necessary for women already known to have metastatic disease. Extrapolating from the data, it looked like more than 7,000 women (based on an estimated 110,000 new cases of breast cancer in 1981) would have unnecessary surgery (including Halsted and super radicals) if they are not staged after their biopsies confirm diagnoses of breast cancer, but *before* further treatment is done.

The reports from the American College of Surgeons gave me exactly what I needed to present my point of view, as a patient, at the June 5 NIH Consensus Development Conference.

Dr. Dao had been right about the Halsted. Except for Dr. Urban, there was unanimity among all the other panelists that the Halsted should no longer be considered the treatment of choice. At the end of the long and tiring day, some last-minute compromising was done on the exact wording to be used in the final recommendations. Had I not listened to Dr. Dao's sage advice, there would have been no paragraph saying:

"It was also the consensus that a two-step procedure should be done in most cases, i.e., a diagnostic biopsy should be studied by permanent histologic sections before definitive therapeutic alternatives are discussed with the patient."

Presurgical staging, per se, was not given the time nor the space I hoped it would have, but the report did say, "Selection (of treatment) in the past appears to have been based on . . . tradition rather than (being) tailored to a patient's stage of disease. . ." Although this is not a clear-cut recommendation to stage for extent of disease, it is nonetheless a hint that the practice of the past should be changed.

My contribution to the Conference was incorporated into its final recommendations. The two-stage procedure, the "raging controversy" in both *Breast Cancer* and in the first edition of *Why Me?* is a controversy no more. It has been accepted by the top level of the medical/surgical establishment, and we women can now sit back and wait for the ancient and sacred one-stage tradition to die.

But presurgical staging, wider use of aspiration biopsies that do not scar and disfigure our breasts, and routine estrogen-receptor assays are battles we still have to fight.

Happily, the national trend toward reducing medical costs goes hand-in-hand with doing aspiration, instead of surgical, biopsies. This trend can be seen wherever pre-paid health medical plans, health-maintenance organizations, and government hospitals are battling inflation. Of course, there will always be some women whose individual problems, such as deep-seated masses in large breasts, dictate surgical biopsies. But for the vast majority of lumps, bumps, and thickenings, a fine needle attached to the end of an ordinary hypodermic syringe can be placed into the mass with little or no discomfort.

If it is a cyst filled with fluid, this will be apparent immediately. The surgeon will be able to withdraw whatever liquid is inside. The shell of the cyst will collapse as soon as the fluid is removed, just the way a balloon deflates when it is punctured by a pin. Then the fluid should be analyzed by a pathologist who has subspecialized in cytology—the study of individual floating cells.

Since most women under the age of thirty are apt to have such benign cysts, aspiration biopsies are the most sensible way to establish a diagnosis at low cost and with a minimum of disfiguring scars. The prick of the needle fades and is gone by the time a woman returns home from the doctor's office, and a positive diagnosis from a cytological examination of the aspirated fluid is as accurate as a permanent, paraffin study of tissue.

"The problem is that there aren't enough cytologists in the country to make aspiration a routine diagnostic procedure," Dr. Cecil Fox, a cell specialist at the Armed Forces Institute of Pathology, told me. He had just returned from a tour in Sweden's Karolinska Institute where surgical biopsies are done only as a last resort, just as it was in Edinburgh. Enthusiastic about what he had learned abroad, Dr. Fox had brought back literature and photographs to launch his own crusade for more aspiration and less surgery. To his chagrin, the European data made no impression here.

"It's a vicious circle," he said. "Unless there's more business for cytologists, no one doing tissue pathology will bother to learn how to examine separate cells. And so long as there aren't many cytologists around, surgeons will use that as an excuse to keep on cutting out every lump in an operating room."

Finally, Dr. Fox turned to women to try to turn the tide, and Anne Kaspar, a member of the board of the National Women's Health Network, the Women and Health Roundtable and a health writer for many feminist and general women's publications, planned to write some articles advocating aspiration biopsies. Unfortunately, the conservative era ushered in by the 1980 Presidential election diverted the attention of all feminist organizations to salvaging the 1973 Supreme Court decision on freedom-of-choice in obtaining abortions, and the crusade for aspiration biopsies is on a back burner.

So the United States is still far behind in this regard. At the end of 1974 in every country I visited in Europe—England, Scotland, Sweden, Finland and the Soviet Union—as well as Japan, where I went in 1976, aspiration biopsies were the first course of diagnostic action. If a mass is solid and no fluid can be obtained, surgeons abroad use a wide-bore needle that actually carves a bit of tissue out of the lesion.

I asked Dr. Bernard Fisher, chairman of the NCI's National Surgical Adjuvant Breast Project, why this situation exists here.

"I use needle biopsies whenever I can," he told me, "but you can't trust a negative on a solid tumor. It's like a pregnancy test: if it's positive, you can be sure the diagnosis is right. But if it's negative, a woman can still be pregnant, but her pregnancy just hasn't shown up in the test yet.

"We know that most breast tumors aren't made up of only malignant cells," he continued. "They're heterogeneous and can have benign spots as well as malignant ones. If a Tru-cut needle happens to hit a benign area in a blind biopsy, you'd wind up with a dangerous false negative."

Because of this, Dr. Fisher said, he proceeds with definitive treatment, if an aspiration of any kind results in a positive diagnosis. "No woman can be a little bit pregnant," he explained.

But he always removes any suspicious solid mass, even if the needle biopsy tells the cytologist it is "nothing." Dr. Fisher suggested that most surgeons in the United States distrust the results of an aspiration biopsy for the same reason.

"If a negative diagnosis still means the mass has to be removed surgically," Dr. Fisher continued, "most guys would decide not to bother with a needle-biopsy in the first place."

However, Dr. Fox is convinced that the reason is simply that medical insurance companies pay much less for an aspiration done in a surgeon's office than they do for a full-scale operating room procedure.

There is probably truth to his argument. Surgical fees vary

considerably around the country, depending on the local cost of living and other factors. Most insurance companies, however, base their rates on one national measure, called the California Relative Value Scale (CRVS). It tells just what the name implies, the relative values of different medical and surgical treatments so that insurance-company clerks and bookkeepers will have some idea of what each procedure ought to cost. The CRVS uses proportions, not dollars, which allows the scale to be applied to any geographical area. (Manhattan has the highest actual fees for most procedures, Montana the lowest.)

After interviewing many general surgeons, I decided that the big profits come from those little twenty-minute operating-room biopsies, not from lengthy mastectomy surgery.

My brief twenty-minute biopsy earned the local surgeon who did it $200, not counting another $30 he got for my office visit and his attempt to aspirate the tumor. (The same fee is charged regardless of whether the mass is malignant or benign.) Although only one lump of every ten that go to biopsy turns out to be malignant and requires a mastectomy, ten diagnostic operations are performed to find that one cancer. Based on my surgeon's fees, that adds up to $2,000 for about 200 minutes of work—or $10 per minute. No surgeon in his right mind will give up that kind of easy money without a fight.

But a prominent Washington, D.C., surgeon (who must remain nameless, for obvious reasons) gave me another opinion.

"I don't think it's the money at all," he said. "Most oldtimers don't want to become students again. You don't just stick a needle into a mass as if you're giving a shot of novacaine. You've got to know how to do an aspiration, and most surgeons who have been in practice for twenty or thirty years don't want to spend their vacations and money learning how to do something they don't have to do. I think that's at the heart of the problem.

"Until women stand up for their rights and start demanding that aspirations at least be tried," he continued, "there's no reason for my colleagues to change."

So again, changing the way medicine is being practiced is up to us consumers. Women must realize that there is an alternative to the disfiguring and expensive scalpel in most instances, and—as my anonymous source said—we will have to stand up and insist on our rights to a needle biopsy before an operating-room date is made.

Several times I have mentioned a test I did *not* have in 1974, because it was then being done only at cancer centers: the estrogen-receptor assay or ERA. I have described how I carried my tumor with me from Maryland to Buffalo, carefully preserved in a bottle of formaldehyde, because I thought a breast-cancer specialist would need it in addition to the pathologist's slides. When I handed him the bottle, Dr. Dao shook his head.

"This doesn't do me any good now," he said. "I must have fresh or frozen tissue."

I was too panicked to ask him what he was talking about, but he thought I knew about the estrogen-receptor assay and had brought the tumor with me to have it analyzed.

After the mastectomy, Dr. Dao continued to talk to me as if I knew all about his research.

"If there was cancer in your nodes," he said, "there was not enough malignant tissue for me to assay its receptors. I must have at least a gram of tissue for that."

He told me he was happy that he saw no cancer in any of my axillary nodes, but he was sorry he could not do the ERA—just in case I had trouble later. Still groggy from the anesthetic, I paid little attention to the details of what he said. I was so relieved to hear that my axillary nodes looked negative that nothing else mattered.

At that time, the estrogen-receptor assay was still experimental and had not yet descended to the community-hospital level where my biopsy had been done. Now, the ERA is no longer experimental and even medical insurance companies are covering it (a sure sign that something is not experimental!) But the ERA is still, unfortunately, not routine in most general hospitals in the United States. Because the easiest time to do it is when the biopsy is done, women must know about it before they even walk into a surgeon's office.

When I presented my petrified tumor to Dr. Dao, he said he had to have "fresh or frozen tissue" to do the test. This means arrangements must be made with the surgeon and/or hospital pathologist to have the specimen frozen to minus 73 degrees Centigrade within fifteen minutes of its removal from its blood supply. (Although there are now some experimental methods for doing the ERA on less than a gram of tissue, it is better to have this much, if possible.) Women must insist that a cup of liquid nitrogen or ordinary dry ice is in the operating room so the mass—benign or malignant—is frozen immediately. If it is benign, the ERA will not be needed. But, if the diagnosis is carcinoma, its results provide the only clues a woman's doctor will have for choosing future treatments if it should be needed.

A brief history of the evolution of the estrogen-receptor assay since 1896 and the importance of the assay are explained in detail in Chapter 10, but women should learn about it when biopsies are discussed. For this reason, I have injected the ERA here, even though it is not at all controversial. Every breast-cancer expert agrees it is vital.

Briefly, the ERA is an indicator telling whether or not a tumor requires estrogens for its nourishment to permit it to grow. Naturally, the more receptors a cancer cell has, the more estrogens in a woman's blood will lock onto the receptor molecules to feed the cancer. This explains why some cancers are more hormone-dependent than others: their cells have more receptors and, therefore, get and retain more estrogens from the blood. Logically, if estrogens nourish the cancer, their absence would "starve" the cell, and it would die. The best way to treat women with estrogen-dependent cancers, then, is either to rid their bodies of as much natural hormone production as possible or to give them an agent that blocks the receptors from attaching themselves to the molecules.

To return to the ERA and the first step—the biopsy.

Once a breast cancer has been assayed, the information is filed away. Again, if no malignant axillary nodes were found and if a woman has no future problems, the ERA data are never needed. The test was a waste of time and money. But if she is estrogen-negative, she must be followed more carefully, because statistics have shown this group has a higher recurrence rate. It is also evidence that endocrine manipulation of any kind—including ovariectomy (removal of the ovaries)—would do her *no* good, and there is no reason to plummet her into a precipitous menopause. If she is ER +, however, her overall prognosis is better— no matter what is done—and she is a good candidate for endocrine adjuvant therapy.

Researchers are also looking for other "markers" that may be clues of either prognosis or treatment. For example the progesterone-receptor assay (PRA) is the subject of a great deal of intensive work in laboratories all over the world.

Although all the potential uses of both assays (ERA and PRA) are still unknown, there is little argument that they are exceedingly valuable aids now and will probably be even more useful as data are accumulated. The ERA, by the way, may also be done using tissue from a metastasis—if the original tumor was not assayed—but it is not always possible to get to it. For example, if spread should be found in the vertebrae, the risk of harming the spinal cord would prohibit doing a marrow biopsy there. This is why it is so important to measure receptors at the time of the initial diagnostic biopsy.

The value of the estrogen-receptor assay has now been firmly established, and scientists are searching for simple methods to get reliable ERA results from small quantities of tissue. Because women today are finding smaller tumors, the necessary gram of tissue required by most current techniques is not always available from a biopsy specimen after enough tumor is removed for diagnosis. One technique for assaying small bits of tissue involves radioactive labeling of cloned antibodies to estrogen receptors, and it is being perfected by Drs. Elwood Jensen and his colleagues at the University of Chicago. They are using space-age-technologies to do this: hybridomas, radioimmunoassays, and chromatography—pieces of modern know-how that are enabling scientists to do research that was impossible to even dream of a decade ago.

In addition, scientists are experimenting with cytological techniques that rely on fluorescene dyes and sugary concoctions to identify estrogen receptors. In June 1979, at a NIH conference on steroid receptors, its large auditorium was packed with scientists from all over the world—most of whom used different techniques. Dr. D. Jane Taylor, coordinator of the NCI's Breast Cancer Task Force feels that no single method has yet been proven to be superior to another.

"At this time," she told me, "I don't think you can honestly write anything about how the ERA should be done, because it may be obsolete before your book is even printed.

"However," she continued, "I do think you should tell women the test should be done and that preparations for it must be made at the time of biopsy—just in case it's needed. It's *our* job to get the right information out to the surgeons and pathologists about how the specimen should be handled and shipped and how the assay should be done."

Dr. Taylor's "our" is the National Cancer Institute and its professional education programs aimed at doctors involved in cancer diagnosis and treatment. As I have said, in spite of efforts made within the last five years to inform the medical/surgical pathological disciplines about the importance of the ERA, it is still not being done routinely.

So it is often necessary for women to do their own checking to be sure their surgeons know about it. Moreover, surgeons often have to be told gently that the tumor must be frozen to -73 degrees Centigrade within fifteen minutes of the removal from its blood supply. Pathologists should know that the specimen must be *kept at this temperature without being thawed* until the assay itself is performed. If the tissue waits longer than fifteen minutes without being frozen, its results may be totally useless. These women will not benefit from the information locked in those molecules of protein.

While the NCI is struggling to find the best way to inform surgeons and pathologists without "intervening in the private practice of medicine," women can assert themselves and insist on their rights.

At one of the semi-annual meetings of the NSABP in 1980, I learned that improper preparation in the operating room is one of the reasons why ERAs are often wrong, even when they are done. Once more, my source of wisdom was Dr. Bernard Fisher.

"When a surgeon sees a grossly malignant mass," he told me, "he'll just cut off enough tissue for the pathologist to use for a frozen-section diagnosis if the woman is going to have a mastectomy at a later time.

"Then, when he schedules the woman for further surgery, he'll proceed with the mastectomy and not send the rest of the tumor down to pathology for estrogen-receptors until the procedure is all finished. That could take three or four hours—maybe more.

"By the time the incision is closed and the breast—with the tumor still inside it—is delivered to the pathologist, chances are that the receptors are dead. Even a woman who is strongly estrogen-dependent would show up as ER negative."

Dr. Fisher told me one of his major teaching chores nowadays is instructing surgeons that the entire tumor must be removed and frozen immediately.

"If the mass is benign," he went on, "nothing is lost. But if the frozen-section diagnosis is cancer, there's already enough tissue in the specimen for a reliable estrogen-receptor assay to be done."

1. A cup of liquid nitrogen or dry ice should be taken to the operating room in advance of any surgical biopsy, just in case the mass is malignant;
2. The surgeon should remove as much malignant tissue as is necessary for both the pathological diagnosis and the ERA *immediately* and not leave the tumor in the breast for removal at a future time during a mastectomy. This operation may take three to four hours, and a tumor's receptors will be dead long before it reaches the pathologist's laboratory.

What else can women do about this problem?
Nothing much.
At such a traumatic time, it is difficult enough to demand that the ER assay be done without adding the burden of telling the

surgeon how to do his job properly. This is clearly a problem the National Cancer Institute must solve—going out into the community and teaching surgeons how to prepare malignant breast tissue for the estrogen-receptor assay.

All we women can do is hope it will happen.

Oncologists are now beginning to use estrogen-receptor levels to help choose the appropriate adjuvant therapy. In July 1981, Dr. Fisher published the results of a two-year NSABP study showing that ER+ women given an antiestrogen, tamoxifen, along with two cell-killing drugs, phenylalanine mustard (L-PAM) and 5-Flourorucil (5-FU) had fewer recurrences than did ER+ women who received no tamoxifen (also known as Nolvadex).

Because women older than fifty (postmenopausal) benefitted most of all, this is especially important: most older women are ER+, and cell-killing chemotherapy has not been as effective in preventing or delaying recurrences in this age group.

This study, and others supporting adjuvant endocrine manipulation, are discussed again in Chapter 11, but I mention it here to stress the importance of doing the estrogen-receptor assay at the time of biopsy. It is one of the newer discoveries scientists have made to help prolong, or even save, our lives.

Who knows what other advances tomorrow might bring? Or next week or next month? Progress is now coming with the speed of light, because pharmaceutical firms and commercial laboratories have discovered that millions of dollars are waiting for the one that finds the ultimate assay—one that will show the presence of microscopic cancers in the breast, nodes or distant organs.

As I have said many times, when there is money to be made, changes come quickly. Women must be ready to insist that their doctors take advantage of whatever new technology that becomes available.

Our breasts—and our lives—depend on it.

9

Psychological Aspects of Breast Cancer: Before *Treatment*

Why Me? necessarily covers again some of the material presented in my first book, *Breast Cancer*—published in September 1975. The reason for changing the title is so complicated that it could—and probably will—be another book, but it can be summarized by one word: "denial." I thought women wouldn't be afraid to be seen buying a book called *Why Me?;* they would not be ashamed to be seen carrying it or reading it on buses or under the dryer in a beauty shop. They couldn't be embarrassed to have it on their night tables next to Drs. Spock and Reuben.

A book called *Why Me?* can be a book about anything.

One of my earliest discoveries of denial came with the publication of the hardcover edition. Soon after it went on sale, the hostess on a TV talk show told me, "I would never have read your book if I hadn't been assigned to do it." A newspaper reporter said, "I put another jacket on it, so I could read it on the subway." In a bookstore, a salesperson told me that several women had asked her to bag the book and bring it to them at the cash register for payment; they did not want anyone to spot them buying it. No longitudinal or latitudinal surveys were needed to show that while women are ready to read about vaginal deodorants, soft bowel movements, and rape, we are not ready for a book boldly titled *Breast Cancer.*

So I knew immediately that the first updating revisions to be made would involve the psychological aspects of this disease *before* breast cancer strikes. Denial is the mechanism that keeps women from learning anything about symptoms; it prevents them from examining their breasts, from going to a doctor immediately, and from accepting treatment when the diagnosis is finally made. In extreme instances, denial can even make it possible for a woman to stop feeling or seeing a symptom entirely!

As I said, the details of denial could fill a book.

Publication of a book makes its author an "instant expert," and to cope with the queries that poured in, I set up a non-profit Breast Cancer Advisory Center (BCAC). The telephone number and address were generously publicized as I toured the country. My partner, Dorothy Johnston, a registered nurse, womaned the telephone and managed the mail when I was away; when I returned, we shared the job. As a result, we have amassed what may well be the single largest bank of knowledge about all aspects of breast cancer obtained from women themselves. For the original edition, I had surveyed 130 women who had undergone mastectomies via a questionnaire. Now, I have verified those data with responses from about 3,000 women (and their men). (Most of the 12,000 + calls and letters to the Center have come from women who have *not* had breast cancer. This, in fact, is the reason for writing this chapter). Statisticians will be stunned to learn that the conclusions drawn from a tiny, 130-woman sample were indeed representative of thousands. For example, women *do* think first of saving their breasts, as a rule, and their lives are but second thoughts. I had been challenged on this point on the grounds that 130 women were not enough for such a statement. But it was also true of the 12,000 + women.

As I said, the first psychological problem I learned about is the incredible denial associated with breast cancer. Obviously, the letters and telephone calls to the BCAC were from women who were *not* denying or they would not have contacted me. But hundreds hinted about mothers, various relatives, and friends who had breast problems but who did not want to know or do anything about them. Many letters were anonymous and, as I learned later, often were written under assumed names; countless telephone callers refused to give us names and addresses for written information.

One of the first anonymous letters the BCAC received was signed simply, "Teenager from Tennessee." The child who sent it wanted to take the Pill to help her catch up with her 34B girlfriends more quickly. Only thirteen, she could not fill out her cheerleader's T-shirt without the help of absorbent cotton. But her mother had died of breast cancer, and she was afraid the Pill might cause breast cancer. Letters from flat-chested youngsters are common.

Teenager-from-Tennessee is an example of another side of the pre-breast cancer psychological story, the side Dorothy and I heard from most: paranoia. And, as her youth shows, fear of breast cancer starts early.

There was nothing more for me to do but try to make the NCI and other breast-cancer educators aware of the problem. Denial, however, is impossible to prove: I have no data bank of letters from women who refused to read my book or refused to call the BCAC. Neither the ACS nor the NCI can count the women who will *not* go to their physicians about a possible symptom of breast cancer. Even the one measurable "avoidance behavior" (another bit of jargon meaning denial)—women's refusal to practice BSE—is often misinterpreted.

For example, at a meeting held in late 1980, the Office of Cancer Communications (OCC) of the NCI reported results of a survey, *Breast Cancer: A Measure of Progress in Public Understanding*. The poll told us that 76 percent of the 1,580 women surveyed thought cancer was their most serious health problem, and 58 percent "specifically mentioned breast cancer as the type of cancer most serious." Yet fewer than 40 percent of the women practiced BSE.

"Did any of the surveyors ask the 60+ percent of the women why they didn't do BSE regularly," I asked.

"The women said they didn't think of it," was the answer.

If breast cancer is the disease they fear most, how could anyone believe more than 60 percent of the women "didn't think of it"?

According to nonscientific, nonrandom polls done by the Breast Cancer Advisory Center, most women do not practice BSE because they are afraid of finding something that will inevitably lead to a mastectomy. Professionals in the business of behavioral modification consider such "avoidance behavior" to be completely normal and rational. After all, women are being asked to do something complex and inconvenient, something that may—if they need a doctor's examination and a mammogram—be expensive and expose them to a small, potential radiation risk. Then, if they were "good girls," did as they were told and find a lump or other symptom, they are "rewarded" by having their breasts removed.

So in spite of all the propaganda by the ACS and the NCI about the need to do this easy self-check, the highest proportion of women who examine their breasts regularly is 40 percent, and this number is achieved only after intensive educational programs that include person-to-person teaching by a physician, nurse, or a volunteer paramedic. A figure of 40 percent is considered to be an excellent score by everyone in the BSE business, but it does not sound high to me.

The ACS and the NCI (as well as dozens of other public and private groups promoting BSE) argue that women do not examine their breasts because they do not know how to do it properly and have no confidence in being able to tell the difference between a normal lump and something new. True believers in BSE insist that better and simpler instruction by human beings (instead of by leaflets and brochures), classes held by health professionals, more publicity, etc., etc., *ad infinitum* will eventually convince all women to examine their breasts every month.

Nonsense.

Until there is a real reward—less surgery—for finding a breast cancer when it is the size of a lentil instead of a lemon, women will refuse to practice BSE.

Here is a letter we received from Kingston, Jamaica, also showing the other side of the pre-breast cancer psychological story.

> Dear Miss Rose Kushner,
>   Greeting to you in the royal name of our soon coming King. On the 21st of January 1981 I have read in the newspaper what you have said about the breast cancer.
>   One night while doing my assignment I take my left hand and feel my right breast, I feel a little lump in it. I jump right up to my mother and tell her to feel it. The following week I went to the cancer society in Jamaica here and they told me to come back about six month time, but I am very scard.
>   My name is Maria. I am 17 year old. It do not hurt me but it scares me sometimes. Please to tell me what I am to do about it. Any is not in my left breast. I haven't had a child so I don't know what is the lump there for. Everytime I remember it I cry about it. Give my love to your family and friends till I hear from you. I think if I read the booklet I will get the full understanding.
>
>   Breast Cancer Advisory Center

>   17 February, 1981
> Dear Maria,
>   I received your letter and would like you to know immediately that the lump in your breast is probably *not* cancer. Although young women your age have been known to get breast cancer, it is so rare that doctors call it a "medical curiosity."

I am also sending some information from the National Cancer Institute in the United States and some material the Breast Cancer Advisory Center publishes. Unfortunately, there isn't much around for young women to read about lumps and bumps in the breast that are *not* cancer. I will tell you, though, that breasts are parts of your body that do a lot of things, and it is common to have strange lumps—especially around the time of your monthly period. The most common growth young women get is a "cyst." This is a hard ball filled with water, and it is harmless. If you live near a hospital, go to the department of gynecology (the doctors who take care of women), and ask for someone to examine you. Most of the time, all that has to be done for a cyst is to poke a needle in it (it only hurts a little bit) and all of the water inside will come out. Cysts like this might go away by themselves or they may stay for a long time. But they never do any harm. Another lump young women often get is "fibroadenoma." This would have to be cut out, but the doctor would give you something so you would not feel anything.

The best place to go for breast examinations is to a hospital—*not* a private, ordinary doctor. At hospitals, there are usually specialists who take care of only women's problems, and they know more about what to do. I don't think you have to worry about cancer at all, but you must be sure to keep seeing someone. Don't just forget about it. BUT DON'T BE SCARED!

I hope this helps.

> Sincerely yours,
> Rose Kushner, Executive Director
> Breast Cancer Advisory Center

How does the 17-year old in Jamaica know she probably has nothing to worry about? Racks in drug stores, supermarkets, libraries, and doctors' offices are jammed with literature about BSE, but there is little else. This is especially true for young women and teenagers, because they are at low risk of breast cancer—although they do get more than their share of lumps.

In 1979, I went to a conference in New York and heard some magazine editors describe the kinds of articles they wanted us to write for them. No one mentioned breasts except for stories with tips on how to keep them firm and beautiful. When I got home, I called the editor-in-chief of *Redbook* Magazine to ask why he had never published anything about breast cancer. *Redbook*, I was told, is aimed at a "target audience" of women under the age of thirty-five. The implication was that these younger women don't worry about breast cancer. In less than an hour, I sieved through some of the letters to the Center (by then, about 8,000), cut the names and addresses off of twenty, Xeroxed the letters, and mailed the package to the editor of *Redbook*.

My cover letter was rather sharp, because these were *not* letters from scared young women looking for information: all were from women who had already had one or two mastectomies, and all of them were younger than thirty.

I heard nothing from *Redbook*'s editor-in-chief, but I did receive a letter from an associate editor who told me the magazine had already commissioned an article on "just this topic." To my surprise and disappointment, when the *Redbook* story was finally published, it was just another humdrum inspirational message about the value of breast self-examination. There was not a line of real information in the entire article. However, in the September 1981 issue of the magazine, I was delighted to read the cover story about breast cancer, one of the best overviews of all aspects of the disease I've seen in a woman's publication.

Anyone who has contact with young women's groups like the Boston Women's Health Book Collective that published, *Our Bodies, Ourselves*, the National Women's Health Network, the Women and Health Roundtable, Women's Health International, and the hundreds of small, self-help feminist organizations scattered around the world knows how much young women want to know about breast problems. But there is little available for them from the medical establishment. They are urged to examine themselves from the time the pink buds on their chests begin to sprout; then, if they should find something suspicious, they are given no help except, "Call your doctor immediately."

Older women are not much better informed. When I found the lump in my breast in 1974, the major problem was the medical profession's resistance to giving real nuts-and-bolts information about alternatives and options to women. This situation has changed dramatically in the years since, and most physicians and surgeons no longer behave as if M.D. meant Mystical Deity. The majority (especially the younger ones) are willing to explain what they do and why they do it. The real medical "censors" now are the editors of all media who want to repeat surefire, upbeat themes that will not offend advertisers or scare anyone away.

Editorial tastes, however, are paradoxical. For example, it is rare for newspapers, magazines, television, and radio to discuss a breast problem that is *not* cancer, even though this is true 90 percent of the time. At the end of 1974, when both the wives of the president and the vice president of the United States—Betty Ford and Happy Rockefeller—were diagnosed to have breast cancer, their operations were banner-headlined. Everyone on earth was exposed to daily reports of their recoveries, and Mrs. Ford's ability to toss a football only a few days after her breast amputation became a well-publicized advertisement for her Halsted radical mastectomy.

But when Mrs. Rosalyn Carter had a benign lump removed from her breast in April 1977, her two-stage procedure was summed up in twelve column inches by the Associated Press—twelve column inches of type buried deep inside the Washington Post. Mrs. Carter's benign biopsy was not brouhahaed by Barbara Walters, Walter Cronkite, John Chancellor, or David Brinkley. Benign diagnoses are not newsworthy; cancer is.

Denial, paranoia, and frustration are the most basic psychological problems women face when they must cope with the problems of breast cancer. Anxiety—especially among women tagged "high risk" because of family history and/or cystic breasts—is another. And, as I have pointed out, there is no lower age limit: Anxiety about breast cancer may be present in children.

But what about women who have faithfully followed the edict, "Thou shalt examine thy breasts" and have found a symptom? Where can they turn for help beside their friendly family doctor or OB/GYN?

The medical establishment—including physicians, surgeons, the ACS, and the NCI—as well as many private organizations like the Young Women's Christian and Hebrew Associations, have long recognized the emotional needs of women who have had mastectomies and have had to adjust to living with only one or no breasts. So has the professional and lay press. I stopped long ago collecting books, scientific papers, and articles or watching television shows about women's rage, lost body-image and self-esteem, sexuality, and the other psychological problems "outsiders" think all mastectomy patients have after surgery. There is now too much being said and written about "coping" with the loss of a breast.

But there is still almost nothing about the terror and fear women endure before they have any reason to worry at all; there is little "coping" support to help women who have found symptoms but who do not know whether or not they actually do have breast cancer.

I was guilty of this sin myself. When I wrote *Breast Cancer* at the end of 1974, I had no idea of the magnitude of the problem, because I had been lucky. Living near the NCI, I had dozens of experts to question via a local telephone call and could ransack every bookshelf in the library from 8:00 a.m. to midnight. Most women do not have these advantages, but I knew nothing about their grief until the avalanche of letters and calls to the Breast Cancer Advisory Center began to pour in.

The NCI is estimating that there will be about 110,000 new cases of breast cancer diagnosed in 1981. Since two of every ten symptoms found by women themselves turn out to be harmless, this awesome and awful statistic means that almost 600,000 women will go through the agony of waiting, wondering, and worrying in this single year alone. Every woman who finds a symptom goes through the same hell—until the final diagnosis is made by a pathologist.

If there are still doubts about the high level of terror women have about developing breast cancer, I can point to the thousands of women *without* breast cancer who are asking for prophylactic mastectomies to prevent the disease. This grotesque phenomenon is not something from Dr. Strangelove or George Orwell; it is happening all over the world. During the last months of 1980 and into 1981, women in the United States were bombarded by articles in newspapers and magazines giving the pros and cons of procedures where healthy breast tissue is removed and replaced with an implant. Amputating a healthy organ to avoid cancer may seem to be melodramatic or even ridiculous. But when women read that they have an almost 10 percent chance of developing breast cancer in their lifetimes and that breast cancer kills one-third of all its victims, this "preventive" surgery is more understandable.

How can women be helped to cope with the psychological problems they have before a diagnosis of breast cancer? My answer was to expand the Breast Cancer Advisory Center and begin a program named NURSUPPORT to offer personal assistance to women being treated in the Georgetown University Hospital's Vince Lombardi Cancer Center in Washington, D. C. NURSUPPORT was short-lived, but the oncological nurses at Georgetown helped more than 400 women while it existed. I think its success is proof that large, organized programs like the ACS's Reach to Recovery or the Y's ENCORE—now both exclusively for women who have already had breast surgery—should begin to do pre- as well as postsurgical counseling.

Neither group will change its policy, however, until the medical profession understands that having medical information and knowing what must be done and why are, in themselves, the beginning of rehabilitation. Until this "novel" concept is accepted, women's psychological problems will continue. Surgeons have written or called me to report that informed patients recover from surgery more quickly with fewer physical and psychological problems. Yet there is still no organized, national program to help women make this first step in their reach to recovery.

The June 5, 1979, Consensus Development Conference recommended that the two-stage procedure become the diagnostic technique "of choice" so that women be given some time after a biopsy to get other opinions and to look into options. There is little point in giving a woman time between diagnosis and treatment if nothing is offered to tell her what her options are.

As I said at the beginning of this chapter, adapting to the loss of a breast is hard for many women. But it is strawberry shortcake in comparison with the psychological traumas she had to endure before that final treatment decision was made.

Does this sound unbelievable coming from a woman who has lost her breast?

Of course it does! Who would dare suggest that the emotional problems a woman must endure before a mastectomy are worse that the ones she will undergo being forced to live with one breast? Or with none?

After years of being challenged on this, I have prepared a scenario to describe what usually happens between the time a woman faithfully follows everyone's instructions to practice breast self-examination, finds a symptom, and that far away day when she finally knows where she stands. The example I am using is a forty-year-old woman of average risk: she has no particular reason to suspect she has any higher probability of developing breast cancer than the average American woman does.

Let's start with two women who do BSE religiously and have periodic professional examinations. Obviously, there can be two outcomes. One—like the vast majority of women—will never find a symptom but will continue to wait, watch, and worry for the rest of her life.

Or, as in the other's case, a symptom is found. If this happens, she has five possible options. One is to do nothing at all. While this may seem outrageous, there are women who find lumps, thickenings, and nipple discharges but who simply decide to ignore them; and this inaction (denial???) may also have two outcomes. The cancer may spread, resulting in eventual death from metastatic breast cancer, or it may never grow at all. There are documented cases where untreated breast cancers *never* reached the point where they became a threat to life. These women went through normal life spans with the carcinomas alive, but static, in their intact breasts.

Some women (and their numbers are few) "self-refer" directly to a surgeon: they do not visit a family practitioner, internist, or gynecologist first. By going straight to a surgeon for biopsy, they eliminate much of the expense as well as the anxiety of waiting.

Here, however, is what the average woman in this country does if she finds something suspicious in her breast: Not wanting to seem panicky or paranoid, she waits a menstrual cycle or two to see if the symptom goes away before calling the doctor. Most women go through this earliest period of waiting, watching, and worrying without telling even their closest friends or relatives. Most, as a matter of fact, feel their husbands or lovers should be protected and will confide in others before telling them.

This behavior also has two outcomes. The symptom may disappear, leaving our friend with months and years of continued waiting, watching, and worrying. Or the symptom persists and, she calls her doctor when one or two cycles have passed with no change. This is usually her gynecologist or, less often, a family practitioner.

Although it should be rare for a physician to tell a forty-year-old woman that a palpable breast lump is "nothing"—regardless of her risk status—it, unfortunately, happens all too frequently. So, one outcome of visiting the doctor may be a diagnosis of, "Don't worry about it. Go home and relax."

She may go home, but it's unlikely she will ever relax. Instead, she will do her monthly BSE, wait, watch, and worry for the rest of her life—or until she finds another potential symptom of breast cancer.

On the other hand, the doctor may not dismiss her immediately but may tell her to return for another examination after another menstrual cycle or two. This common course of physician inaction involves still another agonizing period of waiting. But, in some cases, the reward for the worry is learning that the symptom has disappeared—that it must have been some cyclical cyst. If the lump is still felt, the patient is usually sent onward up the diagnostic ladder to a radiologist for a mammogram.

More waiting and worrying.

Who an "onward" referral is, by the way, depends on a doctor's philosophy. Gynecologists and family practitioners usually request mammograms and would most likely send all forty-year-old women with persistent breast masses to radiologists before referring them to surgeons. Most surgeons, however, would feel that any such lesion would have to be removed—no matter what the breast X-ray indicated—and might not bother to order mammograms. And if they did, it would usually be to show whether or not something else that could not be felt is hiding in the breast. Or, if the breast is large, an X-ray could show exactly where to put the point of the scalpel.

In any event, all women who are sent "onward" by their gynecologists or family practitioners must make new appointments and then wait and worry until they are fit into the specialists' busy schedules. After mammograms are taken, they must then wait and worry again for the results. Of course, some women learn with delight that the lump is clearly a benign cyst. Relieved, they return to years of BSE, waiting, watching, and worrying.

But this is unlikely in the case of a forty-year-old woman, even if the breast X-ray shows nothing. If the doctor can still feel something in the breast, the patient will inevitably be sent on to a surgeon. If the mammogram does have a suspicious spot, she will certainly be told to see one. Sooner or later, all women with any continuing, persistent symptom of breast cancer must end their odysseys on a surgeon's examining table.

Since every visit to and examination by a doctor costs time, money, and involves endless waiting, the obvious question is, "Why doesn't every woman start with a surgeon in the first place?"

It is estimated that about ninety percent of all women in the United States, who use any doctor at all, go first to their gynecologist for everything. Naturally, they will go to them first, *not* to a surgeon, with a breast problem. (Men, by the way, generally go to an internist or family practitioner for their primary health care.)

So all the women who began by visiting their gynecologist or family doctor—after months of BSE, watching, waiting, and worrying (and perhaps a few hundred dollars spent for fees)—finally arrive at the surgeon's office. It would be rare indeed for a surgeon to tell a woman, aged forty, who has a persistent breast mass, to go home and forget about it. And, since all of these women were referred by other physicians, such a likelihood is even more remote.

The next step will most likely be a biopsy of some kind.

Now, before a woman with a breast-cancer symptom has even had a diagnostic biopsy, the anguish and anxiety she feels is at its peak. She has, as a rule, waited and worried for weeks before reaching this critical time, counting the minutes and hours for a "slot" on the operating-room schedule.

The most typical procedure prevalent in the United States

today requires admission to a hospital for a surgical biopsy under general anesthesia. The surgeon removes the entire mass or a section of it and sends it for a "frozen section" microscopic examination by a pathologist. If cancerous cells are found, most surgeons immediately proceed with so-called definitive treatment, usually a modified radical mastectomy (total mastectomy with an axillary dissection). Women who go through this ordeal do not have to agonize while this study is done, because they are blessedly asleep. Surgeons often use this "kindness factor" to justify combining diagnosis with treatment. And of course, there are women who prefer this combination, and they willingly sign the hospital's admission forms giving permission for a mastectomy if cancer is diagnosed by this quick-freeze diagnostic method. They have already endured so much that it takes little persuasion on the part of their surgeon to "get it all over with at once."

But "kindness" is not the only factor to be considered. First of all, as I explained in Chapter 8, presurgical staging technologies have become more reliable (and are getting better and better all the time) and can detect micrometastases that might be hiding in other organs. Scans, X-rays, and elaborate blood and urine studies cost money; there is also the question of needless exposure to radiation. So, obviously, staging every one of the 500,000 + women admitted for a breast biopsy every year, in the United States alone, is out of the question. Yet without these examinations, there are bound to be thousands of unnecessary mastectomies.

If the biopsy shows the lump is a harmless fibroadenoma or papilloma, the emotional trauma ends immediately; all the psychological pain is over . . . until the next months and years of BSE, watching, waiting, and worrying must begin. However, for those women who do have malignancies, there is no chance to get second opinions on their diagnoses nor do they have the vital time to investigate alternative treatments. This is why the NIH recommended that the diagnostic biopsy be separated from further treatment—to give women time. Unfortunately, however, the single-stage procedure is still the most common one used in this country today.

Even though the trauma of waiting for the diagnosis is avoided by those women who sign one-stage permission papers, they must still wait two or three days to learn about the status of their lymph nodes. Usually, the surgeon uses this waiting period to do the all-important staging scans and X-rays to determine the extent of disease, those examinations explained in Chapter 8 that should have been done *before* any mastectomy was even considered. As a result, some women will be told they already had metastatic disease in another organ and that their breasts were lost for no good reason. Chemotherapy must be started as soon as possible.

Some women will have negative axillary nodes and can breathe a sigh of relief as they look forward to reconstructive surgery. But if any trace of cancer has invaded the nodes, these women must also expect a year or so of adjuvant chemotherapy.

All of these women are still in the hospital, convalescing. Having suffered profoundly, none is yet "coping" with the loss of a breast or even "coping" with cancer, in the jargony "psychosocial" sense that has become so popular with health professionals.

While there are still thousands of surgeons in the United States who refuse to separate diagnosis from further treatment (and many women do want to "get it over with"), there has been considerable change since June 1979. As I said earlier, going this route means an extra period of emotional trauma for women— waiting for the permanent-section pathological diagnosis. But the advantages of being able to get second opinions on the diagnosis, look into alternative treatments, and, above all, be staged before a breast is perhaps removed unnecessarily would seem to outweigh this disadvantage by far.

For women whose surgeons believe in giving them a waiting period, the waiting and worrying scenario is identical to the one I've just described. Some will be told the mass was benign, after agonizing two or three days; some will have cancer and will then have to be staged while they wait to decide what to do next (but there will be no unnecessary mastectomies this time!); some will have mastectomies (all modifieds, by the way, for this scenario) and will learn they had either positive or negative nodes. But, they must usually wait for days or even as long as an anxious week for these results. For the women found to have malignancies in their axillas, adjuvant therapy is the next step; for the lucky ones with negative nodes, it is convalescence and contemplation of possible plastic surgery.

Again, all of this emotional trauma has happened *before* the patient has even had a moment to worry about the psychosocial problems of coping with life singlebreastedly.

Before going on, let us see what happens to women whose surgeons believe in trying aspiration biopsies before resorting to the scalpel. These are still uncommon in the United States, but the practice is catching on, especially in large medical centers. As hospital costs soar and as women begin to object to having numerous biopsy incisions, aspirations will undoubtedly be done more frequently.

So some surgeons will attempt to withdraw fluid from their patients' lumps with a fine needle. Or, if it is a solid tumor, they may be able to carve a specimen of tissue from it with a Tru-cut, wider-bore needle.

Some women will have fluid-filled cysts, hollow balls that collapse the instant they are punctured by the hypodermic needle in their surgeons' office—no hospital stay needed at all. Relieved immediately, they must nonetheless return to more years of BSE, waiting, watching, and worrying.

A few women will have suspicious-looking fluid, however, and specimens must be sent to cytologists for expert examination. Again, they are left waiting for the results of still another diagnostic test, but there are no sutures to remove or any incision to heal. Come what may, their only scars are almost invisible dots on the skin that soon will fade and disappear. Of this small group of women, some will learn the suspicious-looking fluid was clear of any unusual cells; others will be told their lumps' fluid contained "atypia"—cells that were abnormal and *might* be precursors or premalignant. All of these cytology reports bring women back where they began: BSE, waiting, watching, and worrying.

A few aspiration-biopsy results will show the presence of cancer, and these women must then wait for reports from laboratories, radiologists, and nuclear-medicine departments to find out if they are candidates for further treatment. As with the women who were biopsied surgically, a few will already have disseminated disease, so limited surgery to remove the entire tumor and chemo- or endocrine therapy will be prescribed for them. Most will not have any evidence of distant metastases, of course, and —like their sisters who had surgical biopsies followed by a waiting period—they will be faced with a vast array of available treatment options that must be investigated before they know enough to make a truly informed decision.

Should they have modified radical mastectomies to "be sure"?

Should they be trendy and opt for a lumpectomy and irradiation?

Would they really be playing Russian Roulette if they had only a lumpectomy and nothing more?

What about the axillary nodes—all or some?

How about entering a randomized trial where the decisions are made by a computer? This may seem far out . . . but is it? With so many unknowns and uncertainties, it might be a relief to let a superintelligent mechanical brain do the picking and choosing.

Many surgeons in Massachusetts and California, states that legally require them to explain all available alternatives to women after a diagnosis of breast cancer is confirmed, argue that few women are capable of coping with the probabilities, benefits, and risks of making their own treatment decision. This, plus the "kindness factor" I mentioned earlier, was and is the foundation of surgeons' requests that these laws be rescinded. So far, the legislatures have stood firm and have refused.

But surgeons may be right in saying that participating in treatment decisions adds to the enormous emotional burdens of breast-cancer patients, because they must cope with decisions the doctor would otherwise make for them. Some women, it's true, may not be capable of doing this.

And I did not even extend this scenario to include the complete menu of treatment options now available with their accompanying anxieties: less-than-mastectomy procedures, with and without irradiation of the preserved breast, with and without adjuvant therapy. I have also not mentioned the options of having a surgical biopsy under a local anesthetic, either as an in- or out-patient. To have done so would have made this scenario longer than a William Faulkner epic saga.

But I hope my point has been made. All of these women have yet to face the world "coping" with a singlebreasted life; none has yet gone through weeks of radiation or months of adjuvant therapy—each having its own set of emotional trials and tribulations. I only want to show the pain and anguish women endure *before* any primary treatment is completed. It's about time the medical/surgical establishment, the National Cancer Institute, and the American Cancer Society realize that more time, talent, energy, and money should be devoted toward helping women during this critical period. Coping with life after primary treatment is—for most women—far less traumatic than what we had to endure between the time we found that terrifying lump or thickening and its ultimate treatment.

10

Surgery: Toward Freedom of Choice

"A whole book about breast cancer? I don't believe it." I had just turned down her third party invitation. "What's there to say you haven't already said? You've written articles about the different operations. What in the world will you fill—"

"Surgery is just the beginning." I broke into her flood of questions. "It's nowhere near as important as—"

"Losing a breast isn't important?" she cried. "You must have forgotten what *you* went through, or you couldn't say that."

She was right. I had forgotten. In less than a year, I had forgotten my horror at being suddenly confronted by the prospect of losing a breast. The awesome, awful ordeal—the mammograms, the thermograms, the research into choices of surgery, the rush to Sloan-Kettering, and finally the flight to Buffalo, to Roswell Park. The pain of the surgery, the agony of that first moment naked and unbandaged before a mirror, stuffing cotton balls into bras, the first time Harvey saw the incision—how could I have forgotten so much so quickly?

But, as I wondered, my belly tightened and I felt the fingers of dread creep along my skin. No, I had not forgotten. Those clammy conditioned reflexes will probably be with me forever. But the mastectomy itself had become less important. By learning so much about breast cancer as a potentially fatal disease, I had put the surgery itself in its proper perspective—the beginning of treatment.

The blazing "breast-cancer controversy"—lumpectomy versus mastectomy, modified radical versus Halsted radical—is no longer the real burning issue of breast-cancer treatment in the

United States. As Ann Scott had said so poignantly in her televised interview, most women believe that the decision about surgery is the end of their problems. Afterward, they think, as soon as they have bought the "stupid prosthesis" and learned some cosmetic tricks, life goes back to normal. Few women realize that mastectomy simply marks the beginning of at least five years of intensive care and examination, five more years of close medical supervision, and a lifetime—a long and healthy one, it is hoped—of constant vigilance for signs of recurrence or metastasis.

I called my friend back to explain. "There are so many other things wrong about the way women with breast cancer are treated," I told her, "that the kind of surgery at the beginning doesn't seem as earth-shaking to me as it did."

Ann Scott was uppermost in my mind. "There's not enough good follow-up," I told her, giving details.

She remained quiet for such a long time that I thought we had been disconnected. Then she spoke. "It does make 'What kind of mastectomy?' sound like a huge tempest in a small teapot, doesn't it?" She forgave me for again missing her party.

Burning issue or not, some kind of surgery must be the first step in breast-cancer treatment. Here is a brief description of the possible alternatives, from the least to the most extensive.

1. **Lumpectomy (tylectomy, and local excision).** Essentially, a lumpectomy is an excisional biopsy. The entire lump is removed, along with a little surrounding tissue. Unless the tumor is very large, the breast involved should look the same as the other one afterward.

2. **Partial mastectomy (segmental resection, wide excision, and wedge resection).** The tumor and a considerable portion of the surrounding breast tissue are excised, along with overlying skin and underlying fascia. The axillary lymph nodes may also be removed, making this a "partial radical" mastectomy. The breast will be somewhat smaller, but still there.

Obviously, what the cosmetic results of these minimal procedures will be depend on the size of the tumor and the size of the breast it is in. A lumpectomy involving a large cancer in a small breast would look like a partial mastectomy; a small tumor taken from a large breast may cause only a slight dimple.

Breast Cancer was written before the dramatic effectiveness of adjuvant therapy was accepted in early 1976. The above procedures were described in it without telling the importance of removing at least a sampling of axillary lymph nodes for pathological examination. Even a cluster of a few microscopic invasive cells in the breast itself can—albeit rarely—spread to the nodes, and it is imperative that women in such a situation be given adjuvant therapy. So although the actual surgery done to the breast itself is "minimal," some nodes must be removed.

If the tumor was located near the axilla, these nodes can usually be excised through the same incision. However, if the cancer is far from the underarm area, a separate incision is usually required.

3. **Total (or simple) mastectomy.** Both terms describe the same operation, but the NCI is recommended that the word "total" be used. It is more precise surgical nomenclature and describes a specific procedure: removal of only the breast. Axillary nodes and pectoral muscles are left intact, although some women have a lymph node or two in the "tail of the breast," and these, of course, would be removed with the mammary tissue. If these "tail" nodes are malignant, the axilla may be irradiated or chemotherapy may be used. This procedure is usually reserved for elderly or unwell women who have medical problems that prohibit more extensive surgery. It may also be performed if a woman has evidence of metastatic disease, but has pain, an infection, or other local problems in the breast.

    Another situation where a total mastectomy is performed is one where a diagnosis of *in situ* noninvasive carcinoma or hyperplasia is found. As I will detail later in this chapter, whether or not these cells are true precursors of cancer ("premalignant") is now being hotly debated.

4. **Modified radical mastectomy (total mastectomy with axillary dissections).** All tissues of the breast and most of the axillary lymph nodes are removed. The pectoral muscles are left intact.

5. **Halsted radical mastectomy.** All tissues of the breast, the axillary lymph nodes, and the pectoral muscles are removed.

6. **Supraradical mastectomy or extended radical mastectomy.** The breast, axillary lymph nodes, pectoral muscles, and the internal mammary chain of nodes are removed. To get to these, sections of rib must be taken out as well. Some surgeons used to remove the supraclavicular nodes which are in the angle where the neck joins the shoulder. These procedures are rarely done today.

7. **Subcutaneous mastectomy.** A semicircular incision is made in the crease where the lower part of the breast meets the body

(an "inframammary" incision), and the skin and its underlying tissue—the nipple intact—is lifted up. All breast tissue is scooped out, and an implant is inserted to replace it. This procedure should not be done if cancer is present! It is being performed prophylactically to prevent breast cancer in high-risk women, and its use is highly controversial. More details are given in Chapter 13, where I discuss breast reconstruction—reconstructive mammoplasty.

In all of these procedures, the surgeon can excise and examine at least one or two of the axillary lymph nodes to see if the disease has spread beyond the breast. Although salesmen of various kinds of equipment claim a particular piece of apparatus can diagnose malignant nodes, none has yet proven to be as reliable as a pathologist's microscope. There is no way to know a breast-cancer patient's real physical condition without the "radical" part of a mastectomy—the removal of some or all of the axillary lymph nodes.

In September 1974, Dr. Bernard Fisher reported the results of an NSABP study, begun in 1971, involving 1,765 women. After three years, patients randomized into the group treated only by total mastectomy had the same recurrence and survival rates as those who had Halsted radical mastectomies or total mastectomies followed by irradiation of their lymph nodes. (These women have been monitored ever since 1971, and their comparative survival rates are still identical.) This was evidence that excising axillary nodes is not therapeutic and doesn't affect survival, although there are still surgeons who believe taking out all the nodes they can is "getting it all out." But the data clearly show that counting malignant nodes is a staging test to see if the disease has already spread beyond the breast. The NSABP statistics are evidence that invasion of the nodes per se is not a reason for their removal: the presence or absence of cancer in the axilla is a signal that micrometastases may be present elsewhere in the body. Because of this, adjuvant therapy of some kind must be started as soon after surgery as possible. What that adjuvant therapy should be depends on the woman's estrogen-receptor status, whether she is pre- or postmenopausal and her general physical conditions. Adjuvant, as well as drug therapies for advanced disease, are discussed in detail in Chapter 11.

What is the difference between the Halsted and the modified radical (or total mastectomy with axillary dissection) as far as the patient is concerned?

On paper, not much. On the body, however, there is an enormous difference. The Halsted operation "seems to have been designed to inflict the maximal possible deformity, disfiguration, and disability," according to Dr. George Crile. "The incision," he wrote in his book, *What Women Should Know About the Breast Cancer Controversy*, "extends nearly vertically up over the shoulder so that the scar is impossible to hide. The removal of the muscles of the chest wall cause a depression below the collarbone that cannot be concealed unless a high-necked dress is worn." Dr. Crile continues, in this gruesome vein, about "skin paper-thin," "sloughing of the skin," *ad infinitum*. For all the unnecessary ugliness and discomfort of the Halsted, the results of these two radicals—in terms of years—are about the same. (I must mention that many of the women I interviewed said their Halsteds were not as horrible as Dr. Crile painted them. A great deal of the cosmetics, apparently, depends on the surgeon.)

An American Cancer Society policy statement in 1974 declared that "recommendations for treatment of a breast cancer should be made by the physician" and that "the patient and selected members of the family should be thoroughly advised by the physician about the proposed surgery and its rationale; this being the essence of informed consent."

Nowhere did the policy statement hint that a woman might have opinions or desires different from those in the statement or from those "advised by the physician" or that she had the absolute right to decide for herself. While I chose to give up my breast and nodes to have a better chance of surviving longer, every woman—once told of the differences in risk—should be allowed to have a lumpectomy or anything else she wants, even if her surgeon or her husband or family disapproves.

One of my reasons for visiting European cancer centers was that I suspected breast-cancer surgery would not be as extensive in countries where more women were practicing medicine than in the United States. Also, I wanted to see if care was better under socialized medicine than under our fee-for-service system. Both hunches were right, but in reverse order of the importance I had given them. The "economic motive" had much more to do with the amount of surgery performed than did the number of women on the medical staff.

But having more women on hospital staffs did have an effect on the patients and on male doctors. It could not have been a coincidence, for example, that in late 1974, Moscow's oncology institute—where an all-female medical staff directed both breast-cancer research and treatment—was in its fourth year of clinical trials of partial mastectomies. Although Professor Sviatukhina thought radical mastectomy offered the best chance for a cure, she was nonetheless willing to do lesser surgeries on women who wanted them and whose tumors met certain criteria. Her male boss, Academician Professor Nikoli N. Blokhin, the director of the institute, had apparently given Professor Sviatukhina *carte blanche* to do as she saw fit.

At the Royal Infirmary in Edinburgh, the chief of the breast service was Professor Forrest, whose concern for his patients was as sensitive and sympathetic as any woman's could have been. (In staff conferences, he invariably asked about patients', husbands, children, and family problems as well as about their medical status.) Under his direction, the breast-service staff (three-fourths female) did no radical mastectomies at all. The practice was to do simple (or total) mastectomies, with irradiation of the nodes postoperatively if there was reason to think the cancer had spread beyond the breast. The results were as good as those from radical mastectomies where axillary nodes are surgically removed. Professor Forrest had used this treatment for seven years in Cardiff, Wales, before moving to Edinburgh, and those patients are still being followed. As it is now in most countries, ever since adjuvant therapy has become routine for node-positive women, a sampling of women's axillary nodes is now being excised to see if such treatment is necessary.

At Stockholm's Karolinska Institute, Dr. Westerberg, of the Breast Section (a two-thirds female staff), told me the custom there was to try to persuade reluctant women that radical mastectomy was best in terms of a possible cure. She smiled. "However, it is, after all, their bodies to do with as they see fit. If we do not succeed—and often we do not—we do as the patient wishes. Over the years, there have been quite a few young women who have had only the tumors removed, and most are doing well. While we do not advise it, we most certainly permit it."

The attitude at Royal Marsden and Guy's hospitals in London was the same.

On the other hand, in Leningrad's oncology institute, the chief of surgery, Professor Riurik Melnikov, was a staunch defender of the Halsted radical, and so were all the other men on his surgical staff. Their salaries were paid by the government, and they earned nothing extra for doing more extensive surgery. Professor Melnikov told me he had used the modified radical several years earlier but had poor results and returned to the Halsted. Naturally, his younger surgeons followed their chief's preference.

When comparing treatment, even in countries with nationalized medicine and many women doctors, however, another important variable has to be considered—stage of disease at the time of diagnosis. For example, when I visited Hungary in the summer of 1980, I went to the Oncology Institute high in the hills of the Buda side of Budapest. There, I was able to talk with Dr. Istvan Besneak, the chief of cancer surgery. Trained in the United States, Dr. Besneak frequently went to Western medical conferences and knew about the latest advances elsewhere.

"We have a very low incidence in most of Hungary," he told me, "perhaps because our country is primarily rural. Yet our mortality rate is quite high in relation to the rest of the world."

He shook his head. "Last year, there were only about 1,600 cases reported through our registries, and all came here for treatment. In Hungary, few women are diagnosed early enough to even consider minimal surgery for a moment. I wish I could, but most of my patients came to the Institute far too late. Ulcerated, painful, and infected breasts must be removed. There is no alternative; I wish I was able to get women with tumors smaller than the size of a walnut."

Dr. Besneak said he would certainly welcome the chance to do lumpectomies with or without irradiation, if Hungarian women came to him early enough to be candidates for such treatment.

"Women in our country are simply not as aware of the early symptoms," he said. "Until they come for treatment at earlier stages, the only surgery that offers any hope is mastectomy."

Could this kind of stage-at-diagnosis factor be responsible for variations of treatment between Moscow and Leningrad? When I was in the USSR in 1974, it had not occurred to me to ask Professor Sviatukhina what the criteria were to be eligible for lumpectomy in Moscow. Did women go to an all-female breast department earlier? Was there more emphasis on early-detection in Moscow, because its oncology institute had more women on its breast-cancer staff?

I wish I had known enough to ask these questions, because I may never have another chance.

From everything I learned, it appears that different pathological types of breast cancer could be treated differently. For example, Japanese women—who have low breast-cancer incidences—also have relatively "benign" cell types like medullary, tubular, and comedo carcinomas. Such slow-growing, sluggish cancers could probably be treated with minimal surgery as effectively as with mastectomies of one kind or another. Yet I did not meet one surgeon in any of the major cities of Tokyo, Osaka, Kyoto, or Nagoya who would consider doing less.

Nor did I meet one female surgeon in Japan, although I met

several women active in laboratory research into various aspects of the disease.

In 1974, however, even where women predominated on breast-cancer staffs, some kind of mastectomy was the preferred operation in all of the countries I visited. (Unfortunately, I did not go—and have not yet gone—to France, where radiotherapy has been a primary treatment almost since the discovery of radium by Madame Marie Curie.) The feminine impact was seen primarily in more interest in trying lesser operations where tumors were small and no palpable nodes were present. Women doctors also have more empathy with the emotional problems a woman faces at such a time. Having a physician who can empathize and sympathize with breast amputation, because they too have breasts must be exceedingly supportive, emotionally. Decisions must be made, benefit-risk ratios weighed, and having a knowledgeable, understanding woman to explain and answer questions cannot help but benefit women facing the loss of a breast.

What does the American Cancer Society say about the different surgical treatments of breast cancer?

In 1974, the ACS, a conservative organization that moves with the speed of a senile snail, had issued a policy statement clarifying its stand on the question. "Pending clear proof," the statement said, "that equally good results can be achieved by limited procedures less than mastectomy, the American Cancer Society believes the public should not be misled into accepting less proven methods." These "proven methods," according to the announcement were the Halsted radical and the extended (or supraradical) mastectomies. The Society also gave its approval, albeit with words indicating some reluctance, to the modified radical.

Anything less—lumpectomy or segmental surgery—was playing Russian Roulette.

But the American Cancer Society is now changing. Although no new policy statement has been officially issued, subtle movement can be seen in the ACS' point of view about the treatment of breast cancer. At its annual Science Writers' Seminar, held in Daytona Beach, Florida in March 1981, the ACS gave definite support to the many clinical trials now being carried out all over the country to compare radical mastectomy with lesser surgery, with and without postsurgical irradiation. Medical writers attending the Seminar interpreted this as a major shift from previous ACS support of extensive surgery.

This statement was, in my opinion, a "delayed reaction" to the 1979 NIH Conference. As I related in Chapter 8, this Conference marked the official funeral of the Halsted radical mastectomy.

The panel also recommended that there be a separation between the diagnostic biopsy and further treatment, both for the sake of the patient and to permit continuing research to compare any mastectomy at all with segmental procedures with and without irradiation of the breast. While the ACS' change of heart did not mention the two-stage procedure, this is implicit in any mention of a comparative clinical trial. If women are to have their breasts removed automatically as soon as a pathologist breathes a diagnosis of cancer, there would be no chance for them to even consider another alternative.

Actually, even the NIH's recommendation was a "delayed reaction" in terms of other countries' treatments. Segmental surgery followed by irradiation has been the rule, rather than the exception, in France for early breast cancer for decades. And, as Dr. Bernard Pierquin told the June 5 Conference, surgeons there do not always do a "tumorectomy" at all. They merely do an incisional biopsy to get a definite diagnosis from the pathologist and—if it is cancer—the radiation therapy is begun immediately. The rest of the tumor is not even removed. While this sounds risky and reckless, the proof of the pudding is that while France and the United States have almost identical overall incidence rates, breast-cancer mortality rates in this country have been considerably higher for years, according to the American Cancer Society's own mortality table, "Cancer Around the World."

This is not the only example of the considerable variations of the treatment of breast cancer—all of them having no apparent impact on mortality. For example, more than thirty-five years ago, Professor Sakari Mustakallio, a Finnish radiologist, began removing the breast but leaving the lymph nodes, using irradiation to destroy any suspicious ones. Occasionally, if the tumor was very small, he removed only the growth. After twenty-five years of these conservative procedures, Professor Mustakallio analyzed his results and found no difference between them and those of the various radical surgeries.

In 1948 Dr. Robert McWhirter had begun doing the same kind of nonradical mastectomy with irradiation at Edinburgh's Royal Infirmary with the same results: no significant difference in either the five-year or the ten-year survival rates. Then, in Cardiff, Wales, Professor Forrest began his clinical trials with simple (or total) mastectomy plus irradiation, the treatment he is continuing at the Royal Infirmary in Edinburgh.

Dr. Maureen Roberts explained the Royal Infirmary practice. "When the breast is removed, one node—the one that is in the tail of the breast, closest to the axilla—is removed and examined by serial dissection." This, she said, means that the entire node is sliced and examined, instead of only a sliver or two. "If that node is negative," she continued, "the patient is discharged and nothing more is done. However, if the node has a carcinoma, she is given X-ray therapy. Our results have been equal to or perhaps a bit better than at hospitals where radical surgery is the rule."

Of course, this was in 1974, before adjuvant therapy made it imperative that axillary nodes be examined and not destroyed by X-ray.

At the Karolinska Institute in Stockholm, just across the North Sea, Dr. Westerberg must have had some advance information in 1974. Just as earnestly as Dr. Roberts argued for irradiation of the axillary nodes instead of surgery, she believed they had to be removed.

"It is absolutely necessary," she insisted. "The reason is really quite simple. The nodes must be examined to know if the disease has spread and, if so, how far. Future treatment depends on having this knowledge, and there is no way to be certain unless at least twenty or twenty-five are removed and studied."

Nodes are not invaded by cancer in any particular sequence, she explained. There are "skipped nodes" and "transverse nodes" and other ways for cancer to by-pass the one or two in the tail of the breast. "It's quite possible that the nodes removed and studied would be free of disease, while others were malignant," she said. "One or two nodes are not enough."

The controversy about the number of nodes that must be removed is still far from resolved. Data pro and con keep pouring out of cancer hospitals all over the world. When I first learned about this medical argument, the conflict made no sense. "Who cares about them?" I asked Dr. Bernard Fisher, one of the National Cancer Institute's consultants, at a press conference. "The nodes are invisible. The important parts are the breast itself, first of all, and then the pectoral muscles, second."

Then I learned one good medical reason for the concern about removing as few nodes as possible. I met a woman with "milk arm"—lymphedema.

This serious complication of an axillary dissection is due to two factors. When removing the nodes *en bloc*—in a continuous section—the surgeon must also cut out the lymphatic vessels connecting them if the axilla is to be thoroughly cleared. In addition, other, uninvolved lymphatic vessels in the regions must be severed. The degree of circulatory damage resulting from this operation can be limited if the surgeon is especially skilled and well-trained. Otherwise, the loss of the vessels that channel lymphatic fluid from the hand are blocked. With nowhere to go, the fluid fills the vessels of the arm, causing the swelling and pain.

One woman I met was so grotesquely misshapen she did not want to show me her arm. Confined to long sleeves forever, she also suffers from a twisting, grinding pain that has persisted long after her mastectomy.

I have since learned from hundreds of letters and telephone calls to the Breast Cancer Advisory Center that radiation therapy also may cause lymphedema, and even small samplings of axillary nodes often damage enough lymphatic vessels to contribute to women's developing milkarm. For these reasons, getting rid of the Halsted radical mastectomy and replacing it with segmental surgery and axillary samplings followed by irradiation may *not* eliminate the incidence of lymphedema at all. As a matter of fact, lesser surgery with irradiation done by radiotherapists not specially trained to treat breast cancer may actually result in more cases. The problem is serious enough to have included a section on hand-care in Chapter 14.

Before discussing breast-cancer surgery any further, it is important to explain a term—clinical trials (CTs)—that I have used and will often use again. The words also appear frequently in newspaper, television, and radio accounts of new drugs and surgical treatments. Usually, however, no explanation is given to tell the meaning of a clinical trial.

Essentially, it is a scientific method to compare various technologies and treatments (medical and surgical) by case-matching large numbers of people who have a particular problem. Patients are assigned, at random, to different groups—each treated (in the case of medications or surgical procedures) in a different way. Generally, one group (the "control") will get something that has been accepted as "standard." However, when drugs are compared, the control-group may be given a placebo, a "drug" by mouth or injection that is made of a useless substance. Depending on the number of comparisons to be made, the second, third, or fourth group receives a different treatment that has already been tested for safety and effectiveness in small groups of humans or in animals.

"This is the age of clinical trials," *Science* magazine reported in an article about an NIH conference held on October 3-4, 1977. "They are not only coming into increasing use but they are becoming increasingly sophisticated, increasingly costly, and many now involve enormous numbers of participants."

According to *Science,* clinical trials were also controversial.

"A decision to start a large-scale clinical trial is a decision to commit a great deal of money and effort over a long period of time—often as long as a decade—in the hope of deciding whether a treatment or preventive measure is worthwhile . . . ," the article said.

Although critics usually acknowledge the statistical sense and speed of evaluating different drugs and procedures by well-designed and well-controlled clinical trials, they argue that all CTs are neither well-designed nor at all controlled.

Dr. Emil Freireich, a biostatistician at the M. D. Anderson Cancer Center in Houston, is one of the most vocal opponents of large-scale clinical trials.

"As soon as a patient or doctor agrees to participate in a trial," he told me, "true randomization flies out of the window, because they are already 'self selected.' The only way to really have a randomized trial is to force Patient A to be in one group and Patient B to be in another. Dr. A and Dr. B must use specific, assigned treatments for these patients, no matter what. If a patient reads an informed-consent letter and refuses to sign it, that trial includes only people who agreed to sign it. And if a doctor refuses to use a certain drug or do a certain operation, because he or she doesn't think it's appropriate for a specific case, the trial includes only doctors who agree to put patients into the next slot—whatever it may be.

"That," he said, "automatically destroys the concept of randomization."

The reason I go into such detail about the controversy swirling around the value of randomized clinical trials is that we women are its victims. While the doctors argue, we must sit back and wait for their results to learn whether or not a mastectomy is ever necessary. Is segmental surgery—with or without irradiation of the preserved breast—all that needs to be done to treat early breast cancer? Or any stage of the disease?

Dr. Bernard Fisher and the members of the NCI's NSABP firmly believe there is no other way to get the answers to these questions. In a paper published in 1978, he wrote:

"One of the major medical advances of our time has been the introduction of the prospective randomized clinical trial as a mechanism for clinical problem solving. It provides the ultimate opportunity to obtain answers to biological questions of importance which can be gotten in no other way."

A "prospective" clinical trial uses "contemporary" controls. This means that procedures done in the past, with archaic techniques and antiquated equipment in the years before sophisticated devices permitted women to be diagnosed earlier, are ignored. Instead, new patients are randomized either by a computer or on an A, B, C, odds-or-even, or 1, 2, 3 basis.

Dr. Dao is one of the thousands of surgeons who refuses to randomize women in his surgical trials, because like Dr. Freireich, he believes there is no such thing as true randomization.

"As soon as a woman even decides to go to see a doctor," he insists, "she is no longer randomized. She is part of a group that is seeking treatment. Who knows how many women select themselves to obtain no treatment at all? From the moment a woman picks up the telephone for her first appointment, she is not part of a random sample."

Again like thousands of other surgeons, Dr. Dao also does not want to randomize *himself*.

"I do not want to be forced by any protocol to perform a procedure I do not think is safe," he explained. "For example, I do local excisions with axillary dissections in selected cases, but I do not think irradiating the breast afterward is necessary. In my opinion, the importance of multicentricity has been overdone, and I am more afraid of the possible dangers of large doses of X-ray than of the relatively small risk of having another cancer growing somewhere else in the breast."

If he were a participant in one of the NCI's clinical trials, he said, some of the women would have to be randomized into sections requiring postsurgical irradiation. For this reason, he has steadfastly refused to be involved in any of the randomized clinical trials.

At another end of the treatment spectrum, radiation therapists, like Dr. Samuel Hellman of the Joint Center for Radiation Therapy in Boston and Dr. Robert Goodman at the University of Pennsylvania Medical School, also reject participation in clinical trials. They and their radiotherapy colleagues believe expertly done irradiation of the breast after the removal of the tumor is equivalent to a mastectomy and refuse to be a part of any study where women must be randomized into a section where their breasts will be amputated.

In March 1981, I spoke at a meeting held in the Fox Chase Cancer Center in Philadelphia, and Dr. Goodman was also on the program. He told the audience of social workers, "I don't see any justification for my being involved in any study where one group of women will have their breasts cut off." I've also heard him say this before groups of physicians and surgeons in other cities; Dr.

Samuel Hellman and other radiation therapists, who feel the same way, have also said this publicly.

These breast-cancer experts who reject randomized clinical trials are not alone. Dr. Fisher is often chagrined—and more often, angry—about "doctors who know what the right treatment is." He readily confesses his own ignorance and wonders aloud how so many of his colleagues can be certain they know the answers without sufficient supporting data. He made his position clear in the introductory paragraph of the paper I cited earlier:

> "Despite these virtues (of randomized clinical trials), the vast majority of surgeons in this country have failed to become involved in or support clinical trials for a variety of unconvincing reasons, thus impairing the rapid and orderly attainment of definitive information so necessary to . . . the care of many thousands of patients."

We women are the patients or would-be patients he is referring to, and this is why I called us the "victims" of the clinical-trial controversy. The NSABP study (Protocol B-06) is divided into three sections. In one, the women have total mastectomies with axillary dissections (the procedure known in the past as the modified radical mastectomy). Women in the second section have segmental surgery (the tumor and a margin of healthy tissue) and axillary dissections, followed by irradiation. If malignant nodes are found, adjuvant therapy is given. Those patients randomized into the third section will be treated by segmental surgery and axillary dissections *without* irradiation. Again, node-positive women receive adjuvant therapy.

Protocol B-06 has been trying to accrue 2,000 women since June 1976, and there are more participating surgeons in Canada than there are in the United States. Incredible as it seems, by the time Protocol B-06 was five years old, fewer than 1,000 women had been recruited in both the United States and Canada.

Another NCI-sponsored clinical trial is underway at the Clinical Center of the NIH itself in Bethesda, Maryland. This study began in April 1979 and requires only 300 women to yield those "statistically significant" results. Unlike the NSABP study, this one has only two groups: half of the women will have total mastectomies and axillary dissections *plus* reconstruction as soon as the operation can be done. The second group is treated by lumpectomy (less tissue is lost than in segmental surgery) followed by irradiation of the breast. The immediate area where the tumor was located is given a "booster" of radiation by way of radioactive implants to destroy any residual cells that might have been left behind. Treatment, travel and living expenses as well as long-term follow-up care are free.

More than two years after the study's birth, only about sixty-six women had been recruited, even though Montgomery County, Maryland—where the NIH is located—has one of the highest breast-cancer incidence rates in the country. (This NCI study is open to all residents of the United States. I mention Montgomery County only because the required 300 patients could have been obtained locally, and long ago, if surgeons there would cooperate.)

This is the surgical dilemma we women are facing; the year 2000 will have come and gone, and we will still not know whether or not breasts must be amputated to treat breast cancer.

But we cannot blame the absence of data entirely on doctors, because women also do not want to be randomized. Even though we may know intellectually that there is no "best," most women rebel at the idea of having our treatment chosen by a computer. (I must stress, however, that many women have told me they are so bewildered by the many permutations and combinations of today's treatment options that they actually welcome having an electronic brain make their decisions.)

To me, the requirement for randomization is difficult to understand, because I agree with both Dr. Dao and Dr. Freireich: as soon as a woman makes up her mind to see a doctor, she is already "self-selected." Besides, I know many surgeons (and chemotherapists) participating in so-called controlled clinical trials who, for various reasons, decide a particular patient should not be put into the next available "slot." Instead, they give her whatever treatment they think is appropriate for her situation "outside of the protocol." I am no statistician, but it seems as if such "cheating" must do something to affect a clinical trial's results. Is randomization really necessary? Obviously, doctors' refusal to randomize and women's refusal to be randomized is responsible for the absence of those critical data.

One factor in the clinical-trial controversy I have not mentioned concerns the use of "historical controls" rather than "contemporary controls." Many scientists believe a new drug or procedure can be evaluated by using past records of patients who have been matched for (in the case of breast cancer) age, size, and location of the tumor, stage of disease, etc.

Dr. Allen Lichter, the radiation therapist in the NCI trial, believes this is impossible. "There have just been too many changes," he explained. "Mammography can now pick up microscopic cancers that could never have been found ten years ago. We have better treatment, women are more aware . . .

"There's just no way to use old records; we've got to use 'contemporary controls' so the comparisons are made using today's technology."

In *Breast Cancer*, I anticipated the clinical-trial problem, writing:

"Such trials must certainly be held some time soon . . . but who would do them? And how many women, apprised of the relative risks of radical mastectomy, which are known, and of partial mastectomy or lumpectomy, whose risks are a total blank, would give their informed consent for the so-called lesser surgery?"

I followed this question of mine with one I had frequently been asked by surgeons: "How, in good conscience as a physician, can I randomly assign a woman to be treated by a technique that is unproven and could be very dangerous? There is, after all, a time-tested alternative—radical mastectomy."

Little has apparently changed since then, except that the "time-tested alternative" is no longer the Halsted. The clinical-trial dilemma is still with us, and we women share the blame for not entering trials.

Earlier, when I described the various kinds of breast cancer, I mentioned the rare inflammatory carcinoma, a disease whose symptoms are swelling, intense pain, and redness. Many doctors consider this to be inoperable because it is so widespread throughout the lymphatic system. However, I have found references to several cases of inflammatory carcinoma in which the breast was treated with irradiation or drugs, which alleviated the symptoms enough to make mastectomy possible. None of the women had lived very long after the surgery, but they did gain a few comfortable years. Any woman with any kind of "inoperable" breast cancer—any person with cancer—ought to be given the chance to opt for some extra time on earth. Freedom of choice does not apply only to the *kind* of surgery, but to the right to have surgery at all. When doctors automatically pronounce someone "inoperable," they are playing God. And they do play God too often.

Not long ago, many surgeons would not perform a mastectomy on a woman under thirty. According to statistics going back to 1851, young women had shorter survival rates after mastectomy than older ones, so why operate? This do-nothing attitude persisted for decades. In 1958, a controlled study was finally done of

550 women under thirty on whom mastectomies had been performed. Some differences were found that made their cancers more lethal, but many of them did live a long time after surgery. Fortunately, since then surgeons have been giving young women their fair chance at life.

For decades, surgeons refused to operate on women during pregnancy or while they were nursing. Breast cancers are so well fed by hormones at those times, the argument ran, that the pregnant woman would probably die before her baby was born. Another reason for declaring these women "inoperable," Dr. Dao told me, was that the extended radical, or supraradical, mastectomies done routinely in the past were so "formidable" as to make the surgery itself too dangerous to consider. Sometimes, with an early pregnancy, abortion was recommended instead, in the hope that a sudden reduction in the hormone level would stop the cancer's fast growth. It was found, however, that an abortion, without mastectomy, made no difference.

But the problem had never been studied experimentally. Then mammary carcinomas were induced in mice, half of which were impregnated, half not, and mastectomies were performed on all of them. While the over-all survival rates of the pregnant mice were lower, some of them lived long enough after surgery to show that mastectomies are worth doing during pregnancy. As a matter of fact, some of the experimental animals lived to a ripe old mouse age. Most breast-cancer specialists now treat pregnant and lactating women exactly as they treat all their patients.

Many surgeons also feel that an elderly woman should not undergo a mastectomy, especially a radical. Some only irradiate the breast and axilla; others remove just the breast and irradiate the nodes. Here again, I think the woman should make the decision herself.

Curiously, while surgeons in the United States seem to have no qualms about declaring certain patients "inoperable," in other cases they do mastectomies when the surgery is clearly useless—when the cancers have already metastasized to other organs. As Dr. Roberts, in Edinburgh, stated so emphatically, "If a cancer is found to be metastasized during the preoperative staging examinations, the woman should be put on chemotherapy immediately and no mastectomy should be permitted at all. There is *absolutely* no medical justification for these procedures." In 1974 these were the only unnecessary mastectomies I found in my months of research.

Mammography has changed all of that, because it is so supersensitive it can find abnormal and atypical cells that *may*, someday, become malignant. This has led to unnecessary surgery.

Of course, there are atypical cells everywhere. In the brain or in deep-seated organs like the liver, pancreas, and ovary, they are never observed unless they do become malignant. In organs like the cervix, mouth, and lower intestine, the cells can be easily seen. Because doctors can keep abnormal cells under constant observation in these latter organs (and have no way of knowing about them in the first group), surgeons are not so quick to remove them unless an invasive cancer is actually diagnosed.

With atypical breast cells, it is a different story. When a mammogram shows something abnormal and a surgical biopsy is done, everyone (including the patient) is afraid to risk doing nothing more than the biopsy, just in case . . . The most common of these questionable "cancers" is named lobular carcinoma *in situ*.

I first stumbled across this non-cancerous carcinoma in 1977 when the report of the BCDDPs showed that several hundred women were treated with some kind of mastectomy because their biopsies had this diagnosis (although these were not related to the "66 benigns" that received so much publicity). Who would think that anything with the awful word "carcinoma" in its name was not lethal? Yet some cancer experts refuse to call this non-invasive growth "carcinoma" at all. Instead, they have named it "lobular neoplasia."

Dr. John Bailar, the NCI hero who blew the whistle on the excesses of the BCDDPs was the person who explained that these were probably just as nonmalignant as the masses that had actually been found to be benign.

"Sometimes ductal carcinomas *in situ* may become invasive in time," he told me, "even though that's rare. The Latin words *'in situ'* literally mean 'in place.' By definition, these cells shouldn't invade, and so a true lobular carcinoma *in situ,* or LCIS, should never invade. There are two characteristics that all cancers must have: they contribute nothing whatsoever to the body's functioning and they invade healthy cells to make them malignant too. If abnormal cells don't have these two characteristics, they are not really cancer. As a matter of fact, if malignant axillary nodes are found after a diagnosis of LCIS, the mass was usually misdiagnosed by the pathologist."

When I read the report of the Commission on Cancer of the American College of Surgeons in May 1979 to prepare my testimony for the 1979 Conference, Dr. Bailar's comments came back to me loud and clear.

According to the final report, published in February 1979, 462 *in situ* carcinomas had been found among the 24,136 cases studied. No lumpectomies were reported. About 58 women (12.6%)

had wedge excisions, while 192 women (41.6%) were treated by total (or simple) mastectomies—removal of the breast with or without a sampling of the axillary lymph nodes.

In spite of the fact that lobular carcinoma *in situ* never invades, 202 women—almost half of all so diagnosed in the survey—were treated by some type of radical mastectomy.

Lobular carcinoma *in situ* accounted for about 2% of the diagnoses, but there is no way to really know how many of these "cancers" are present in women's breasts. They are always microscopic—cannot be felt—and are discovered coincidentally when another mass is biopsied. Only rarely, if ever, do they show up on a mammogram. However, based on studies of breasts removed for invasive cancer and on examinations of women autopsied due to deaths from other causes, pathologists guess that non-invasive "cancers" like lobular carcimoma *in situ* make up about 4-5% of growths found in the breasts of American women.

In the past, lobular carcinoma *in situ* of the breast was not the surgical dilemma it is today. Microscopic clusters of any atypical cells were never discovered unless they grew to the size where they could be felt. But now that mammography is being used, lesions too small to be palpable can easily be seen, and while lobular carcinoma *in situ* does itself not appear, the others do. If these should be invasive cancer, there is no dilemma: something must be done to treat the malignancy, and the *in situ* is dealt with at the same time. But what should be done about lobular carcinomas *in situ* that accompany cysts, fibroadenomas, papillomas, or other benign growth has become the subject of much controversy.

By the end of a 1980 conference on this issue at the NCI, it was agreed that there are actually four types of "minimal" breast cancers:

1. Lobular carcinoma *in situ* —cells that are always microscopic, non-invasive, and found with another benign or malignant mass;

2. Intraductal (within a milk duct) carcinoma *in situ* —cells that are visible on mammography and which may or may not invade other tissues;

3. Invasive clusters of real cancer smaller than 0.5 centimeters (about a quarter-inch), tumors that—in spite of being tiny—may already have spread to the axillary lymph nodes;

4. Hyperplastic or overly large, atypical cells that, in experimental mice, if untreated, are frequently the beginning of a "continuum" to become invasive.

Now that mammography and other early-detection techniques are discovering growths that cannot be felt, more and more of these atypical and non-invasive lesions are going to be diagnosed. What are women to do when faced with this "doctor's dilemma"?

Some women may decide to take the safe route of 100% cure and choose to have a radical mastectomy, but others may want to keep both of their breasts and live with some uncertainty for 10 or 20 years, should a second cancer develop. For these women, the solution is to find a breast-cancer expert who believes that local excision and frequent follow-up are all that is needed.

When a "minimal breast cancer" is diagnosed, it is apparently *not* like being a little bit pregnant, and women need all the information and help they can get.

At the end of all my research and interviews, I was suddenly hit with a devastating thought. All surgical innovations—including those of Drs. Crile, Hellman, Goodman, Fisher, Veronesi, Lichter, etc., always use radical mastectomy as the yardstick for measuring "success." To be as good as, or even better than, the radical is the goal—from Professor Mustakallio in Finland in the 1940s right up to the experts at the National Cancer Institute today. It seems as if the results of radical mastectomy were spectacular to make it the criterion all other procedures are measured against. Unfortunately, the overall survival rates of radical mastectomy are far from spectacular: a fifty-fifty chance of living longer than ten years after surgery.

I remember the precise moment when the thought chilled me. I was standing in the air terminal in Edinburgh with Professor Thomas Symington of London's Chester Beatty Research Institute. We were waiting for the shuttle flight back to London when I turned to him, shaken.

"Isn't anyone looking for something with *better* results than we have from radical mastectomies?"

He seemed stunned by my question and pondered it a few minutes before answering.

"It's probably that surgery has gone as far as it can, my dear," he said softly. "The place to look for an end to breast-cancer death is not to the scalpel."

It was a sobering idea that put all the controversies about "What kind of surgery?" into proper perspective.

The treatment of breast cancer with the knife has gone as far as it can go.

11

When Surgery Is Not Enough: Chemotherapy, Anti-Estrogens, and Hormones

HISTORY

About fifteen years ago, a friend of mine was diagnosed to have breast cancer. She went through the usual general-hospital routine of mastectomy, ovariectomy, and weeks of intensive X-ray treatment. For almost three years, she managed to hang onto life, although she had to go through periodic, increasingly frequent stays in the hospital for "shots of cobalt."

One night, Harvey and I met a mutual friend at a business meeting.

"How's Lil?" I asked. "She sounded so bad the last time I talked to her that I've been afraid to call again."

He shook his head sadly. "She's back in the hospital. They've put her on chemotherapy. That's the last resort."

Harvey and I nodded. "When they start using drugs," Harvey said, "I guess that's the end of the line."

Less than two decades ago, chemotherapy was the "last resort" for breast-cancer patients—the "end of the line" in general hospitals in the United States. We have come a long way in the years since then. Now, when examination of the axillary nodes shows the cancer has spread or if a recurrence appears, chemotherapy is the first resort—even in community hospitals, by community physicians.

As I detailed earlier, ancient medicine-men used "drugs" of all kinds—especially caustics—to fight cancer, but their use was discarded in favor of surgery when anesthetics were developed in the early 1800s. Then, after X-ray was discovered, this agent was added to the scalpel. Drugs were simply dropped from the arsenal of anti-cancer weapons for a few decades.

Dr. Paul Ehrlich, inventor of the "magic bullet" against syphilis, was the scientist who opened the first door to modern cancer chemotherapy. In 1910, he proved that alkylating agents could destroy cancer cells. He thought carcinoma was caused by invaders like infectious organisms, and he tried to kill them in the same way—as if they were microbes that lived separately outside healthy cells. Without the technical know-how provided by the electron microscope and decades of basic research into the biology of malignant cells, it was impossible for him to know that this theory was wrong.

The first "drugs" used to fight breast cancer were estrogens, but it was a negative use of the female hormones: women's estrogen factories, their ovaries, were removed surgically. Of course, ovariectomy (or oophorectomy) was not considered "chemotherapy," and it still is not by most doctors and patients. Yet decreasing the level of estrogens by removing their producers is as much "chemotherapy" as giving a drug like androgen, a male hormone to counter the female hormones in the blood stream.

It might be said, therefore, the age of chemotherapy for breast cancer began in 1896, when Sir George Beatson discovered that removing ovaries sometimes retarded or even regressed the progress of the disease. This operation became a routine postmastectomy procedure, but it was done empirically—no one knew why it worked. The results were unpredictable: some women improved; some did not.

The work done by the University of Chicago's Dr. Charles Huggins, a 1966 Nobel Laureate in medicine, provided the first clue explaining the unpredictability. He wondered why some young women whose ovaries had been removed still had enough circulating estrogens in their bodies to continue to have menstrual periods. Huggins' research showed that the adrenal glands also produced female hormones, and he suggested these too be removed (adrenalectomy) in breast-cancer patients who developed recurrences or metastases.

As the years passed, it was found that many women did not respond at all to any surgical estrogen manipulation. The theory—now a known fact—evolved that not all breast cancers are stimulated by estrogens, that is, not all are hormone-dependent. Therefore, only tumors that are definitely dependent on estrogens for growth are affected by the removal of ovaries and/or adrenal glands. But surgeons had no way of knowing what kind of tumor a woman had, and most of them routinely performed ovariectomies on all premenopausal women immediately after radical mastectomy if positive axillary nodes were found. After Dr. Huggins proved the adrenal glands also manufacture estrogens, surgeons began to do prophylactic adrenalectomies on postmenopausal women with positive nodes to try to prevent recurrences and to slow the growth of metastases.

Often, however, even ovariectomy plus adrenalectomy did not reduce estrogen levels in the bloodstream to zero. The pituitary gland, deep inside the brain, continued to release another hormone, prolactin, which, in the presence of estrogens, scientists knew was important to the growth and nourishment of a breast cancer. But, at that time, they did not understand how or why. This hormone is always present in a woman's body and is secreted in large quantities after childbirth to trigger milk production. Yet lactating women, even with these elevated prolactin levels, rarely develop breast cancer. Nonetheless, the pituitary gland was blamed for contributing to the development and growth of a breast cancer, and—until scientists discovered that every cell in a woman's body secretes small quantities of estrogen, the "extraglandular" process, described in Chapter 4—many experts felt that the pituitary gland should be removed in an operation called a hypophysectomy. Because this is major cranial surgery, however, and poses a considerable risk, it was never done by ordinary general surgeons. The most obvious alternative was to prescribe androgens in the hope that they would counteract the effects of any estrogens secreted by any gland. These various endocrine manipulations—surgical and medical—helped about half of all breast-cancer patients in some way.

Let me repeat again, the surgical procedures listed here are in this chapter on chemotherapy because any "ablative" operation that stops secretion of a substance performs the same function as giving a medication that, somehow, cancels out the effects of that substance in the body. This is why the term "endocrine" or "hormonal" manipulation is used—it covers both medical and surgical methods for eliminating (in the case of breast cancer) the effects of estrogens.

By the middle of the twentieth century, then, scientists knew that—while hormonal manipulation improved about one-third of all breast-cancer patients—it was totally useless in another one-third. The remaining third responded unpredictably, and there was no way to know which woman was in which group.

By the early 1950s, breast-cancer experts began to question routine prophylactic oophorectomy, because the results were so poor. In 1961, the National Cancer Institute (through the National Surgical Adjuvant Breast Project) began a study following more than 300 women whose surgeons had removed their ovaries at random. At the end of thirty-six months, the data showed no difference in the number of recurrences or in the mortality statistics between the two groups. Dr. Bernard Fisher, chairman of the NSABP, concluded that ". . . there is no clear-cut circumstance in which the use of oophorectomy is indicated as an adjunct to the primary treatment of what is today considered to be operable breast cancer."

However, he continued, "The worth of oophorectomy as a therapy in advanced cancers cannot be denied, (because there is) a remission rate of 25-30 percent when ovaries are removed, if a recurrence should develop in premenopausal women."

As a result of this study (duplicated elsewhere with the same conclusion), prophylactic oophorectomy was abandoned, and the surgery was reserved for women who developed second cancers. Done after a recurrence appeared, doctors reasoned, if the second cancer regressed, this would be a sign that the tumor was hormone-dependent and that the patient would probably benefit from adrenalectomy as well. However, if there was no improvement, removing the adrenal glands would do her no good.

On the basis of trial-and-error, many scientists concluded that all breast cancers are hormone-dependent to a greater or lesser degree when the tumors (*not* the patients) are young and that some kind of endocrine manipulation should help every woman with early breast cancer. This view was never widely accepted, however, and treatment of high-risk women with positive axillary nodes as well as of women with metastatic disease continued to be ad lib until the 1970s.

Everything was tried. Some women improved when they were given additional estrogens; some became worse. Other women responded to hormones like cortisone or prednisone; still others to male hormones. The helter-skelter and contradictory effects of various steroids on breast cancer in pre- and postmenopausal women became evidence for the case arguing that there are actually two different kinds of breast cancer, depending on the age of the woman.

As time went by, even women who improved after ovariectomy or any other kind of endocrine manipulation eventually reached a point where their cancers grew at about the same rate as those in women who did not have surgery or any other hormonal treatment. Such clinical findings, plus laboratory data from animal experiments, showed that all breast cancers eventually become autonomous—hormone-independent. With this information, breast-cancer specialists realized that even when tumors were strongly hormone-dependent, endocrine manipulation was not enough, and the search for "something else" continued. Basing their experiments on Dr. Ehrlich's original ideas about alkylating agents, pharmacologists tested drug after drug, hoping to find one that would destroy malignant cells with minimal side effects.

The major discovery grew, as I have said, out of war and the development of nitrogen mustard as a biological-warfare weapon. In 1946, scientists discovered that mustards shrank cancerous tumors in mice. Then, in 1948 it was found that leukemia victims were helped by the first of the antimetabolites—aminopterine. Using this as a precedent, some specialists began to try drugs for breast cancer—but only as a last resort when all else failed. And the "all else," just a few decades ago, was radical mastectomy, oophorectomy, adrenalectomy, X-ray (usually cobalt), and, in certain instances, both male and female hormones. Hormonal treatment alone was still trial-and-error, because there was no way to know which of the women would be helped.

Everything on earth has probably been tested at one time or another for its effect on cancer. Certainly, few substances from plants and even from marine life have not been used on experimental animals to see if they can destroy the cancer without also killing the hosts. Unfortunately, most that are effective are so lethal they fail this critical test. Going back to the analogy of cancer and the war in Vietnam, the "medicine" we gave that country was too strong to attack only the invaders. B-52 bombers, massive artillery, napalm, and defoliants were too random and indiscriminate to hit just the "enemy": hundreds of thousands of helpless, innocent people were killed or wounded as well. In the end, the country was destroyed by the medicine. This can also happen with anticancer agents.

There are, however, about thirty drugs that have been found safe to use in cancer treatment. Of these, a dozen or so are effective against different breast cancers, and so, in addition to hormones of one kind or another, the anticancer pharmacopoeia grew to include alkylating agents, antimetabolites, mitotic inhibitors, antibiotics, enzymes, and miscellaneous "random" synthetics. Most of the drugs that affect cancer cells either stop cell reproduction altogether or kill the malignant cells during that one vulnerable time when DNA molecules are twinning. Unfortunately, there are always healthy cells twinning at the same time, but—except for certain fast-growing tissue like bone marrow, blood, and intestinal lining—these grow more slowly and are not affected by the drugs.

When my friend was put on chemotherapy, drugs were used only when all else had failed. To the surprise of many, some of the drugs resulted in complete or partial remissions; some caused enough improvement in cases like hers to convince scientists that they might be more effective if they were given earlier as "adjuvant" or "helping" therapy immediately after surgery, before recurrences actually appeared.

Two major research advances preceded the decision to begin trials of adjuvant chemotherapy. One was proof that the presence of cancer in the axillary lymph nodes was almost a sure indication that the disease would recur. The second, most important advance, involved meticulous studies of "cell kinetics"—the precise way to measure doubling times of cancer cells—by Dr. Howard E. Skipper of the Southern Research Institute in Alabama. His milestone-setting work showed that drugs worked best if the tumor-burden was small. In other words, if a single dose killed, for example, eighty percent of all cancer cells in an animal's body, it was theoretically possible to achieve a 100 percent cell-kill, if enough of the drug was given over time. Naturally, the fewer cells present, the better the chance of ultimately achieving that 100 percent cell-kill. This supported the concept of giving adjuvant chemotherapy to women when there were no symptoms of spread—except for malignant axillary nodes—after surgery.

Spectacular results from trials done in the early 1950s with leukemic children who received combination chemotherapy added impetus to the move.

Armed with data from animal experimentation and the children's study, the NSABP began to give women with one or more positive axillary nodes (separated into groups of 1-3 and four or more) adjuvant chemotherapy in 1958. It was a "double blind" study of an alkylating drug, Thio-TEPA (TSPA), in which half of the 826 women received the drug while the other half were given a placebo. After five years of follow-up, there were significant differences in the survival rates of the drug-treated premenopausal women who had more than four positive lymph nodes. This group ordinarily fares badly in terms of recurrence rates, but the trial's results showed the young women randomized into the TSPA group not only lived longer, they also had fewer local recurrences. These differences still persist, more than twenty years after the TSPA trial began.

Then, a second study using another drug, 5-Flourourocil (5-FU), was begun in 1961. Again, the results showed that premenopausal women who had more than four positive axillary nodes did better than those in the untreated group. However, the differences were not as dramatic as those of the Thio-TEPA trial.

These two pioneering studies marked the beginning of two

major changes in the treatment of breast cancer (indeed, of all cancers): 1) the advent of large-scale comparative clinical trials as a way to test the efficacy of different treatments and 2) the routine use of some kind of anticancer agent as a "first resort" for women at high risk of recurring. However, such adjuvant therapy was still only being used in specialized cancer centers by research-oriented physicians and oncologists.

It took a long time (since 1961) for the word about chemotherapy to filter down from the NSABP and cancer centers to the average family doctor, but when it finally did, it was no shower—it was a downpour. On February 19, 1976, the prestigious *New England Journal of Medicine* published results of an NCI-supported study of adjuvant chemotherapy done in Italy. Carried out by Dr. Gianni Bonadonna of Milan's National Cancer Institute, the research showed that high-risk women (that is, those who had one or more malignant axillary lymph nodes) developed fewer recurrences and had longer disease-free periods if they were given anticancer drugs immediately after surgery. The difference was far more dramatic in premenopausal than in older women, but postmenopausal women also had better results if they received the drugs. The time of follow-up was too short to be statistically significant, but the Bonadonna results were widely advertised by both the professional and general media. Almost overnight (in terms of the way medical change usually takes place), the concept of giving "positive-node" women some kind of adjuvant therapy after surgery became routine.

As I said earlier, the first anticancer drug was an alkylating agent, nitrogen mustard—a component of poison gas developed as a weapon during war. Refinements were made in the basic formula, and alkylating drugs widely used now for breast cancer include phenylalanine mustard (L-PAM, Alkeran) and cyclophosphamide (Cytoxan). Thio-TEPA, the first drug used as an adjuvant, is also an alkylating agent, but it is no longer used much in the United States, although I found it was still prescribed in some of the European countries I visited. All are cell poisons whose molecules attach themselves easily and quickly to various substances inside the cancer cell. Alkylating agents act so much like radiation that they are often called "radiomimetic agents," radiation imitators. Their effectiveness stems from the fact that malignant cells twin so much more frequently than normal cells do that, they can be killed more rapidly. Because drugs reach their target without affecting as much healthy tissue as X-ray and can also attack occult micrometastases local radiation treatments do not reach, systemic drug therapy is more effective.

A second group of drugs used against breast cancer is called "antimetabolites," and Methotrexate and 5-Flourourocil (5-FU) are the most popular. These are "Trojan Horses"—counterfeiters that sneak inside a cancer cell's membrane disguised as nutrients and fool it into using them. Because they are fake foods, antimetabolites cause massive indigestion that interferes with DNA duplication and either kills or sterilizes the cell. Like alkylating agents, these drugs also destroy healthy cells in the process of division and may cause considerable toxicity. Occasionally, a "rescue factor" or antidote is used after massive doses to counter the effects of these drugs on healthy tissue.

Another way to attack a cancer cell is simply to prevent it from twinning. The substances that do this are "mitotic inhibitors" (from mitosis, cell division). Two descendents of the common periwinkle plant, vinblastine sulfate (Velban) and vincristine sulfate (Oncovin), are such drugs. By preventing mitosis, these substances sterilize the cancer cell. Because many women cannot tolerate their toxic neurological side effects, mitotic inhibitors are not used for breast cancer as frequently as other drugs are.

A potent tumorcidal antibiotic, Adriamycin, was approved for general use about fourteen years ago. Developed in Italy, Adriamycin has been shown to be remarkably effective against a large number of tumors that were among the most stubbornly resistant to chemotherapy, and these include advanced breast cancers. Most oncologists give Adriamycin in combination with other chemotherapeutic agents, but it is one of the few drugs that is effective alone—either as adjuvant therapy or for advanced disease. As a rule, it is given by injection, and nine sessions (or courses), three weeks apart, are the maximum most women are likely to receive.

As it is in most of life, there is nothing good in cancer therapy without a bad side too. Almost all anti-cancer agents have general toxicities, but Adriamycin may also affect the heart. Blood tests and electrocardiograms must be used to monitor patients. But even if no problems occur, the time limit for Adriamycin is about six months. (Of course, if any problem does arise, the drug is discontinued earlier.) From letters and telephone calls to the Breast Cancer Advisory Center since September 1975, I have the reports from hundreds of women who told me how a shot or two of Adriamycin almost miraculously stopped the bone pain, chest fluid, or other symptoms of recurrent disease they had been having. Unfortunately, if they developed signs of cardiotoxicity or when their six months of treatment were up, the drug had to be stopped.

Both the National Cancer Institute and Adria Laboratories, the manufacturers, are searching for a way to get rid of the cardiotoxicity, and trials of a "second generation" Adriamycin, a formula of the drug modified to remove these side effects, are underway at the Sidney Farber Cancer Center in Boston. So the heart's trouble with this drug may soon be a thing of the past.

There are several other tumorcidal antibiotics that seem to be promising. Two were developed in Japan—Actinomycin D and Bleomycin. Surgeons there often put these directly into a woman's body before the incision is closed. Dr. John Macdonald, an associate director of the Division of Cancer Treatment at the NCI, told me neither substance has been effective in treating breast cancer in this country. He suggested that the reason for this odd situation might be due to a difference between the kinds of cancers Japanese and Western women develop. As I said earlier, Japanese women not only have lower incidences, but when they do get breast cancer, it is usually a less virulent type than we have in the United States.

Another antibiotic is mitomycin, but its toxicity is so severe that it is still being tested only in animals and in some cases of far-advanced disease. Except for minor variations, however, the concept of combination chemotherapy has now circumnavigated the globe. A woman with breast cancer in Iceland, South Africa, or New Zealand is likely to get the combination developed by Bonadonna in Milan, by Cooper in Buffalo, Falkson in Pretoria, or Powles in London.

How did all of this happen so quickly?

Because of the severe side effects of large doses of these anticancer agents, scientists were facing an impenetrable stone wall in 1960. One problem was timing: to do its lethal work, a tumorcidal drug must attack a malignant cell while it is twinning. But since all cells are not in the S-phase at the same time, even a large, toxic dose of a single drug could destroy only a relatively small percentage of cancer cells one time.

The complex cell-kinetic mathematics worked out by Dr. Skipper was valuable in solving this problem. He proved that using several drugs, each having a different toxicity and modus operandi, would have a greater impact than single drugs used one at a time. The answer turned out to be a "chicken soup" recipe: the combination of Cytoxan, Methotrexate, and 5-FU (CMF) introduced by Bonadonna et al. Combining drugs that work either simultaneously or sequentially, have individual side effects, are effective for varying lengths of time, and that use different methods should—logically—be better and less toxic than single drugs used alone. But scientists were leery about loading a curable woman's system with more than one potent, potentially dangerous substance.

The successful results of combination chemotherapy in treating children with terminal leukemia at the NCI during the 1950s finally convinced oncologists that the same technique should at least be tried in women with advanced metastatic breast cancer. At about the same time, newer data about cell kinetics showed how vital it is to hit cancer cells at precisely the right time, and this too strengthened arguments supporting such a trial. In the clinical trials with the young leukemia victims, the chicken-soup attack had worked. Several drugs were given in smaller doses—some together, some in sequence—and an unexpected number of the children improved. Dr. Paul Carbone, then the chief of the Division of Cancer Treatment at the NCI, Dr. Steven K. Carter, and others at the Institute set three criteria a drug must meet to be considered suitable:

1. It must be an effective anticancer agent by itself. In larger doses, each drug in the "soup" must be able to kill cancer without help from any other agent;
2. There must be no overlapping toxicities, that is, no two drugs whose major side effects are the same—liver damage, for example—can be included. This is essential to prevent the possibility of one drug's compounding the toxicity of another;
3. All drugs must be able to do their killing job on an intermittent or interrupted basis, so continuous administration is not required. The patient must have time between doses to permit her body to recoup and regain strength.

Getting the clinical trials set up for treating women with advanced breast cancer took time, but finally they were fact, not fantasy. And, when the two-, three-, and five-year data were analyzed, Dr. Carbone and his group announced to the world that the chicken-soup worked! Women who thought they were doomed went into complete or partial remissions.

As I said earlier in this chapter, the success of these trials of combination chemotherapy against metastatic disease triggered the first adjuvant chemotherapy programs carried out by the NSABP. The rest is now history: combination chemotherapy has proven itself.

There are still many questions, however. How many drugs should be given? Current NCI and NSABP trials are using only two cytotoxic agents, in some cases combined with tamoxifen—the antiestrogen mentioned in Chapter 8—or various substances that might boost the immune system. The "Cooper Regimen" (introduced by Dr. Richard Cooper in Buffalo in the late 1960s) is composed of five drugs: CMFVP, the "P" referring to prednisone—an adrenal hormone thought to influence the growth of some kinds of breast cancer. Some chemotherapists believe in "aggressive" treatment and zap patients—especially premenopausal women—with every anticancer agent in their arsenals, at maximum tolerable doses.

Are three drugs better than two? Are five better than three?

How about six, seven, or eight?

No one knows yet.

So, before going any further, I want to stress that, at this time, there is no known "best" for all women, either as adjuvant therapy or for recurrent disease. The dozens of chicken-soup recipes being tried everywhere in the world are all relatively new and *all* of their findings are still preliminary. True, the published results of some are most encouraging and make wonderful headlines, but none has been used long enough to know its effect on long-term survival rates. This is the only yardstick: whether or not a treatment prolongs life.

Moreover, it is unlikely that there will ever be one therapy that is "best" for all women, because there are too many variables: the age of the woman, her estrogen-receptor status, the kind of cancer she has (i.e., its cell type and nuclear grade), the stage of her disease when it was diagnosed, the strength of her immune system, her overall physical condition, etc. All of these factors play important roles in helping to make any anticancer therapy successful.

So even though there seem to be almost monthly proclamations about some new, "spectacular," "monumental," or "miraculous" combination that will save tens of thousands of women's lives, these must, unfortunately, be taken with a huge box of salt. The Italian trials did not get started until the early 1970s, and the others have even shorter track records. Common sense tells us that these "breakthroughs" are actually hopes based on early results.

Otherwise, why would so many expensive comparative clinical trials, using so many different agents (with and without X-ray, with and without immune boosters, with and without antiestrogens, with and without hormones), still be going on?

An excellent example showing how misleading early results can be occurred in late 1974. On September 30, Dr. Bernard

Fisher told an international conference at the NCI that a trial of phenylalanine mustard (L-PAM) as adjuvant therapy for 250 women in 37 institutions showed dramatic differences in recurrence rates. Although the alkylating agent produced longer disease-free periods in premenopausal women who had positive nodes, there were also differences in the postmenopausal group. Mrs. Betty Ford (then fifty-six years old), who had a mastectomy only two days before the meeting, had positive nodes, and the new wonder drug was prescribed for her.

In no time, L-PAM was being given out like jellybeans in the White House.

After all, it could be taken by mouth, had virtually no side effects, and was relatively inexpensive. As time went by and more data accumulated, however, the lines on the graphs showing the differences in recurrence rates began to merge, and at the end of five years, there was virtually no effect at all for postmenopausal women. At about the same time, the 1976 announcement about CMF came from Milan, and the combination was so superior (even in premenopausal women where there was still a difference) that L-PAM is no longer used alone but only as part of a regimen with other substances.

In breast-cancer treatment, at least ten years of follow-up are essential before anything, including surgery, can be evaluated. Because the two-year results of the L-PAM trial were preliminary and showed benefit to older women as well as to younger women, thousands of postmenopausal patients were given the alkylating agent and were unnecessarily exposed to possible problems.

The L-PAM trial is also an excellent illustration of another difficult medical problem. How are new anticancer agents to be tested in humans? The NSABP trial had been a double-blind study—neither the patients nor their doctors knew who was getting what; half of the women received the real drug and half a placebo. When the "code" to the trial was broken and the difference in recurrence rates was announced, there was a great storm of criticism about the medical ethics of such a study. The women who were given the placebo had recurrences because they had fallen into certain slots, critics charged, while the lucky women who accidentially fell into the L-PAM slots benefited at the expense of their less lucky trial mates. (I was told [but could never verify] that several of the women in the placebo group threatened lawsuits against the NCI, despite having given their informed consent and having been told all the details of the clinical trial before it began.)

Of course, no one knew for two long years that L-PAM would

have the results that were announced on September 30, 1974: the outcome could just as easily have been that the "victims" were those women who were given the drug and *not* the placebo. For that matter, the real long-term results are still unknown: there are data linking long-term use of alkylating drugs with the development of leukemia. So it is possible that after another ten years, the "lucky" women will be the ones who fell into the placebo slots, after all.

I am going into such detail about the problems of relying on preliminary data, because hardly a week goes by without some "breakthrough" or another being hailed in the press as the cure for breast cancer. As the excitement over interferons (discussed in Chapter 12) as well as the L-PAM study clearly shows, early results can be misleading.

So far, I have discussed adjuvant therapy for node-positive women only in terms of using cytotoxic drugs, the conventional "chemotherapy" most people think of in this sense. This is why, for the purposes of this discussion, I am taking some license with standard jargon and including antiestrogens and male and female hormones under the broad umbrella of "chemotherapy." I will also use such prophylactic therapy synonymously with treatment for recurrent or advanced disease, because the agents being used are identical for both groups. So are the recommended dosages: the maximum the patients can tolerate.

The major differences between treating high-risk women and those with visible disease are 1) that there is still no way to measure the success or failure of any adjuvant regimen except that a recurrence does or does not develop, and 2) that there is good reason to believe preventive adjuvant therapy will be curative. Unfortunately, at this time, no drug or combination of drugs has been known to cure anyone whose cancer has returned, although there are signs that disease-free intervals *are* being lengthened by chemotherapy. No woman with breast cancer needs to write her Last Will and Testament anymore just because she has many positive nodes or develops a recurrence. Even more important, no doctor should erase her from his ledger. The modern age of chemotherapy has started a new ball game!

Leaving cytotoxic drugs for a few pages, I would like to catch up with the progress made in using endocrine manipulation. When the manuscript for this revised chapter was in first draft, the information about the application of estrogen-receptors to treatment was based on "soft" data. In medical jargon, this means the results did not come from large, controlled, and randomized clinical trials. The reason I had no "hard" data is simply that none were available: I had collected the success stories from doctors who treated patients on a case-by-case basis, depending on their own situations, or from scientists who were studying a relatively small number of women.

In early March 1981, however, at a chemotherapy conference in Tucson, Dr. Bernard Fisher announced the results of the NSABP trial mentioned earlier (and subsequently published in the *New England Journal of Medicine*, July 2, 1981). About 1,900 women were divided randomly into two groups: one was given L-PAM and 5-FU; the second received the PF and tamoxifen. Their ER status was not taken into account for the randomization. Two year recurrence rates were compared and their ERAs correlated. It was then found that the postmenopausal, ER+ women (older than fifty), who had one to three positive lymph nodes and who were given tamoxifen, had less than half of the recurrences than did the ER+ women in the same age and lymph-node group who had not received the antiestrogen. Older, ER+ women with four or more malignant nodes, who received tamoxifen did even better. Women younger than fifty did not benefit from the antiestrogen, regardless of their ER level or nodal status.

Critics charged that it was too soon to make a judgment, but Dr. Fisher pointed out that 80 percent of all recurrences appear during the first two postoperative years and that—if nothing else—the trial proved that tamoxifen increased disease-free intervals and would probably prolong the women's lives.

Of course, I have warned against getting excited about early, preliminary two-year results, and—if I did not have other success stories—I would urge caution too. But the NSABP data are, as far as I can see, the final seal-of-approval that reinforces what I had already written: women who are ER+ do better if some kind of endocrine manipulation is part of their adjuvant regimen.

Long before 1981, adding hormonal therapy of one kind or another to symptom-free, positive-node women was being hotly debated at meetings, conferences, and in medical journals. Many breast-cancer specialists have been treating ER+ premenopausal women with ovariectomy and postmenopausal women with either tamoxifen, adrenalectomy,* or both ever since the estrogen-receptor assay was developed. For example, Dr. Charles A. Hubay of the Case-Western Reserve Medical School in Cleveland had already presented 45 months of follow-up com-

---

*In its September 3, 1981 issue, the New England Journal of Medicine reported optimistic results of another substance for estrogen-positive women: aminoglutethemide (Ellipten). This drug functions as a "medical adrenalectomy," since it stops adrenal production of estrogen.

paring cytotoxic chemotherapy alone with the same three drugs plus tamoxifen. The trial involved about 400 women, and those who were ER + did significantly better after almost four years if they received the added antiestrogen. Conversely, the ER + group *not* getting tamoxifen had more recurrences during the same period. There was no difference in the relapse rates of ER − patients in either group.

Other experts, Drs. Olaf Pearson, William McGuire, Eugene DeSombre, and my doctor, Thomas Dao, were also using the ERA to help decide what kind of adjuvant treatment patients should receive, long before the NSABP results were made public.

In the spring of 1979, a head-to-head conflict between the two schools erupted at the annual convention of the American Society of Clinical Oncology (ASCO). Conflicting data were reported about the relative merits of endocrine manipulation compared with cytotoxic chemotherapy, and the only clear-cut information was what I mentioned in Chapter 8: that the estrogen-receptor assay was useful for predicting prognosis, because ER + women, as a rule, do better than ER − women, no matter what treatment was used.

The conflict suddenly seemed to put a brake on the trend toward increased use of the ERA to help choose appropriate adjuvant treatment. Combinations of cytotoxic drugs became routine, even for women whose tumors were strongly estrogen-dependent. Oncologists believed the longer disease-free periods reported by Hubay and his group were not due to better adjuvant treatment but to the fact that ER + women simply have less aggressive cancers.

The prestige and clout of the NSABP study should reverse the current trend of putting all women with positive nodes on the same combination of cell-killing drugs, regardless of any personal, individual factors like ER or menopausal status.

What does this complex controversy mean to women?

There is little point in doing the ER assay if its results are ignored, especially since cytotoxic agents have certain toxicities that may seriously affect women's quality of life. Baldness, or alopecia, is—to women—the most formidable. After losing one symbol of femininity, their breasts, they must then lose their crowning glories and wear wigs. Some women suffer from acute nausea and vomiting (although marijuana's chief ingredient, delta-9-tetrahydro-cannabinol, THC, has been approved by the FDA to alleviate this problem and is available in pill form). Some women have sore mouths, diarrhea, and begin to get severe headaches. The most serious side effect, however, is the drugs' weakening of the body's defense mechanism, the immune system, and white cell counts must be carefully monitored. If these fall to a dangerously low level, all cytotoxic agents are stopped immediately until enough time has gone by to build up the count again. Otherwise, patients may become seriously ill and even die from a simple cold that gets out of hand.

Of course, the majority of women do not suffer severely and have only mild problems for a day or two. Some women have no side effects at all: they lose not one hair nor do they have a single queasy moment. But many women do. There is no toxicity involved when any kind of endocrine manipulation (including ablative surgery) is used. Tamoxifen is taken by mouth twice a day, and its known side effects occur only rarely: slight cramping at the time a menstrual period would be due ("tamoxifen flare") and a faint rash. True, the substance has been on the market for too short a time to know its long-term effects, but animal data indicate only some problems involving calcium metabolism.

Women who have ovariectomies, of course, go through the menopause immediately, and those whose adrenal glands are removed must take daily doses of cortisone. But there is no toxicity of any kind. Obviously, the benefits of endocrine manipulation are not available to women whose doctors did not arrange for an estrogen-receptor assay or for those whose assays were not done properly.

The NSABP data in the *New England Journal of Medicine* received a great deal of general publicity. Now I am afraid the absence and unreliability of ERAs will result in an indiscriminate addition of tamoxifen to all adjuvant regimens, regardless of whether the women are ER + or ER − . This would help the women whose cancers were estrogen-dependent, but it would be useless (and expensive) for those who will not benefit from the substance.

The NSABP results have not gone unchallenged. Recently Dr. Bonadonna presented updated results from his Milan study, and he feels that the reason postmenopausal women did not do as well in his original trial is that they did not receive large enough doses of the drugs for a long enough time. In the United States, a similar view was published in September 1980 in *Cancer* by Dr. James Holland and Richard Cooper who reported on their five-drug trials. After the Fisher data were published, Dr. Holland told reporters he doubted the long-term effects of tamoxifen would equal those of his drugs. At the Mt. Sinai Hospital in New York, Dr. Ezra Greenspan also believes in aggressive cytotoxic therapy for all women, regardless of their age or estrogen-receptor status.

And so it is going around the world.

I repeat, it should be clear by now that indeed there is no "best" chemotherapy for all women, and every patient's chemotherapy regimen should be individualized to take her own personal variables into consideration.

As I write this chapter, I hear a clock ticking away. Just as the first draft became obsolete within a matter of weeks, this one may be woefully behind the data when *Why Me?* comes off the presses. As I said earlier, we are on the brink of major advances, and even medical journals are having trouble keeping up with progress.

So instead of continuing to tell the story of postsurgical treatment for breast cancer as I have, I will summarize today's state-of-the-art in a list that incorporates what is known at the time of this writing:

1. The estrogen-receptor assay must be done and done properly, as explained in Chapter 8.
2. The probability of cure or a long disease-free interval is greater if adjuvant therapy is begun as soon after surgery as possible.
3. Single-agent therapy—as adjuvant or for recurrent disease—is not as effective as a combination of agents.
4. Available evidence indicates that switching from one combination of agents to another, when a measurable tumor becomes resistant to the first combination, improves metastatic breast cancer. Therefore, alternating drugs in this way after three or more cycles of adjuvant therapy would probably be equally effective against microscopic metastases (when there is no cancer that can be measured).
5. The first three or four cycles of therapy seem to be the most important, and scientists are questioning the value of prolonged treatment. There are data showing that women do not benefit from treatment after the first six courses.
6. So far, disease-free intervals after two-drug regimens are identical to disease-free intervals after multiple-drug regimens.
7. Women whose tumors are ER+ have a better prognosis, in general, and benefit from having some kind of endocrine manipulation.
8. All of the side effects of cytotoxic drugs disappear when they stop being used.
9. The Food & Drug Administration (FDA) warns that all chemotherapeutic agents should be given by someone trained and experienced in using them. Many family practi-

tioners and general surgeons are giving single-agent chemotherapy, but combinations are complex and require stringent monitoring which they may not know how to do.

10. There are no data supporting the use of any immune boosters as part of either adjuvant or advanced-disease regimens. Every study of substances like BCG, citrovorum parvum, levamisole, MER, etc. has shown them to be of no value in the treatment of breast cancer.

11. Although women with no malignant axillary nodes have about a 25 percent risk of developing a recurrence, the NIH has recommended *against* the routine use of any adjuvant chemotherapy in such cases, because the risks outweigh the possible benefits. However, there are some women who are at very high risk of a recurrence (i.e., who have strong family histories or large tumors in one of the inner quadrants of their breasts), and many oncologists are giving this group prophylactic drugs for short periods of time.

12. For unknown reasons, women with one to three positive nodes benefit less from any therapy than do women who have more than four, regardless of their estrogen-receptor status.

I would now like to peer into a crystal ball and try to make some educated predictions about the future of chemotherapy, including all types of endocrine manipulation. Some of these will be repeated in Chapter 17, The Future, but I would like to mention them here as well.

First, of course, there will soon be computerized customtailored therapy after surgery instead of the current fashion of giving women certain combinations simply because they are a particular oncologists's favorite or because they are popular in certain places at certain times. Primary surgery is gradually changing so women are being individualized according to the stage and type of breast cancer they have, and the same changes will occur in choosing adjuvant therapy. Age, estrogen-receptor status, and perhaps other variables will be taken into account when prescriptions are written.

One of these may involve changes of schedule, including adapting therapy to a woman's own biorhythms. Drs. Lawrence E. Sheving of Arkansas, Franz Halberg and William Hrushesky in Minnesota have impressive data showing that "chronobiology"—the study of the way life varies at different times—influences the effectiveness of anticancer therapy. Cancer cells never stop growing and reproducing, but healthy cells slow down or even stop working entirely during sleep. Since the only time any cell can be damaged or destroyed is during the period when its DNA is twinning, drugs' cell-killing properties do far less harm to their healthy neighbors at night when their rates of metabolism are slow.

Another way to custom-tailor postsurgical therapy is rapidly moving from the laboratory to the clinic. In Tucson, Dr. Sydney E. Salmon is at work developing a way to test a drug's effectiveness against a specific cancer cell just as bacteria are cultured to learn which antibiotic will destroy certain strains of infectious invaders. Known as the "clonogenic stem-cell assay," the test— when it is perfected—will do away with the trial-and-error waste of time and money and the unnecessary toxicity patients now encounter. Dr. Salmon has had some success with ovarian and bladder cancer with his assay, and Dr. Daniel Von Hoff is at work in San Antonio looking for ways to test drugs against breast cancer in a test tube instead of in a woman's body.

At a meeting of the NCI's Breast Cancer Task Force in February 1981, Dr. Von Hoff explained that the biggest obstacle in assaying substances against breast cancer is the large number of variables that exist in a woman's body—variables that cannot be put into glass tubes or dishes. Moreover, it is exceedingly difficult to keep breast-cancer cells alive in artificial nutrients long enough to assess the effectiveness of some of the agents. Even a fractional change in temperature or humidity, he explained, can destroy entire colonies.

If private pharmaceutical and medical laboratories were not interested in the assay, its future might be grim in today's economic climate. However, I have been told, a still-anonymous corporation has been interested in investing in the work, and when there is money to be made from anything, the result is speedy progress. So it seems likely that the clonogenic stem-cell assay will be available to help women within a few years, if not sooner.

But even before drugs are chosen for cloning and assaying, they may be evaluated by a computerized program developed in Canada by Dr. James Goldie. Head of the Advanced Therapeutics Department at the Cancer Control Agency of British Columbia, Dr. Goldie and his colleagues have developed a computer program for simulating drug resistance and are using it to design dosages, scheduling and combinations. Undoubtedly, the computer models and simulations for chemotherapy will also be supported by the business community.

Another important area where business has also shown an interest is one I have been referring to as "markers." In breast-cancer treatment, many are needed, and this exciting field of research is detailed where it belongs—in Chapter 17, The Future. But women receiving adjuvant treatment must have one urgently, so I will mention it here.

Until adjuvant therapy became routine, this was not a problem: the effectiveness of any treatment was easily known, because the size of a symptomatic recurrence of cancer can be measured by the pain a woman feels, blood and urine tests, X-rays and scans.

But adjuvant therapy is different: there are no symptoms. The only way to know if the treatment is being effective in postponing or preventing a recurrence is simply that there is none. Women receiving adjuvant treatments feel fine, except for problems caused by the drugs themselves. Yet they must take the medications, because they had positive axillary lymph nodes and are at high risk of developing another cancer somewhere in their bodies. As a result, women receiving such therapy may spend years going through various kinds of hell without knowing if the drugs are doing them any good.

On the other hand, some women have no side effects at all. They never lose a single hair, have not even one twinge of nausea; when everyone else in the family is down with the flu, their immune systems are strong enough to turn them into Florence Nightingales. These women endure a different kind of side effect—sleepless nights of worrying that the drugs are not helping them at all. If they were, the women think, they too would be bald, nauseous, and have low white-cell counts.

Both groups of women must have some crutch to lean on, some way of knowing whether or not their treatment is working. Again, several medical businesses have entered the marker sweepstakes, and the incentive of the almighty dollar should hurry progress along.

Scientists are combining drugs and hormones to fight advanced disease that has stopped responding to standard regimens. Female hormones like estrogens, that are tumor-promoters, are being given to accelerate the doubling-times of women's cancer cells. Then, when the rates of twinning have become more frequent, cytotoxic drugs are administered so they can move in and destroy the artificially active cancer cells. Data from these experiments are sparse, because such trials with humans may legally be done only on patients who have exhausted all proven methods of treatment. Nonetheless, responses to this kind of growth-enhancing hormonal therapy followed by cytotoxic drugs have been cautiously and guardedly encouraging. If adjuvant chemotherapy's research had not begun with the same low-key, careful attitude, I would put this work into Chapter 17, The Future. But computerization, mathematical modeling, cell-kinetic simulation, and all of the paraphernalia of modern technologies are helping scientists decide what might work well and what the best time is for moving in for the maximum cell-kill. In the 1960s, these electronic miracles were not available to help, and adjuvant chemotherapy still managed to evolve from research done with advanced disease. So I am confident history will repeat itself, and in less time.

Radiation may also be made more effective and less toxic to healthy tissue, in large doses, by substances that are either radioenhancers or radiosensitizers. The first group of drugs, radioenhancers, have the capability of magnifying the effects of low doses of radiation, so easily tolerated quantities are able to do more damage and destruction to cancer cells. The second group may protect healthy tissue from radiation doses so large these would not be tolerated otherwise. I will go into more detail in Chapter 17.

There is also a glimmer of hope about prevention. Dr. Pierre Mauvais-Jarvis of the Hôpital Neker in Paris has been giving progestin and progesterone during the luteal phase (an interval of the monthly menstrual cycle) to high-risk young women. After treating about 500 women, women who had to have breast biopsies for a variety of benign masses, with the female hormones, Dr. Mauvais-Jarvis is convinced this may delay or even prevent the development of breast cancer. Of course, these women are now only in their twenties and thirties, and it is too soon to know. But there is hope that he will be right.

Dr. Dao, basing laboratory research on the epidemiological statistic that early age-at-first-birth reduces a woman's chances of developing breast cancer, is trying to find a way to imitate pregnancy's hormonal effects without, of course, resulting in the birth of a baby. So far, he has shown that inducing early pregnancies in mice does confer considerable immunity. The next step is to learn precisely what changes gestation causes and to try to create these changes artificially. Other scientists are looking for safe ways to develop young girls' breast cells, so they begin to produce milk *without* pregnancy. The basic idea is the same: to exploit whatever it is that early pregnancy does to protect women from developing breast cancer.

There may even be that magic bullet against cancer that scientists have been looking for: a safe, easy, and inexpensive weapon that will cure this dread disease with a single volley.

But if not, there will at least be control.

There is still no cure for diabetes, but the mortality rate from this disease has dropped, because insulin is able to keep its fatal complications under control. Something will also be found to keep malignant cells dormant so they cause no symptoms, no pain, and have no influence on our lives.

This is the magic bullet we can realistically expect to have within the next decade.

12

When Surgery Is Not Enough

RADIOTHERAPY

"You can quote me as saying I think all radiotherapy in the post-operative treatment of all cancer will be as obsolete as the buggywhip someday. In breast-cancer treatment, after a radical mastectomy, it is already obsolete except as a painkiller."

This paragraph from *Breast Cancer* (emphatically omitted from the first edition of *Why Me?*) caused me a great deal of trouble. It caused the person I was quoting, Dr. Gerald S. Johnston, a lot of trouble too, because Jerry—a personal friend—was (and still is) the chief of Nuclear Medicine at the NIH, *not* the chief of Radiation Therapy. As a nuclear-medicine man, he had "no right" to tell me what he did. The person I should have interviewed was Dr. P. Ralph Johnson, in Radiation Oncology, but he was then out of town. Not knowing anything about medical/surgical pecking-orders at that time, I called Jerry, never dreaming that it would cause me or him any future problem. After all, the question I wanted answered was not all that specialized.

"Would it be accurate to say that X-ray treatment has absolutely no place in managing breast cancer after a radical mastectomy?"

Jerry pondered it for a moment or two. "This is for the record, isn't it?"

"Yes," I told him. "You're a top authority in the best United States research center. What you say would be a definitive quote to end all quotes."

"Hmmm. That means I have to be very, very careful." He laughed. "You did say treatment, not diagnosis, didn't you?"

"Treatment," I repeated. "I know mammograms are X-rays, and I know they have to be done for diagnosis."

"And you're only referring to a primary breast cancer after a radical mastectomy? I do think X-ray therapy has a place as a palliative in metastatic disease."

"No, I don't mean X-rays to kill pain," I explained. "I'm asking about the prophylactic X-ray treatments women are given to their underarms even after they've had all their axillary nodes cut out."

Another short silence. "I think, then, it is an accurate statement to make. No radiation treatments to the axilla are justified after a radical mastectomy."

"Suppose there *is* a sign that the cancer has spread to a couple of spots in the bones?" I pressed. "Would you recommend X-ray treatments for those places?"

"If there is any sign of bone metastasis, some oncologists put the patient on drug therapy and use X-ray to alleviate pain," he answered. "They believe that, by that time, the disease is systemic—spread through the body—and not local. X-ray is entirely a local form of therapy."

Dr. Johnston said that this opinion was shared by many specialists but that others felt radiation—not drugs—was the treatment of choice for malignant bone spots.

"It's controversial," he smiled.

Another question I asked him was what to do if a woman's tumor lay in the medial (central) part of her chest, an area that usually drains to the internal mammary chain (the lymph nodes along the breastbone under the ribs). In such cases, the axillary nodes may be free of cancer, while the inner ones may be malignant.

"That's another controversial area," he explained. "Many experts think that once these nodes are involved, the disease is systemic and use chemotherapy instead of radiation; others always irradiate inner tumors. No one knows for sure, at this point in time."

"But postmastectomy prophylactic irradiation is still routine after radical mastectomy in most hospitals in the country, isn't it?" I asked in 1974. "Even if all the nodes are negative . . ."

He had sighed. "Well, we sit here in our ivory tower in Bethesda, outside Washington, and plot the ideal. It takes a while for the word to filter down. Sometimes it takes a pretty long while. There's nothing we can do about that."

NIH research, by the way, was and is being done with NIH funding in institutions all over the United States and in many other countries as well. The results are reported to Bethesda and disseminated by publications, conferences, seminars, and various "outreach" programs. But physicians and surgeons cannot be force-fed information. So, unfortunately, Jerry was absolutely right: it can take years for news to "filter down." In addition, under the law that created them, the National Institutes of Health can only "report the results of research." All it may do is disseminate results of research and hope and pray these eventually reach the average family doctor. As far as prophylactic axillary irradiation after radical mastectomy was concerned, the word had been sifting down with the speed of a snail.

Happily, since *Breast Cancer* was written in 1974, routine irradiation of the affected axilla after a radical mastectomy has stopped, even in this country's vast hinterlands. At that time, however, it was virtually a standard postoperating procedure for women to have "shots of cobalt," even though there was nothing to irradiate except healthy tissue!

So even though my information was correct, I had problems with surgeons and radiation therapists, because I used a nuclear-medicine expert as a source, and it was not in his bailiwick to give me an answer.

After my mastectomy, I had also expected the usual twenty radiation treatments and was astounded when Dr. Dao looked as if I had suggested coffee enemas.

"What for?" he cried. "I took out all the nodes I could get to. If there's any disease left I couldn't reach, your immune system will take care of it. All radiotherapy would do is damage normal tissue."

I explained that I had never heard of any woman whose radical mastectomy was not followed by several weeks of cobalt.

"I'll bring you some information to read," he laughed. "Don't judge all of us by what a few people do."

The next day, he came to my room with a briefcase filled with literature.

One was a report titled, "The Role of Roentgen Therapy in Carcinoma of the Breast." Published in *1946*, it gave the results of a comparative trial of two groups of women. Although radiation of the axilla after a radical mastectomy reduced the number of local recurrences, metastases to distant organs occurred more frequently. X-ray had had no effect on the ultimate progress of the disease in either group of women: their survival rates were the same.

For the next fifteen years, scientists all over the world continued to compare the recurrence, metastatic, and survival rates of women with breast cancer who had been given "prophylactic" X-ray therapy to their axillas after a radical mastectomy with the rates of those who had not. All age groups and stages of the disease were studied. The general opinion was that the increased incidence of metastases to other organs after axillary irradiation made routine X-ray therapy risky when the nodes had been removed. Preventing recurrences did not warrant the risk, because new local tumors could be treated surgically. On the other hand, metastases occurring far from the original tumor site might not be found until too late. This was the opinion of many specialists by the early 1960s, but the practice had continued in average hospitals by average doctors in 1974.

Dr. Dao had been wrong when he said "a few" people were doing it. *Most* doctors in the country were giving the order to irradiate axillas.

X-ray was discovered in 1895 by Wilhelm Conrad Roentgen who was awarded the Nobel Prize in physics in 1901 for this work. Doctors soon found that the invisible force could harm external body tissues while it was photographing the bones inside—and could also harm their own bodies while they were taking the films. Scientists studying cancer immediately began to look for the quantity of irradiation that could safely be tolerated by normal cells but would still kill cancerous ones.

Early in this century, the precise workings of the phenomenon were not understood. Scientists knew what happened empirically, without knowing why. They tested various time intervals and dosages without understanding the effects the X-rays were having on cellular operations, normal or malignant. Only since the invention of the electron microscope have scientists learned why X-ray destroys malignant cells without killing all the healthy ones around them.

X-rays are produced in a vacuum tube, when speeding electrons hit a metal plate, and the depth to which they can penetrate depends on the rate of speed at which the electrons strike the plate. Roentgen's 1895 machine has, naturally, been made obsolete by new technical know-how, such as the use of certain "boosters" in linear accelerators, cyclotrons and betatrons to increase the speed of the electrons. There are also machines now that deliver protons, neutrons, mesons, pi-mesons and "heavy ions." These high X-ray technologies make it possible to attack tumors without harming the layers of tissues and organs en route. With such modern equipment, radiologists can home in on a cancer more precisely, resulting in two important advances:

healthy tissue is avoided; X-rays can be aimed more safely at deep-seated organs, like the pancreas.

X-ray destroys malignant cells by attacking them while they are reproducing, during that vulnerable period when their DNA molecules are twinning. Since they reproduce more frequently than healthy cells do, they have more of these vulnerable periods, and more of them are destroyed. In other words, malignant cells are more "radiosensitive" than normal ones are. In addition, some cancers are more radiosensitive than others. This vulnerability is directly related to the rapidity of cell growth.

When irradiation is needed to treat any cancer, radiotherapists calculate how much X-ray to give a patient and what the length of exposure should be, they take into account the kind of cancer it is and where it is located in the body. A great deal of expertise is required to be certain the normal tissues around, above, or below the malignancy receive as little irradiation as possible. This is a tricky process, and radiotherapy is not to be entrusted to anyone except a physician who has received additional training in this subspecialty. Technicians who operate the equipment should also be specially trained and certified. Therapeutic radiotherapy is far more complex than diagnostic radiology (mammograms or X-rays to find bone fractures), and a technician who is trained only to snap the shutter of a sophisticated camera has no business giving X-ray treatments to cancer patients. Computerization of radiation-therapy equipment has taken much of the guesswork out of this form of treatment, but this does not negate the need for an expert.

Some kinds of cancer cannot be destroyed by any dose of X-ray that would not also be lethal to surrounding normal tissues. These are radioresistant, as opposed to radiosensitive, and X-ray therapy is ineffective against them. Muscle, heart, and nerve cells, for example, never duplicate. However, these nonreproducing cells are often overlaid by cancers metastasizing from other organs. These organs may also develop primary cancers arising from neighboring cells that do reproduce—that is, are *not* nerve, muscle, or heart cells per se. The radiosensitivity of such cancers would be like that of the cells of the tumor. Such cancers might, therefore, benefit from X-ray. Cells that divide rapidly—those of the intestines, blood, bone marrow, skin, and hair—are the most radiosensitive, because their DNA molecules are constantly twinning. Since they are so fast-growing, their healthy cells are easily damaged during radiotherapy. This explains why the first side effects of X-ray treatment are usually intestinal upsets, reduction of white blood cells, peeling skin, and baldness.

Not all the cancer cells in a tumor will be in the twinning stage at the same time. Only those in the process of splitting will be affected by an X-ray treatment, and, therefore, only a small percentage of the cancer cells are destroyed during a single therapy session. Timing is as important in radiotherapy as it is in all cancer therapies.

Some tumors may be so deep in the body that even the most modern X-ray equipment has difficulty penetrating them without harming organs in-between or harming the skin. X-ray equipment is always being improved, however, and so are exposure techniques. It is now possible to treat some deep internal cancers with very high-intensity rays, like those I listed a few pages ago, rays that can be focused more directly on the tumor. Also, patients can be rotated during therapy so the same healthy organs are not always exposed. A technique called crossfiring prevents the same tissue from being bombarded repeatedly: rays are aimed at the tumor's site from various angles.

Most breast cancers are relatively slow-growing. But this virtue also means that most of them are relatively radioresistant. On a ranking of thirteen cancers in descending order of radiosensitivity, breast cancer was fifth from the bottom: X-ray treatments were far more effective in destroying eight other kinds of cancer. What this means is that before a mammary carcinoma is touched by radiotherapy, the fast-growing skin, blood, bone marrow, and other tissues near it are bound to have been damaged.

Fear of possible side- and after-effects of irradiation is given as one of the major reasons most doctors in the United States do not refer women for radiotherapy, instead of surgery.

"A mastectomy certainly has disadvantages," Dr. Dao said, "but now with breast reconstruction, these can be minimized, and—most important—we know what they are. With high-dose radiation, no one can possibly know what might happen. If a woman's left breast is affected, the X-rays might burn her heart; on either side, the lungs and esophagus might be injured. I know of women who developed severe lymphedema from irradiation, and I am afraid of it. Surgery is a known quantity to me; X-ray is full of unknowns."

He also mentioned a possible long-term effect—the development of other cancers.

"Too much radiation may damage the immune system, and leukemias and certain rare sarcomas could be triggered by radiotherapy," Dr. Dao explained.

The electron microscope aided scientists in learning why X-rays that destroyed cancer could also cause it. It was observed that a low dose of radiation may damage the DNA molecule during the duplication process without destroying the cell. If the growth gene is the part of the molecule affected, a healthy cell will probably become a malignant one.

Dr. Allen Lichter, the radiotherapist managing the NCI trial, agreed that no one knows what might happen in twenty or thirty years. "All we can do is point to long-term studies like the one done by Dr. Vera Peters in Toronto and say that radiation-induced second cancers haven't happened," he told me. "And she started her trials to compare mastectomy with radiation back in the 1930s, when equipment was relatively primitive."

The equipment used at the NCI, of course, is the most modern available, and as computerized as possible.

"I'd be the first person to agree that, at this point in time, treating breast cancer with radiotherapy is almost more of an art than it is a science," he told me. "Getting a good cosmetic result without compromising a woman's life requires an experienced radiotherapist who knows what he or she is doing. Simply owning a linear accelerator doesn't qualify someone to treat breast cancer."

Dr. Lichter told me many women prefer having a mastectomy to being treated by radiotherapy, because it is much easier.

"When a woman has surgery," he explained, "it's over and done with. In a couple of weeks, nowadays, she's back into her usual routine and might even have already had breast reconstruction."

He continued. "It's a different story if she chooses radiation therapy. She's got to be prepared to come in to the hospital every day for five or six weeks; she's got to expect a more long and drawn-out treatment period. Some women would rather get it all over with as soon as possible, and they don't think losing a breast is too high a price to pay to get the whole business behind them."

When I spoke to a group of oncological social workers in March 1981, Dr. Robert Goodman, a Philadelphia radiation therapist, also pointed out that surgery is cheaper, especially for women who must leave their hometowns for treatment.

"If a woman leaves Maryland," he said, using my own state as an example, "Blue Cross and Blue Shield won't pay the total cost of radiotherapy in Pennsylvania. They pay only five hundred dollars for this kind of treatment out-of-state. That doesn't include the cost of travel, a hotel, meals, and all of the incidentals, of course.

"There's no question, radiation therapy is more expensive if insurance companies won't pay the bill and if women have to leave their homes to get it."

But as far as potential dangers of radiotherapy are concerned, Dr. Goodman agreed with Dr. Lichter in saying that there is already enough information available to show these are minimal, provided the doctor and equipment are top-notch.

To kill a cancer cell, the dosage of X-ray given must be enormous; diagnostic X-rays use relatively tiny doses. A chest X-ray, for example, gives an exposure of about one-tenth of a rad. X-ray and radioactive irradiation both have effects on living tissues that are cumulative, that is, they build up over long periods of time. For example, two rads absorbed daily for six months can have the same effect as a single dose of 360 rads. Ignorance of radiation's cumulative effect explains why, in the earliest days of experimentation, many scientists working with X-ray developed cancer. Even today, no one knows the maximum dose that can be absorbed without harm.

Of course, this is the reason for the "mammography controversy" I detailed in Chapter 7: presumably healthy women were being routinely exposed to low doses of ionizing radiation every year. As I explained in that section, the breasts of premenopausal women are—except for a developing fetus—the most radiosensitive of all human tissue. High-dose X-ray kills cells; low-dose X-ray may damage cells without destroying them. The fear that exposing healthy women to such a known carcinogen was the cause of the national debate that ultimately ended the NCI/ACS Breast Cancer Detection Demonstration Projects.

Palliative radiotherapy usually means a few hundred rads are absorbed during each treatment, and since palliation is necessary only when a person already has cancer, there is little reason to worry about dosage. As always in medicine, benefit must outweigh risk: there is no point in worrying about developing the disease in the future if the pain of an existing cancer can be helped by irradiation . . . low-dose or high.

In the sixty-four years during which X-ray was routinely used after radical mastectomy, many studies here and abroad supported the combination. The reason for the favorable results was obvious. In those decades, a cure was defined as survival for five years after surgery. Since X-ray after radical mastectomy did reduce local recurrences, more women were alive after five years. But metastatic disease can take years longer to appear. When survival rates were checked after ten years, the irradiated women did not fare as well. There were many more skin, marrow, lung, and liver metastases in this group than in nonirradiated women.

In 1961, the NSABP began a randomized trial to finally assess the value of postradical radiotherapy. After almost ten years and more than 1,000 women, Dr. Bernard Fisher reported, "The survival rate of patients receiving irradiation was slightly less than that observed in the [nonirradiated] controls. . . . As the result of this study, which I consider to be the most definitive investigation yet carried out to evaluate the worth of postoperative irradiation, there seems to be no justification for its further use in any circumstances as an adjunct to radical mastectomy in the *primary* treatment of breast cancer" (the emphasis is Dr. Fisher's).

The report was published by NCI in 1970. Reporting results, remember, is all the Institute is permitted to do. Dr. Fisher could not go into every hospital and force general practitioners and general surgeons to read the reports.

In 1962, Dr. Dao and an associate at Roswell Park, Dr. John Kovaric, had already published an account of 354 women they had treated postoperatively, some with radiation, some without. In 48 per cent of the nonirradiated women, lung and skin metastases developed later; within the same period 89 per cent of those who had had radical mastectomies followed by irradiation developed distant secondary cancers. The irradiated women survived the same number of years as the others, but they suffered more bouts of cancer after their surgery.

Although the report was criticized at the time, Dr. Dao has not given X-ray therapy after radical mastectomy since 1962. And since then, a growing body of data—including the NSABPs—supported him. But still the X-ray habit continued around the country.

In a medical journal dated January 13, 1975, obstetricians and gynecologists in the United States were given some stunning "news" from Lausanne, Switzerland. "A Swiss investigator," the bulletin said, "reports that the routine use of local postoperative irradiation of early breast cancer should be seriously questioned. 'In the six controlled trials that have been published so far,' says Dr. Jan Stjernesward of the Swiss Institute for Experimental Cancer Research, 'survival rates were significantly lower among those women who were irradiated than among those who were treated by mastectomy alone'." The news announcement said, "Dr. Stjernesward concludes that stopping the routine use of prophylactic local radiotherapy after radical mastectomy not only could increase the survival rate but also save resources."

Perhaps having the word finally handed down from Switzerland was the reason most doctors in the United States began to pay attention. Whatever the reason, postoperative "shots of cobalt" are now the exception rather than the rule here.

Until the need to count malignant axillary lymph nodes to stage for adjuvant therapy was accepted in 1976, there were studies going on in the United States to study the results of total (or simple) mastectomies followed by irradiation. In one NSABP trial, about 1,700 closely matched women were randomized into Halsted radical mastectomy vs., total (or simple) mastectomy plus axillary irradiation. Although the trial stopped, the women enrolled are still being followed, and so far, there is no significant difference in survival rates between the two groups. Dr. Fisher feels this is definitive proof that the presence of cancer in the nodes is only an indicator to tell the doctor that the disease has already spread beyond the breast itself.

When radiotherapy is given *instead* of a mastectomy, therapeutic dosages to kill breast-cancer (or any cancer) cells usually range from 4,000 to 6,000 rads, given over a period of five to six weeks. In addition to irradiating the preserved breast to be sure all hidden foci or centricles of disease are destroyed, advocates of this method of treating breast cancer often focus the machine's beams on the chest wall, the underarm area (if an axillary sampling showed malignant nodes), or the supraclavicular nodes high at the base of the throat.

There are no hard-and-fast rules about the amount of tissue to be treated in such cases, because therapeutic decisions are usually based on the size and density of the breast and the location and size of the tumor. A woman's age, family history, and the type of cancer cells found may also be factors in the treatment chosen. The important point to remember here is that there are at least fifteen kinds of breast cancer and that there are so many variables between women that no comparisons can really be made. If a woman feels the radiation therapist is planning to expose her to too much X-ray, a second opinion from another doctor will do no harm.

In addition to irradiating the preserved breast itself and adjacent parts of a woman's body, most radiation therapists believe the immediate area where the tumor was located should be given an extra "boost" of X-ray. At this time, the most popular way to do this is threading plastic tubes (catheters) containing radioactive isotopes of certain chemicals through the breast tissue where the tumor had been. Women have told me the idea of having their breasts pierced by tubules, like mini-swords, makes them feel that the procedure will be extremely painful. However, patients who have gone through it assure me that it was, at most, uncomfortable. Doctors who do the procedure give me equal assurances that a local anesthetic is all that is required, unless the woman has unusually hard and dense breasts. According to several reports, the most difficult part of the procedure was being radioactive for two full days—too "hot" to be visited by family and friends.

Another method for giving an extra zap of irradiation only to the tumor's former home is to bombard that area with a potent electron beam. Dr. Leonard Prosnitz, at the Yale Comprehensive Cancer Center in New Haven, advocates this technique rather than the radioactive catheterization. There is, at this time, no known difference between the two procedures as far as survival is concerned. Extra boosters of irradiation are given to be sure any residual cancer cells missed during a lumpectomy or other segmental surgery are destroyed. Most breast-cancer specialists believe that women may have died of metastatic disease unnecessarily after segmental procedures, because nothing was done about such "seeding" in the part of the breast where the tumor had been.

The trial at the NCI uses irridium implants. So do Drs. Samuel Hellman at the Joint Center for Radiation Therapy in Boston and Robert Goodman in Philadelphia. Irridium seems to be the radioactive element being used throughout the world at this time, but I have also read and heard references about the use of cesium implants, another chemical that can be made radioactive for this purpose. In the future, I am certain more advances in technological know-how will be perfected to give only high-risk tissue more irradiation while protecting other parts of the breast from the excess.

The third "arm" of the current NSABP clinical trials will, eventually, show whether or not *any* postsurgical irradiation of the breast is needed. As I explained in Chapter 10, this group of women is being treated only by segmental surgery and an axillary dissection: no radiotherapy is being given at all. At this time, survival rates are equal enough to allow the study to continue. If, after ten, fifteen, or twenty years, there is no difference between the survival rates of these women and of those whose breasts were irradiated, this will be proof that the X-ray treatments were not needed. The results won't be in until the end of the clinical trials, however, so most breast-cancer experts believe everything possible must be done to try to destroy any hidden centricles in the rest of the breast.

While the NSABP and NCI trials are relatively new, some breast-cancer experts have been using radiotherapy instead of mastectomy for a long time on a "self-selected" basis. (This is why their results don't count to statisticians. Self-selection, they insist, affects the accuracy of the data.) I have already mentioned

Dr. Vera Peters in Toronto and Drs. Samuel Hellman, Leonard Prosnitz, and Robert Goodman in this country. Another U.S. pioneer was Dr. Eleanor Montague, a professor of radiation therapy at the M.D. Anderson Cancer Center in Houston. In 1975, she told the Radiological Society of North America that minimal surgery followed by irradiation, in her study, had a recurrence rate of only four percent, while women who were treated by the Halsted radical mastectomy had a recurrence rate of 15 percent. In 1974, the doctors involved in this "unorthodox" kind of cancer treatment were reticent about reporting data. All emphasized the preliminary nature of their short-term results and stressed that distant metastases would take many more years to show up. Nonetheless, they insisted that women who refused to lose their breasts be permitted to have some kind of treatment, rather than have none at all, simply because the data had not had enough years to become "significant."

As time passed, the all-important data began to accumulate and showed impressive results. Women of the world began to be told the truth—that no one really knew the answer yet; much will depend on the results of the clinical trials.

In the meantime, a treatment not long ago labeled as an "un-proven method" (as if any method is "proven") is now in the clinical-trial stage and the trials have been officially endorsed by the American Cancer Society. Dr. Hellman is Chairman of the Board of Scientific Counselors of the NCI's Division of Cancer Treatment, and I—who was, at best, a maverick patient—was appointed by President Jimmy Carter to the National Cancer Advisory Board. The breast-cancer-treatment world had turned topsy-turvy.

As I wrote this paragraph, I could not resist calling Dr. Hellman in Boston to read it to him. He laughed at the wonder of it all, but then he quickly became serious.

"There's still a lot to do," he warned me. "We're not finished yet."

Of course, he is right. For most women in the United States, the struggle to have a finger in their own destinies is far from over: we still have a long way to go.

Until there is a well-trained radiation therapist available to every woman in the United States who chooses this option, the battle must still go on. Being well-trained means the doctor causes no burned hearts, no fibrous lungs and esophagi, no breasts so scorched and hard that women beg for mastectomies to replace them with skin grafts and implants, no arms so swollen because of sealed lymphatics that the women must hide them in long sleeves. Unfortunately, we must still fight to get enough of these experts. The reason is simple economics.

Women usually go first to their gynecologists, and few members of this specialty refer patients with breast-cancer symptoms to radiotherapists. Instead, they refer them to surgeons, and surgeons are trained (and paid) to perform mastectomies. Naturally, radiotherapists must also make a living, and so they set up their practices in communities where they can expect referrals. Without referrals to treat breast cancer, there is no incentive to invest the considerable quantities of time and money to become proficient at treating this disease. Without experience and the proper equipment, they cannot do what we women expect them to do: save our lives as well as our breasts.

IMMUNOTHERAPY

On December 3, 1967, Dr. Christiaan Barnard, the South African surgeon, performed the first human heart transplant in history. He removed the healthy heart of a twenty-five-year-old woman who had died after an automobile accident and put it into the chest of a fifty-five-year-old man, Lewis Washkansky. The patient appeared to do very well, and within a few days television screens around the world were showing him walking around with other patients and giving his wife a long, loving kiss. Eighteen days later, Washkansky was dead of a lung infection.

Less than a month later, on January 2, 1968, Dr. Barnard again transplanted a heart to a man named Philip Blaiberg. This time, however, the patient was kept in isolation. There was no walking around and chatting and no long, loving kisses. In a few short weeks, Dr. Barnard had drastically changed his postoperative procedure. What had happened?

I don't know what went on in Dr. Barnard's mind, but I suspect he got some very strong mail from immunologists who saw Washkansky visiting with germ-infested patients and kissing his bacteria-laden wife. This kind of socializing simply cannot be permitted by a patient who has been given immunosuppressants to enable his body to accept a foreign organ as its own. Every immunosuppressant known weakens the body's resistance to all disease.

Most people are familiar with immunology because of the various vaccinations they have had all their lives. The science was born one day in 1796 when Dr. Edward Jenner scratched his son's arm with secretions from a pustule of a cow suffering from cow-pox. This first vaccination immunized the boy against the small-pox epidemic then raging throughout England. In 1796, Dr. Jenner knew nothing about T-cells, B-cells, macrophages, antigens, or antibiotics. But he did know that anyone who had survived an attack of smallpox was somehow able to resist catching the disease again for the rest of his or her life. He theorized that if a person could be given a mild case of a similar disease, the protective system of the body might be fooled into conferring immunity to the more virulent disease. Medical history shows that Dr. Jenner's theory was correct.

All living things have built-in defense systems to fight off disease, and that is why life has continued on earth as long as it has. Building on this theory of bodily immunity and on the first successful smallpox vaccination, scientists have developed vaccines against many diseases that were once fatal to millions. Most of these are infectious diseases, however, which are passed from one person to another, not diseases that are caused by the kinds of agents suspected of causing cancer.

Reading the section on immunotherapy in *Breast Cancer* gave me the strange feeling that I was reviewing an ancient text from the historical shelf in a medical library. There has been so much exciting progress in the past seven years. But of course the basic principles of immunotherapy have not changed; scientists have developed the technical know-how to use them.

The immune system is made up of the thymus gland, the spleen, bone marrow, and the regional lymph nodes, and they produce such things as T-cells (from the thymus), white corpuscles (also called leukocytes), B-cells (from bone marrow), macrophages (the Greek word for "large eater"), and lymphocytes (from the lymph nodes). There may be others, as yet unknown. Together, these cells identify and target foreign invaders and destroy them. Those of us old enough to remember the Vietnam War can vividly recall the term, "search and destroy." This is exactly what components of the immune system do to defend the body they belong to. In dealing with breast cancer, the most important parts of the immune system are the axillary lymph nodes and their lympho-cytes. But all these are killer cells, which work in different ways as they wander through the bloodstream and lymphatic system searching for and destroying foreign invaders.

Dr. Paul Ehrlich, a bacteriologist by training, whose work has been a forerunner for so much cancer research, first proposed a general theory of immunity in 1885 in Germany. He suggested that the bloodstream carried antibodies—proteins manufactured by various cells—that searched for and either neutralized or destroyed bacterial invaders. He called the invaders antigens. But he and his followers worked on the assumption that cancer, like infectious diseases, was caused by a bacteriumlike parasite. So, although Dr. Ehrlich's hypothesis about the existence of an immune system later proved to be correct, he and the scientists who continued his research made no progress against cancer because they were attacking it the same way they attacked bacterial diseases.

In the years that followed, doctors found that cancer patients, who developed diseases with very high fevers, like malaria and erysipelas,* frequently improved considerably afterward or even had their cancers disappear entirely. Such phenomena led researchers to believe that the antibodies being produced to fight the infections were also effective against cancer. Essentially, 1896—the year this evidence was accepted—marks the year when real research in immunology began, although adequate financial support did not come until almost seven decades later, when kidney transplantation became a surgical reality. In order to avoid rejection of a kidney or other foreign organ, the body and the organ to be transplanted must first be treated with immunosuppressant drugs or irradiation. By suppressing the immune system artificially before surgery, instances of rejection were dramatically reduced. Then, when it was realized that a disproportionate number of kidney-transplant patients were developing cancer, scientists felt this was proof of some relationship between cancer and the immune system. More research was initiated to study the possible link, and immunology became an established branch of cancer investigation.

But what is the exact role played by the immune system? As far as breast cancer is concerned—no one really knows.

For example, cancers seem to be more common at the extremes of life, in the very old and young, when the self-defense system is either immature or failing. Therefore, cancer and immune deficiency must be somehow linked, even though this theory does not explain the development of breast cancer, a disease that usually strikes women in the prime of life.

---

*In 1974, Dr. William B. Coley was listed as an advocate of an "unproven method" (read "quackery"), because he said that patients suffering from the ravages of erysipelas were somehow magically saved from cancer. Now, "Coley's toxins," the results of the work he did to induce bacterial infections to create antibodies against cancer, have moved him from the unorthodox to the pioneer.

"That doesn't necessarily mean mammary carcinoma has nothing to do with the immune system, however," Dr. Tibor Borsos, an NCI immunologist pointed out to me. "It may only mean that we don't yet have the tools for measuring immune-competence or immune-deficiency accurately. Our tests are still new and relatively primitive. There is considerable evidence that the presence of a malignancy in a woman's breast triggers a great deal of immune activity in the regional lymph nodes, for instance. This could certainly be interpreted as an indication of some association."

In reviewing the literature, I learned that many researchers are studying this phenomenon to see if the various types of immune reactivity are "markers" that may give doctors a clue about a woman's prognosis. Dr. Maurice M. Black, a world-famous pathologist working in New York City, has probably done more work in this field than anyone else. He has been collecting results from analyses he has made of women's immune systems after mastectomy and continues to follow the patients' progress. If his predictions, based on these tests, should turn out to be accurate, they will be valuable aids to oncologists in deciding which women are at higher risk of developing second cancers and should be monitored more closely than others. The success of Dr. Black's prognostic tests would also influence the decisons made regarding the need for adjuvant treatment, even if there is no cancer found in the nodes.

In 1974, only one human cell line—the MCF-7—had been successfully kept alive in vitro, that is, in a test tube or Petri dish. Now there are at least fifteen, far more than the lone MCF-7 (Michigan Cancer Foundation, #7) strain of cells taken from fluid of the chest cavity of a woman in Detroit. In addition, methods have been developed to keep whole organs alive in vitro, using various nutrients not known in 1974. Such "explants" make then-impossible experiments routine, because all researchers working in every field of breast-cancer investigation can simply order blocks of tissue from commercial or private laboratories for their experiments. This development—along with the ability to keep more individual cell strains alive in an artificial environment—has opened a new world of possibilities to scientists.

An immunological debate that may soon be settled is whether or not there is an existence of immune "surveillance system." This means simply that cancer cells are always present in the body and that the various immune components wander through and destroy them before they can begin to multiply and cause trouble. If malignant cells do manage to establish a colony somewhere, according to this principle, it is a sign that the defense system is damaged. Although this has not been definitely proven in the case of breast cancer, extrapolations can be made based on the number of untreated women with positive axillary nodes who, nonetheless, do not develop metastases. If there were no such surveillance system, this would not be possible.

And if there were no immune surveillance system, there would be a few survivors of the disease—indeed of any cancer! Moreover, random blood samples taken of patients with metastases of one type or another usually show the presence of living cancer cells. Something must be preventing them from anchoring and establishing new colonies, and that "something" must be the immune system. As I have and will state again, autopsies of older men and women who have died of other causes frequently show breast, prostate, and other cancers that began to grow and simply stopped. The only possible reason for such phenomena is strong resistance by the immune system.

Back in 1974, scientists were still debating whether cancer cells had unique characteristics that could be used for identification. The existence of a tumor-associated-antigen (TAA) on the surface or inside a cancer cell that would then permit them to be recognized and, perhaps even destroyed, was still in doubt. Dr. Lloyd J. Old, of the Memorial Sloan-Kettering Cancer Center in New York, had not yet published the data that proved each cancer cell carried a "foreign label" of its own.

What was theory in 1974 is old-hat now, and all experts know these labels—the TAAs—are as individual as a person's fingerprints. More important, immunologists are studying how to use these TAAs to both detect and destroy the malignant cells to which they belong. Again, we have come a long, long way since 1974. The field of immunology is so dynamic that what I will write today might be obsolete in a few weeks, but the basic principles should be the same. Knowing them is essential for understanding why so much hope (not to mention talent, energy, and money) is being put into the interferons and other biological-response modifiers, hybridomas, and monoclonal antibodies.

But this is getting ahead of the story.

As I said earlier, the major manufacturers of the various components of the immune system are the thymus gland, bone marrow, the spleen, and the hundreds of lymph nodes scattered throughout the body. Some immune factors kill foreigners; others only look for invaders, so they can red-flag a target so different killer cells will home in on it to destroy it in various ways.

Macrophages, for example, engulf and surround the enemy cell and literally eat it up. Antibodies, as I will explain later, may damage a single part of a cell, interfering with its nutrition, for example, or stopping its ability to reproduce. Researchers still do not fully understand the numerous ways immune components do their jobs. Since immunology is essentially an infant science, a great deal must still be learned.

But there is also a great deal that is known. For example, scientists know that the body's Department of Defense is divided into two armed services: the humoral and the cell-mediated forces. The humoral system is like a police station that has cops walking regular beats to patrol their neighborhoods. The policemen check doors and peer down dark alleys to look for possible trouble, while the policemen at the telephone switchboard in the station house mastermind the system. Like these stationary police, the humoral switchboard system sends various substances (beat-patrolling cops) out to circulate in the body's fluids and to roam through the body searching for anything that does not belong there. As soon as a stranger is recognized, these humoral foot-patrolling "police" (antibodies) are "educated" or "sensitized" to identify and attach themselves to specific parts of an invader by a lock-and-key attraction. When this is done, various types of killer cells or phagocytes then move in to attack and destroy the foreigners.

A cell-mediated immune response, on the other hand, goes in to action only when that specific cell is itself a target. Both mechanisms—the humoral and cell-mediated responses—use the same cops-on-the-beat to do the actual fighting: T- and B-cells, macropages, lymphocytes, and antibodies. But each is activated in a different way. As I've said, cells (not only cancer cells) have their own distinctive "fingerprints," antigens, either on the surfaces of or within their cells. When a wandering humoral B-cell recognizes an enemy, it becomes sensitized to that particular target, and immediately begins to divide into groups, or clones, of identical cells. All of the member cells of the clone are programed to identify that antigen and nothing else. This is what is meant by "educated" antibodies.

After the foreign invaders have been destroyed, some of the humoral antibodies remain as "memory" cells, already trained to identify and fight that antigen if it should ever show up again. This is the familiar immune mechanism that protects us from polio, measles, diptheria, whooping cough, etc.

Antibodies may also defend us in other ways. They may actually damage the foreign antigen and, in this way, destroy the cell to which it is attached. Or antibodies may "coat" the invader, interfering with its normal functioning and act as a signal to attracting phagocytes that will then kill it.

But antibodies may be a double-edged sword. There is evidence that the antibody-coat may often protect the invader and actually enhance its growth by somehow causing it to be identified as "self" by the body's natural killer (NK) cells. This theory would explain why healthy, immune-competent women develop breast cancer: their self-defense systems simply do not recognize the coated malignant cells in their breasts to be the enemies they are.

Cell-mediated, rather than humoral, responses occur when a cell of the body is itself the target of the antigens of foreign invaders. The same cloning process of educated antibodies results, and some of these will join humoral B-cells in a "memory bank" for future invaders. But another cell-mediated response is to manufacture proteins called lymphokines as soon as any invading antigens are contacted. Lymphokines may be the most valuable components of the cell-mediated immune system. Not only do they mobilize natural killer cells and direct them to the places where they are needed, but they can prevent the NKs from leaving the scene until the invaders are completely destroyed. Interferons (IF), now-famous lymphokines, also have the capability of stopping viruses from multiplying. During the last years of the 1970s, there was a great deal of optimism about interferons' potential value in treating breast cancer. However, several clinical trials showed that they were ineffective, at least using the interferons then available. If interferons had not received so much publicity, I would end the discussion of them now simply by saying that the future merit of these substances must wait for the test of time. But since they have even made it to the covers of *Time* and *Newsweek,* they cannot be shrugged off as being in an immunological limbo.

First isolated and identified as having antiviral activity in 1957, IFs were neglected as interesting, but too-hard-to-get proteins until 1971. They were neglected and too-hard-to-get simply because the amount of interferon each cell produces is miniscule, and it was almost impossible to obtain enough to treat even one human patient.

But in 1971, Dr. Hans Strander and his colleagues at the Karolinska Institute in Sweden were able to get a large enough quantity of leukocyte interferon to treat a few patients who had osteogenic sarcoma—a rare and virulent bone cancer. Leukocyte IF was extracted from white blood cells by a method developed by Dr. Kari Cantrell of the Central Public Health Laboratories in Helsinki. The conventional production method required 65,000 pints of human blood to produce 100 milligrams of IF, and one doctor I interviewed estimated it would have cost about $10,000 to treat one patient for one month. During the 1960s, Dr. Cantrell, in cooperation with the Finnish Red Cross, had been able to obtain enough white cells to extract interferon for small treatment trials. These involved viral infections as well as certain types of cancers—including mammary carcinoma.

In spite of the expense, trials did go on, and Dr. Strander's study was one of them. His data showed that almost sixty-five per cent of the osteogenic sarcoma patients treated with leukocyte IF were free of disease two and a half years later, as opposed to thirty per cent in the nontreated group. After these results were announced, researchers all over the world began to clamor for a chance to try the substance against other cancers.

But there simply was not enough leukocyte interferon to go around. In 1978, the American Cancer Society announced that it was investing $2 million for clinical research involving the use of this kind of interferon in 200 patients who had one of the four different tumors being investigated—breast cancer was one of them. Subsequently, the ACS allocated another $3.2 million to IF trials. Pressure from constituents pursuaded members of Congress to request that the NCI also invest in the research, and in October 1978, its Division of Cancer Treatment set up a Biological Response Modifiers Program. A large part of the NCI budget, $13.5 million, was allotted to the BRMP, but not all of the money is being devoted to interferons. Other agents known to fight cancer by affecting the actions of the many components of the immune system were to be studied as well.

As far as IFs were concerned, the bulk of the funding was spent to find quicker and cheaper ways to produce the lymphokine. Eventually, several commercial firms were awarded contracts to develop two other types, fibroblast and lymphoblastoid interferon. At its Frederick (Md.) Cancer Research Center—formerly the U.S. Army's Fort Detrick for Biological Warfare Research—the NCI itself began to manufacture interferon, using methods that do not require human blood. (One technique, for example, uses foreskins obtained from circumcisions.)

Early public reports of the four clinical trials involving breast cancer indicated that IF was working well. However, at an international immunotherapy conference I attended at the NIH in May 1980, the mood was all cynicism and skepticism.

"Interferon is emphatically *not* going to be any magic bullet against breast cancer," one of the IF program directors at the NCI told me. "I'm not ready to go public on this yet, but I'm sure we all will soon. The press is raising false hopes and causing a lot of harm."

He told me his telephone rang incessantly with pathetic pleas from women who had read about the "miracle drug" in *Business Week, Forbes* or *The Wall Street Journal*.

"Those are great sources of accurate medical information," he quipped. "There are a lot of people making fortunes overnight on interferon as a cure for cancer." He paused. "Maybe for colds, shingles, or pneumonia, someday. Maybe for some of the malignancies that might be caused by a virus.

"But for breast cancer?" he asked rhetorically. "Not with what's available now. Maybe we'll find a way to change an atom or two, one of these days . . . "

Dr. Dao agreed. Since a group of the women being treated with the ACS leukocyte interferon was at Roswell Park, I could not help but react to the hoopla with apprehension after he told me his opinion of the trials. Like my "anonymous source" at the NCI, I too had a telephone ringing off the hook with calls from women begging for interferon. A medical-writer friend, Maya Pines, was assigned to write an article about the lymphokine at about that time, and she asked me what I thought.

"According to my sources," I told her, "a woman with breast cancer would be better off buying stock in any of the companies jumping on the bandwagon than she would be by taking interferon."

In February 1981, the American Cancer Society held its annual science writers' seminar in Daytona Beach, Florida, and the news about interferon for any cancer was no longer as optimistic.

"I never thought interferon was a magic bullet for cancer treatment," Dr. Frank J. Rauscher, Jr., senior vice president of research of the ACS told reporters. "But you've got to go for broke . . . The jury is still out."

By that time, according to the April 10, 1981 issue of *Science*, the Society had spent nearly $6.8 million to buy IF and the NCI had spent about $11 million. Only members of the New York Stock Exchange and the Internal Revenue Service know how many private dollars were bet on this "magic bullet."

But everyone is still hoping. In mid-February 1981, the NCI began testing 150 patients with advanced disease to determine maximum safe dosages. Other trials were about to begin in medical centers all over the country, using different kinds of interferons against various types of cancer. The most recent advances are now in the development of techniques to produce purified IF using either monoclonal antibodies or various kinds of genetic engineering.

Again, we women must wait for the development of technological know-how, this time to solve the puzzle of interferons. Virtually all progress against breast cancer—its detection, diagnosis, and treatment—has relied on advances in engineering and electronics, as well as on medical findings. Now millions of women all over the world must wait once more to see if a more purified interferon is to be the "magic bullet" for which we have been waiting so long.

As the name of the NCI's Biological Response Modifiers Program indicates, interferons are only one kind of biological-response-modifier—even though IFs have received the lion's share of the money and publicity. There are other substances that have the ability to modify or change the body's response to disease organisms, including cancer. For example, under the broad umbrella of "immunoaugmenting" agents, there are several immune boosters. One is BCG *(Bacillus Calmette Gùerin)*, also known as the Mirayama vaccine. It is nothing more than weakened tuberculosis germs.

There are two principles underlying the use of BCG (as well as other foreign agents). One is the well-known concept of boosting a cancer patient's overall immune response to these almost-dead bacteria, and, by doing so, strengthening his or her natural defenses against invading cancer cells. This is often successful in treating certain kinds of cancer, but it has not been useful by itself against breast cancer. Instead, BCG and other kinds of immune boosters are given in combination with conventional radio- or chemotherapies. This involves another purpose of immunoaugmentation: counteracting the side effects of these therapies.

All known anticancer agents weaken the immune system, and by adding BCG or MER (methanol extraction residue of BCG), C. Parvum (Corynebacterium parvum), Levamisole, or other "nonspecific" stimulators, immunologists try to offset such immune suppression from radiation and/or chemotherapy.

"Immunoaugmenting" biological response modifiers, then, are *not* natural products of the body, as lymphokines are, but are external agents introduced to stir the immune system into action to achieve these two results: destruction (or, at least, inhibition) of cancer cells and opposition to the suppressing effects of other therapies being used. At this time, most immune therapy is nonspecific: the goal is to strengthen resistance to everything foreign that may be in the body rather than to a certain disease. Interferons and interferon inducers (literally, substances that trigger the body's own white cells into manufacturing natural IFs) are, obviously, in this category.

Developing "active specific" immune therapies is a major goal of the NCI's Biological Response Modifiers Program. The groundwork for such immunological manipulations, for both the detection and treatment of cancer, has already been laid. Earlier, I referred to hybridomas and monoclonal antibodies, but the work is still too preliminary to detail in this chapter. It is a hope for The Future.

Interferon is not the only immunological therapy that has made banner headlines around the world. Lawrence Burton, Ph.D. (Zoology) has also managed to snare the print and electronic media, in particular the respected CBS' *60 Minutes* television program. This is one immunological tale I can enjoy telling firsthand, without interviews or library research, because I lived it.

In March 1979, my daughter Lesley and I went to Freeport, Grand Bahama Island to celebrate the end of a tedious writing job of mine and her excellent mid-semester grades. The Breast Cancer Advisory Center had been in existence almost four years, and I had received dozens of inquiries about the Immunology Researching Centre, Ltd. in the Bahamas, so I planned to combine pleasure with business if I could find Dr. Lawrence Burton. Once in the Freeport casino, I discovered this was easy: there is nothing for his patients to do every evening except gamble. Sitting around a blackjack table, I quickly struck up conversations with several of them. As soon as I told them my name, they recognized it from the cancer grapevine and insisted I take up his cause.

"He's all that has kept me alive," an elderly gentleman, I'll call Mr. Smith, told me. "But I hate having to leave the family every couple of months to come down here. I can't understand why they won't let him do what he's doing back home."

A lovely young blonde woman from New Jersey showed me photos of her two children. "I miss them so much," she said. "It breaks my heart to leave them with my mother every time I have to come down here."

When I complimented the Grand Bahama Island for its beautiful beaches and plush hotels, both were bitter.

"Sure, it's a great place for a vacation," Mr. Smith said, "but try living here six or eight weeks. Everything is imported except tomatoes, chicken, and fish. A gallon of milk costs $4.00.

"If Dr. Burton was legal up home," he said angrily, "my retirement health plan would be paying all his bills."

Mrs. Jones nodded. "It's making my family bankrupt for me to live down here," she explained. "It's not the cost of the treatment that's the problem, it's the living expenses."

Even though I had never heard would-be patients talk about the Burton therapy for several years, I had never even thought of the financial hardship living on a vacation-resort island must be.

Packing Lesley's camera and lenses, we hailed a taxicab the next morning and rode over to the Rand Memorial Hospital. There were four women in the waiting room. One carried an arm in a sling; another had a ballooning abdomen. All of them were complaining about their rents and the astronomical cost of living in Freeport. Since I had called for an appointment, Lesley and I were ushered into Dr. Burton's cluttered office within a few minutes. A huge computer terminal took up most of his desk. The stocky, gray-bearded zoologist looked like everyone's ideal grandpa.

"I got my Ph.D. in zoology from NYU in 1956," he began without any help. "I was a Navy corpsman in World War II, and I'm fifty-four years old."

He smiled at me as I madly tried to keep up with him.

"Is there anything else you want to know?"

"Yes, as a matter of fact," I answered. "What are you doing here that you can't do in the United States?"

"Absolutely nothing!" he barked. "I never touch a patient. I've never given a shot or taken blood pressure. All the medical treatment given is done by medical doctors. All I do is read the computer print-outs."

"There must be something more," I insisted. "Why are you here and not back in New York?"

"It's a long story," he began. "Back in 1973, I started to use a blocking factor in Great Neck, New York. It looked pretty good, and I went the orthodox route and went to the FDA to get an INDA—an investigational new drug application. And I got it too . . . BBINDA #844."

"What happened?"

"I couldn't get permission to go ahead," he explained. "They wanted to know how many immune components I got from a liter of blood. They asked what my results were with cat leukemia. Who gave a damn about cat leukemia? I wanted to cure people."

"What's your blocking factor?" I asked. "Every immunologist has a different one."

"Alpha proteins."

"But what are they?"

"My wife, Esther, has everything written down," Dr. Burton

told me. "She's home sick today, but I'll send them over to your hotel tomorrow."

After filling me in on more of his past problems with various cancer bureaucracies, Dr. Burton took Lesley and me on a tour of his impressive computerized laboratories.

"Everything is the most modern and the best," he said proudly. "I work here with the blessing of the Bahamian government. But I would like to go home. My kids are all grown, and let's face it . . . I get homesick."

"There isn't anything you can be doing that someone isn't doing at the National Cancer Institute," I told him. "Everybody has some kind of blocking factor or immune component they're taking from or giving to cancer patients. I can't believe what you're doing couldn't be done in New York, so all of these people didn't have to spend so much money."

He agreed. "It costs them a lot more to fly and live here than it does to get my treatment."

At that time, the costs at the Burton clinic were $2,200 per month.

"All I'm drawing is $30,000 a year, and my wife works for nothing," he said. "I'm not doing this for the money."

After shooting four rolls of film, Lesley and I went back to the hotel. I was determined to "decriminalize" Dr. Lawrence Burton.

The next day, nothing arrived. I telephoned.

"Esther is still not feeling too well," he explained. "Tomorrow."

But nothing arrived the next day either, and we were to leave Freeport the following morning. I telephoned again.

"Esther's still not well," he told me. "I'll mail it to your house."

When I returned home, I called Dr. Jeffrey Schlom, an NCI immunologist, and described what Burton had told me about his type of cancer treatment.

"I think the problem might be that he is a zoologist and not an immunologist," I said naively, "and he's embarrassed to admit that he doesn't really know what he's doing or why whatever he's doing works."

"You might be right," Dr. Schlom said. "I'm sure I could figure it out. Write and tell him I'm interested and that there's no conspiracy just because he's not an M.D."

Instead of writing, I telephoned and offered Dr. Schlom's help.

"I'm sending all the material right up, Air Mail," he responded. "You ought to have it in a couple of days."

That was in March 1979. (I have yet to find out what Dr. Burton's immune components are.) Fewer than two months later I watched *60 Minutes* with intense fascination. Picking and choosing only those fragments of film that said what the program's narrator wanted the message to be, he was able to make Lawrence Burton emerge as a maligned and persecuted hero, exiled to Freeport because the National Cancer Institute does not really want to find a cure for cancer.

Knowing that some of the resources of the NCI had been unofficially offered (and ignored) by Burton only six weeks earlier, I stared at the screen in disbelief. Later, I learned that Dr. William D. Terry, the NCI's chief of immunology, had been interviewed for several hours and had painstakingly detailed the situation. On-screen, Dr. Terry was the heinous villain for a total of, at most, four minutes. The producers had set out to show the Cancer Establishment to be an exclusive society, closed to unorthodox approaches, and that is exactly what the vast viewing public saw and heard.

In October 1980, Lawrence Burton attended a conference in New York, and one of his living patients called to ask me to "stand up" for him. I told her to ask him for his "formula" or "recipe" or whatever he termed the immunological procedure to be. After describing my unwarranted enthusiasm the preceding March, I suggested she relay a few words about the embarrassment Burton had caused me.

"He backed down," I told her. "He never has sent me what he promised. There's really no reason for him to be an outcast, unless that's the way he wants it to be."

I doubt that she believed me.

In July 1981, the legislature of Florida passed a bill that would have given Burton nine months to demonstrate the value of using "human blood fractions for the control or cure of cancer"—the treatment he has been using in Freeport. Although both the state's House (101 to 3) and Senate (27 to 11) supported giving Burton legal permission to practice "immunoaugmentative therapy," Governor Bob Graham vetoed the bill. Several doctors in the state legislature told reporters that passage would have made Florida, "the snake-oil capital of this country."

Burton's supporters, however, feel that freedom-of-choice for cancer patients will eventually win approval, and he will be allowed to practice in Florida.

Whatever it is that Burton has been doing in the Bahamas, it cannot be any more unorthodox than immunological procedures that are being done all over the world. Of course, these are used only when all conventional and "proven" methods have failed, but according to Burton, he steadfastly refuses to treat anyone except terminal cases. The following cases would, however, qualify.

For example, in Bristol, England, twenty-five patients with a very malignant kind of bladder cancer had chunks of their tumors inoculated into pigs. When tests showed that the animals had developed antibodies against the malignancies, samples of their blood were injected into the patients. The doctors managing the experiment hoped that the antibodies produced by the pigs would unite with the patients' own killer cells to fight off the cancer. Of the twenty-five patients—none of whom would have lived longer than a year from the time of diagnosis—one-third were still alive after more than a year. In other cases, the bladder tumors disappeared, but the patients died of metastases already established before the pig-cell treatment. One patient was still alive two and a half years afterward.

This cross-inoculation method seemed to be most effective when combined with X-ray treatment given about six weeks after injection of the antibodies. The Bristol team was very cautious in its report and emphasized the extremely small size of the sample, but the experiment could be a milestone. If cross-inoculation using an animal as the intermediary incubator should be successful with bladder cancer, the same kind of procedure might also be useful against breast cancer.

Along the same line, some success—*very limited* success, but *some*—has been achieved in cross-transplantation of cancers. Patients with different kinds of cancer exchange bits of their tumors with each other. Where this has been tried, the immune systems have manufactured large numbers of lymphocytes, which have reacted strongly to the new, strange invaders, and the donated cancers did not "take." While the added boost of lymphocytes in the recipients' bloodstreams did not destroy their own tumors, there was enough improvement to convince some scientists that cross-transplantation merits further trials. On the other hand, opponents fear that exchanging cancers is almost "Hitlerian."

Everything published about new anticancer treatments and every expert I talked to about either chemotherapy or immunology had one constant, common refrain: "Science does not promise miracles."

A miracle, by definition, is "an event or effect in the physical world deviating from the laws of nature." The "laws of nature" I have described here are those that involve breast cancer, and a cure would be a deviant event. What I want is this kind of deviation from the laws, something like a Salk vaccine, some "white magic" from the research laboratories. But experts are senstitive to any talk of miracles or magic. Understandably, nothing in medicine is more cruel than fostering false hope. A way either to prevent or to cure breast cancer is impossible to predict, and we cancer patients know that well enough. We also shy away from talk—or even thoughts—of miracles.

But still, we expect them.

13

Reconstructive Mammoplasty

It seemed as if only a few minutes had gone by when a strange, harsh buzz tore into my sleep. I jumped out of bed and saw the fire alarm light blinking furiously with each buzz. Still only half awake, I opened the drapes and looked down. Black smoke was coming out of a window a few stories below my seventh-floor hotel room, and fire engines were parked in front of the building. "FIRE" suddenly penetrated my brain, and my sleepiness vanished. Quickly, I put on my underwear and slipped the prosthesis into the empty left cup of my bra. Frenzied with fear, I pulled on a pair of slacks and a suit jacket. Because I stumbled over them, I put my shoes on but left everything else behind except my eyeglasses.

I had never been in a fire in my life. And, although I hadn't been in a fire drill since high school days, I did know that elevators shouldn't be used. The stairways were well marked, and I soon found myself hanging onto the bannister that was guiding me in a calm, but packed, line down to the lobby. Some people had had the foresight to dampen a washcloth or handkerchief before leaving their rooms, and these were plastered over noses and mouths to keep out the sharpness. I hadn't been smart enough to do this, and the fumes cut into my lungs like scalpels. Finally, we reached the doors to the lobby and burst out. Almost in unison, we coughed and gasped to get rid of the acrid black smoke and replace it with crisp night air that came into the large room from opened doors.

The hotel staff had already set up coffee urns, and newspaper and TV people were wandering through the lobby to interview us evacuees. I found a chair and sat down, sipping coffee and talking to a young couple who had thrown coats over their night clothes. (I don't think the man had anything underneath at all!) We were interrupted by a reporter who had attended my lecture.

"Pardon me," he said. "Aren't you Rose Kushner?"

"Yes, I am."

"I was at the Baptist Hospital this afternoon," he said, "and I thought you were you."

"Yes," I laughed. "I don't wear eyeglasses onstage. . . ."

He interrupted me as a photographer's flashbulb went off behind him.

"I'd like to know why you bothered to get dressed when the emergency signal went off," he asked.

I looked around, startled by his question. Sure enough, most of the evacuees were just covered by a coat or robe and were wandering around in a state of undress. The only people in the lobby, besides me, who were wearing reasonable amounts of clothing were guests who had come in after the alarm had gone off or hotel staffers, firemen, and members of the media.

It was a good question. I should have put on my robe, my specs and rushed to safety without worrying about being underdressed.

Why, indeed, had I taken the time to put on clothes?

The answer was simple: this "well-adjusted" mastectomee wasn't going anywhere publicly with one breast. This "well-adjusted" mastectomee had a serious, subconscious self-image problem.

The fire occurred on February 2, 1977 in Jacksonville, Florida—a great place to be while the snow was stacked up high in front of my house up north. I had arrived the day before at the invitation of Dr. Curtis M. Phillips, the chief of oncology of the Baptist Medical Center, to talk to the hospital's nurses and anyone else interested in listening to a couple of hours about breast cancer. Although he was chief of the cancer unit, Dr. Phillips' big interest was reconstructive mammoplasty—plastic surgery after mastectomy to replace breasts with implants. He had perfected a unique way of doing this and wanted to show me the operation.

The surgery was performed successfully, and my luncheon talk had a standing-room-only audience. Because the hospital's public relations department had arranged for television coverage and newspaper interviews, the program had received a lot of advance publicity. I remember chuckling about the absurdity of it all: developing breast cancer had made me a "celebrity."

After a long, leisurely bath, I crawled into bed, exhausted from the wear-and-tear of the day's activity and fell asleep immediately. That's when all hell had broken loose! Fire alarms, fire trucks, smoke, flames, mind-curdling terror as I blindly felt my way along the bannister to the clean air of the hotel lobby.

As soon as I pulled my head together from the shock, I realized the reporter's question hit a raw nerve. I made up my mind to investigate Dr. Curtis' reconstruction mammoplasty for myself. I had been *so* sure I didn't need it.

In the operating room, I had teetered on a box to be tall enough to look over Dr. Curtis' shoulder and see what he was doing. Just the way I had seen it in the television show *M*A*S*H*, the doctors and nurses did a lot of kibitzing over the anesthetized body on their table.

"Ever think about getting this done yourself, Ms. Kushnuh?" Dr. Curtis asked. The mask over his mouth muffled his southern drawl.

I shook my head. "No. I just don't feel like being cut again unless its absolutely necessary."

"Haven't had a single lady yet that wasn't glad she did it," he said. Dr. Curtis' back was toward me, and he couldn't see the firm shake of my head and the slight shudder that went through me at the mere thought of having another operation.

"No way would I voluntarily get on another operating table, Dr. Curtis," I insisted. "Besides I had such good surgery that I can wear a bikini. There's absolutely no reason . . ."

"Think you all are makin' a mistake, Ms. Kushnuh," he said. Never missing a stroke, Dr. Curtis had continued making precise slashes with his scapel while a surgical resident quickly cauterized the small blood vessels to stop the flow into the incision. "I've heard that story lots of times, Ms. Kushnuh," he had continued, "and all my ladies tell me afterward that they never knew how much difference it would make to them and their loved ones to put that little old bag of jelly under the skin where it belongs."

"No, Dr. Curtis, thank you," I said firmly. "My husband doesn't mind at all. And he'd be afraid that it might hide something growing underneath. After all, it hasn't even been three years since my mastectomy."

I had apparently touched a sore spot by mentioning the business of having an implant mask or hide a recurrence. The dialogue ended abruptly.

I had, of course, known about breast reconstruction (as reconstructive mammoplasty is usually called) long before going to Jacksonville. But, as I said, I was smugly complacent about my own id and ego and had never even suspected my body-image, sense of womanhood, or "wholeness" had been affected by the loss of a 32A breast. And my short, neat, vertical incision had never stopped me from wearing even the most plunging decolletage.

So, as I had told Dr. Curtis, I never wanted to see the green sheets of an operating suite again, unless I absolutely had to. Dr. Reuven Snyderman, one of reconstruction's early pioneers, and I had been on several programs together, and he—a plastic surgeon—assured me that the operation was not a "cosmetic triumph" even when it was done by an expert. He had also shown me before-and-after slides of his patients and of women treated by some of his colleagues. The baseball-like protrusions that frequently resulted were so unlike breasts that reconstruction hadn't seemed to be worth the money and pain involved.

But the fire and everything that could have happened gave me second and third thoughts. As soon as I could, I paid a visit to the NIH Library to study the "literature." Surgeons had been trying to rebuild breasts lost to breast cancer for decades. Before 1962, such operations involved moving tissue from women's abdomens and buttocks to their chests by different techniques done in separate operations. It was expensive, painful, and time-consuming.

Then in 1962, Dr. Thomas D. Cronin, a professor of plastic surgery at the Baylor Medical School in Houston, developed a procedure for inserting a silicone-gel implant under the skin. Silicone padding, of course, had been used for years to make flat chests more buxom—augmentation mammoplasty. (Everyone old enough to remember Carole Doda and the first topless dancers in San Francisco or the spectacular Dagmar on the Johnny Carson show can probably recall the huge balloons appended to their upper torsos.) However, so little was known about breast cancer's biology in those years that most doctors were afraid to use silicone implants after a mastectomy. For example, Dr. C. D. Haagensen, a world-renowned breast-cancer expert is reported to have called the operation "madness."

In December 1976, after breast reconstruction was becoming popular, he was still against plastic surgery, claiming that too much tissue had to be left during the original mastectomy to accommodate an implant. He felt that anyone who would do reconstructive mammoplasty for the sake of cosmetics was risking the patient's life. Dr. Haagensen called the procedure "unconscionable."

Although Dr. Haagensen's well-known opinions about radical breast surgery had not made him one of my favorite experts, his objections to mammoplasty made me think twice. After all, he *did* know a lot about breast cancer. So, for the time being, his warning turned me off and I filed the idea away.

But it was not forgotten.

Every time I had a chance, I questioned people in the Breast Cancer Task Force of the NCI about any potential dangers, and I also asked Dr. Dao to look into it for me. At the time, he was against reconstruction for still another reason.

"Nobody knows what the silicone might do about causing a sarcoma of the chest wall," he told me. "Nobody has ever studied this. Why take any chances?"

He was afraid, because the Silastic™ (silicone pressed into a sheet) bag holding the gel is porous, and molecules of the silicone are known to pass out of the implant into the body.

These worries about silicone were aggravated by a letter I received from a woman who had had her breasts made larger by augmentation mammoplasty several years earlier. She had been in an automobile accident, and the steering wheel had punctured the implant. Although her doctors believed she was lucky—the implant had cushioned her ribs and protected them from being fractured—she was finding globules of silicone under the skin of her legs, belly, back, and arms. She said her surgeon could do nothing except remove the more unslightly lumps and leave the others alone. One more thing to worry about.

But I couldn't forget my behavior at the Jacksonville fire. No matter how much I learned about its problems, it was impossible for me to forget breast reconstruction.

At the end of 1977, the Breast Cancer Task Force sponsored a special session on reconstructive mammoplasty, and several plastic surgeons and pathologists came to Bethesda for the meeting. They brought samples of some of the different implants, and, for the first time, I learned that the Silastic™ bag does not have to be made with silicone-gel but can be filled with saline—just sterilized salt water.

I don't remember who recommended saline, but I can see him clearly in my mind's eye. He pointed out that saline had several advantages over its competitor. First, there is obviously no reason to worry about migrating molecules, because the body is composed almost entirely of salt water. Secondly, saline implants are less likely to develop the hard, postoperative shells (the technical name for these is "contractures") that sometimes grow around silicone-gel implants. In addition, the size of the new "breast" can be adjusted easily by putting just enough saline into the tiny valve of the implant to match the second breast. Since my external prosthesis was a bit larger than my remaining breast even though it was Size 0, the smallest made, this feature was important to me.

Of course, anything that has advantages usually has disadvantages too. The cosmetic results are not as good with saline, I learned, because there's no way to give a bag of water any kind of solid shape or form. Also, the skin over the saline-filled implant has a tendency to crease or wrinkle with the water swishing around in the bag underneath. But this can only be seen in the nude.

I did not, by the way, learn about all this from doctors but from women who had had the saline procedure done. Jean Zalon, a patient pioneer who wrote a book called *I Am Whole Again,* gave me a lot of information, and several other women permitted me to see their saline-filled breast mounds. Everyone was happy with her miraculous, new-found cleavage.

"They're lopsided and uneven, but I don't care what I look like when I'm naked," one told me. "All I know is that it's soft and feels like the real thing."

As I researched the question more and more, there were fewer and fewer reasons *not* to have the reconstruction. Dr. Dao had left me plenty of skin to accommodate the small size of either a saline or silicone implant, and—in spite of his fears of my growing another cancer—there were absolutely no data from animal studies showing that microscopic migrating molecules of silicone had ever caused a malignancy. I also checked with radiologists and was told that, with certain changes of position, excellent mammograms could be taken. So any recurrence under the implant could be found without any trouble.

What convinced me most, though, was that I couldn't find (and have not, to this day) a single woman who was sorry she had decided to have this plastic surgery. Even when serious complications required additional operations or if the "breast" looked as if someone put a baseball under the skin, all of the women I talked to were unanimous about their happiness with breast reconstruction.

"My external prosthesis was always somewhere around my waist or my shoulder when I swam or played tennis," one explained. "Now I don't have to worry at all. I've always got the comfortable feeling that my breast is on my chest where it's supposed to be."

Another woman told me she didn't at all miss the sweat and itching she had always had during the summer. "That's over now," she grinned. "No more talcum powder and flannel squares between my skin and the prosthesis to absorb perspiration."

I myself remembered an incident in a discount dress shop when the prosthesis had fallen out of my bra as I bent over to pick something up from the floor of the mass dressing room. I'm still embarrassed when I think of the little girl who yelled, "Look Mommy! That lady's booby fell down." Everyone turned to stare, and I never went back to that bargain house again.

There was no question about my going ahead with reconstruction anymore, but, as far as the silicone vs. saline was concerned, I still didn't know what to do.

In March 1978 (I took my time, in spite of the fire), the Breast Cancer Task Force invited someone from the FDA's Bureau of Medical Devices and Appliances to discuss that agency's data about long-term use of internal implants. It turned out that the Bureau had not gone into business until August 1976. All products that had been in use before then had been given automatic approval under a "grandfather's clause," and breast implants fell into that category. So neither the silicone-gel nor saline implants had been evaluated for safety by FDA scientists and would not be unless a complaint was made about them. (Follow-up of the tens of thousands of women who have had augmentation mammoplasty, by the way, is out of the question unless they agree to let the world know they had not been generously endowed by nature, but by plastic surgeons.) The doctor from the FDA did consider the Task Force's question to be an official "complaint," and said he'd recommend that research be started. But obviously, the answer would not be available for years.

By that time, I was champing at the bit to have my breast reconstructed so I could join the constantly growing number of prosthesis-free women. So even though there wasn't (and still isn't) a shred of evidence that silicone-gel is harmful in any way, I opted for saline and found a plastic surgeon who used this type of implant—Dr. Bernard Scott Teunis in nearby Bethesda, Maryland.

After spending more than a year researching and interviewing, getting the implant was almost an anti-climax. I went to the hospital early one June morning, was body-painted with a purple magic marker (to show where the bottom edge of the implant should be to be level with my other breast in a bra) and got a shot. It was a combination of Valium and Demerol that put me into a sort of twilight sleep: I felt no pain but was conscious enough to cooperate. Before the operation, I wondered why I would need to cooperate, but when I woke up from the one-hour operation, I knew. The upper part of my torso was encased in a stiff, long-line bra, and it would have been impossible for Dr. Teunis to put it on a dead-weight anesthetized body. He had to have me conscious enough to slide my arms through the steel-like straps and sit while it was zipped up.

Wearing that harness during a torrid week in June without a bath or shower turned out to be the worst part of the whole operation. By the time I left home for the first postoperative checkup, it was so rancid that I threw it into the first public trash can I passed.

My recovery was, as doctors say, "unremarkable." For a couple of weeks, the implant seemed to be too large and too high, but Dr. Teunis and my "patient-consultants" told me this was normal. Everyone said massaging with cocoa-butter cream would help the implant settle into place more quickly. In the meantime, I unpacked my bathing suit and gleefully ripped out the polyester falsie I had sewn into the left cup. With the same hysterical joy, I detached the down-filled "puffs" stitched into my nightgowns since the Jacksonville fire. By the time we went to the beach for the Fourth of July weekend, I had already forgotten what it was like to hide my scar whenever I had to bend over.

But probably the most exciting sensation was being able to feel elbows when they bumped into me in a crowd. For almost four years, I'd been feeling bumps second-hand: I knew an elbow was poking at me only because the prosthesis was moving. There was no direct contact with me. Now, all of a sudden, those elbows hurt. It was great!

Later, I was asked by the National Cancer Institute to write a booklet for women about breast reconstruction. It answered most of the questions I've been asked about reconstructive mammoplasty, and I'm including much of it here as a fitting end to my personal saga.

"BREAST RECONSTRUCTION"
Creating a new breast contour after mastectomy

Breast reconstruction, also known as "reconstructive mammoplasty," is the procedure used by plastic surgeons to create a natural-looking breast shape by inserting an implant under the skin and muscles of the chest when a breast has been removed, most often to treat cancer.

Breast reconstruction has become increasingly available in the United States within the past few years.

Why?

Because many changes occurred almost simultaneously to make the procedure safe, relatively simple, and inexpensive:

- New materials that are not easily rejected by the body were developed;
- Breast-cancer surgeons began using techniques that save more muscle and skin (to cover the internal prosthesis);
- Plastic surgeons improved procedures;
- Many medical insurance plans began to pay part of the cost as postoperative rehabilitation.

As a result, more reconstructive mammoplasties have been done since 1977 than in all the previous years since the procedure was introduced in 1962.

Although using implants after mastectomy is relatively recent, they have been used for breast enlargement in tens of thousands of cases, all over the world, since the 1950s. So far, the Food and Drug Administration (FDA) and the National Cancer Institute (NCI) have found no evidence that breast implants are harmful.

This is *not* true of injections of any kind. Breast enlargement by injection can be dangerous, and the FDA has warned physicians, surgeons, and the public that this should not be done. While an FDA warning does not have the force of law (disobedience is not illegal) and carries no penalties, a physician or surgeon giving such injections could be subject to civil suits.

Enlarging breasts by the use of covered implants, however, has been done for decades, and—aside from the routine risks and complications of any surgery—there have been no known harmful effects. But all women considering breast reconstruction after cancer surgery should be aware that the practice in these cases is still so new that there are no long-term statistics available from large numbers of women. Only time will allow enough data to be accumulated so researchers will be able to evaluate reconstructive mammoplasty thoroughly. It is always possible that knowledge learned during the next ten or fifteen years will show problems not yet recognized.

WILL PEOPLE THINK IT IS VAIN TO WANT BREAST RECONSTRUCTION?

Having any kind of plastic surgery procedure is a personal decision and is dependent on how important it is to have a defect corrected. There are many celebrities who have exploited features—large noses or projecting ears—that would be painful disfigurements to other people.

Plastic surgeons feel that if physical defect is impairing a person's well-being and emotional health, this is a good enough reason to try to correct it. Where purely cosmetic surgery is involved, the American Society of Plastic and Reconstructive Surgeons (ASPRS) recommends careful analysis (or professional advice) to see if the physical defect has wrongly been blamed for an emotional problem. This, of course, is rarely the case in breast reconstruction, because an organ has been amputated.

It is always possible that friends and relatives may consider reconstructive mammoplasty to be "vanity." Not too long ago, having teeth capped, wearing contact lenses, and tinting hair were also considered "vain." If having an internal implant is important to a woman's personal view of her "body image" and sense of wholeness, the opinions of others should not affect her decision. There is no need to tell anyone.

IS SOMETHING WRONG WITH WOMEN WHO DON'T WANT A BREAST IMPLANT?

According to statistics from the National Cancer Institute and the American Cancer Society, there are about 1,000,000 women in the United States who have had one or two mastectomies. There are no accurate statistics available about the number who have had reconstructive mammoplasty, but the ASPRS estimates that—by the end of 1978—the number done in the entire country totalled fewer than 15,000. Obviously, therefore, women who have *not* chosen breast reconstruction are in the majority. If having an internal implant is unimportant to a woman, there is no reason for her to consider it.

WHAT DOES A RECONSTRUCTED BREAST LOOK LIKE?

There is no way for a woman to know exactly how she will look after reconstructive mammoplasty, because each case is different. But it will usually look round; it will not be tapered. Like most plastic surgery procedures, breast reconstruction is "custom tailoring," and few specific details can apply to all women. Perhaps the only part of the procedure that is consistent in every case is that the mastectomy scar cannot be eliminated, although its appearance may be improved. Some plastic surgeons insert the implant by reopening the original incision, while others believe a new one is required. At this time, there are no data to support either opinion.

Another point that must be stressed is that the "breast" created by inserting an implant of any kind under the chest wall *does not* look like a natural breast. Manufacturers have improved the materials used for breast implants, and plastic surgeons have developed better techniques. As a result, today's reconstructions look more natural than they did in the early years of the art. Nonetheless, any woman expecting her "new" breast to match the remaining one exactly—in either size, shape, or slope—will be disappointed.

On the other hand, plastic surgeons report that few women who choose breast reconstruction regret their decisions, in spite of the unavoidable differences. Several books and many articles have been written by women whose breast reconstructions were—by ordinary cosmetic standards—mismatched and asymmetrical. Yet, as one woman put it, "It's better than the alternative."

IS THERE ANYTHING THAT CAN BE DONE TO RECONSTRUCT A NIPPLE?

Women who have been told that they have breast cancer, but who have not yet had a mastectomy, may discuss the possibility of saving the areola and the nipple with their surgeons. This procedure is referred to as "banking," and the pigmented tissues are usually grafted onto the lower abdomen or groin for eventual placement on the breast-mound. But there have been some cases reported where the banked nipples contained hidden cancer cells in the ducts. For this reason, many surgeons now believe banking the nipple is risky. Everyone agrees the nipple should *not* be saved if the tumor was located close to the areola.

Women who had mastectomies in past years and whose nipples were lost, or those whose doctors believe banking is hazardous, may have a substitute nipple constructed in several ways. Dark skin from the labia (the skin around the vagina) or from the upper thigh can be grafted onto the mound. Or, if the areola of the remaining breast is large enough, it can be divided and shared with the "new" one. Surgeons can make an erect nipple by taking a small piece of cartilage (usually from the back of the ear) to be put in the center. There have also been cases where plastic surgeons have recommended tatooing an areola on the mound. An erect nipple can then be made by using ear cartilage, as described above.

IS EVERY WOMAN WHO HAS HAD A MASTECTOMY A CANDIDATE FOR RECONSTRUCTION?

According to the ASPRS, enough techniques have now been perfected so that a breast-mound can be created for almost every woman who has had a mastectomy—even if the surgery was extensive. However, in such cases, it may be necessary for the reconstruction to be done in several complex and expensive stages involving skin, fat, and muscle grafts. In addition, women who developed much postoperative scarring or whose skin was seriously affected by X-ray therapy might need additional grafts to correct these problems.

Inserting an implant under the pectoral muscle can frequently be a one-day procedure. On the other hand, the steps required to correct defects resulting from operations where the chest muscles and much skin were removed are more time-consuming, costly, and may involve considerable pain. Even though experienced plastic surgeons have developed the techniques to perform such breast reconstructions, many women may not feel the procedure is worthwhile.

If the initial mastectomy places a woman in this category, she may benefit from discussing the advantages and disadvantages with someone who has had such a multiple-stage reconstruction. Plastic surgeons often have patients who are willing to discuss and share their experiences with others. After hearing several points of view, women may decide that reconstructive mammoplasty is not for them.

WHAT ARE SOME OF THE ADVANTAGES AND DISADVANTAGES OF BREAST RECONSTRUCTION?

Rebuilding a woman's breast after it has been lost to cancer is still so new and the number of patients so small that researchers have not yet been able to evaluate the benefits of the procedure scientifically. However, these are being studied.

Many breast-cancer experts believe breast reconstruction will save thousands of women's lives. They feel women who know about the procedure will not delay and postpone seeing their doctors when they find a symptom of cancer, if they know an artificial breast can be created. Obviously, this opinion will only be tested by time.

Psychologists and psychiatrists are comparing groups of women who have and who have *not* had breast reconstruction to determine whether there are any measurable differences in their attitudes. So far, the scientific data are preliminary, but anecdotal evidence indicates that women who have had reconstructive mammoplasty regain former feelings of "wholeness," restored self-esteem, and have less anxiety about having had to lose a breast.

From a woman's physical point of view, the chief advantage is convenience. Having the prostheses under the skin, instead of lying above it, women know their artificial breasts are invisible and cannot be displaced by vigorous activity: minor skin problems caused by contact with the covering of the implant cannot occur. It is less awkward to shop for clothing, because—in a brassiere or slip—no saleswoman will notice any difference, and it is easier to be fashionable because there is no need to hide a prosthesis.

As stated earlier, data about the psychological effects of breast reconstruction are too preliminary to be evaluated. By the same token, emotional disadvantages—like emotional advantages— are still uncertain. There are some indications that women who expected the reconstructed breast to be exactly like a natural breast suffer from disappointment and depression when they discover that this is not so. Although these reports are anecdotal, there have been enough of such cases that many plastic surgeons insist that women postpone reconstruction for a period of time after their mastectomies are performed. They believe most women will not be able to appreciate the reconstructed breast unless "they have had nothing there" for at least six months after their mastectomies.

This opinion is not shared by everyone, however, and some cancer and plastic surgeons are combining the mastectomy and insertion of the implant in a single operation. In some hospitals, the physical effects (incidence of infection, blood-clotting problems, rejection) and the psychological effects of this simultaneous procedure are being compared scientifically.

In addition, plastic surgeons are comparing various kinds of implants to attempt to reduce the incidence of one disadvantage of reconstructive mammoplasty: contracture. A contracture is a firm, fibrous shell that sometimes forms around the implant as the body tries to reject a "foreign" substance. This shell may result in a "baseball" appearance and may also be uncomfortable or even painful.

Another possible complication of breast reconstruction is "sloughing"—the skin of the chest wall literally peels away, and the implant is rejected. Sloughing usually occurs if much underlying tissue was removed during the mastectomy itself. Plastic surgeons have devised techniques to avoid this problem by grafting healthy skin to the chest *before* the implant is inserted.

If a contracture should develop, it sometimes softens, is gradually absorbed by the body, and disappears. Frequently, the plastic surgeon may be able to move it by hand to break the shell so the implant can assume its normal shape. In severe cases, the capsule (shell) may need to be removed surgically. Plastic surgeons believe contractures are caused by reactions between the body and the implant, and this is why research is continuing to find other materials.

HOW IS RECONSTRUCTION PERFORMED?

Because reconstructive mammoplasty is so individualized, specific details do not apply to every woman. But, in general, an incision is made in either the original scar or in another location, and the implant is inserted under the skin and pectoral muscles so it is firmly in place. (Women whose muscles were removed during their mastectomies have usually had muscle-grafts prior to this stage.) Plastic surgeons attempt to match the remaining breast in size, shape, and position, but success depends on the initial surgery. For example, the location of the tumor determined the site of the original incision, and the size of the tumor was probably a deciding factor in the quantity of tissue that was removed.

A reconstructed breast should be judged by its appearance in a brassiere or bathing suit—not by the way it looks with no clothing on. For this reason, the lower border of the implant is usually level with that of the other breast when it is raised by an uplifting garment. When consulting a plastic surgeon for an opinion, a woman usually will be told how the procedure will be done in her individual case. She will be told where the implant will be inserted, and, frequently, the plastic surgeon will show her photographs of former patients. By talking with her general surgeon and the plastic surgeon, seeing some photographs and, perhaps, seeing someone's reconstructed breast, a woman will get a better idea about her own situation.

TYPES OF IMPLANTS

A variety of implants are available. All of them use Silastic® as the outer material that will come in contact with the body. Shaped like a breast, the sacs usually contain silicone-gel, saline, or both. An implant gaining in popularity is filled with gel but is covered with a layer of polyurethane foam. Undoubtedly, manufacturers will develop others as research continues.

All of these implants have the feel of a natural breast and are, as far as is known, inert—silicone does not appear to react with any body tissues. Those filled with gel are sealed by the manufacturer and are sized according to standard measurements. Implants to be filled with saline are usually inflated in the operating room through a small valve.* Each type of implant has advantages and disadvantages for different women, and the choice must be made after consultation with an experienced plastic surgeon.

HOW SHOULD A PLASTIC SURGEON BE CHOSEN?

The NCI's Cancer Information Service (CIS) and the American Cancer Society (ACS) try to keep lists of all specialists cancer patients may need, and women should consult the CIS or ACS in their areas for the name of plastic surgeons who have experience in breast reconstruction.

In addition, general surgeons usually know such specialists, and in some cities, the yellow pages of the telephone directory have physicians divided according to their specialities. The American Cancer Society's RENU program is actively supporting breast reconstruction, wherever practical, and state or local divisions and units may have lists of names. Women may also contact the American Society of Plastic and Reconstructive Surgeons directly for names of Board-certified members in their areas:

American Society of Plastic and Reconstructive Surgeons
Suite 800
29 East Madison
Chicago, Illinois 60602
(312) 641-0935

However the decision is made, women should feel free to ask questions about every aspect of the procedure as it applies to them. This pamphlet has been written by the National Cancer Institute as a guide in preparing a list of questions to ask, but the details of breast reconstruction must be decided for you and your personal situation.

HOW LONG SHOULD A WOMAN WAIT BEFORE HAVING BREAST RECONSTRUCTION?

For physical as well as psychological reasons, opinions differ as to the required length of the waiting period between a mastectomy and reconstruction of the breast. Most surgeons feel that

---

*My saline implant began leaking in September 1981, and—by that time—their high "deflation rate" had already taken them off the market. It was replaced by a tightly sealed "double-bubble" implant, containing a tightly sealed silicone core floating in salt-water.

before reconstruction can be attempted, the first incision should be well healed and the skin easily movable and elastic. Moreover, many breast-cancer experts believe that women should wait at least eighteen months to two years to make sure the cancer doesn't recur; some believe women should wait as long as five years.

On the other hand, some cancer specialists believe no delay is necessary to insert the implant when the breast is removed. If the cancer should return, they feel, any treatment could be given with the implant under a woman's skin. And, of course, there are opinions between these extremes.

CAN RECONSTRUCTION BE PERFORMED WHEN WOMEN ARE RECEIVING RADIATION THERAPY?

As explained earlier, extensive postmastectomy radiation therapy of the chest may require skin grafts from other parts of the body, because the X-ray treatment can reduce the blood supply to and elasticity of the surgical site.

Radiation therapy *after* reconstruction, however, is given to treat a skin recurrence just as if an implant were not in place.

CAN RECONSTRUCTION BE PERFORMED WHEN WOMEN ARE RECEIVING CHEMOTHERAPY?

Most experts believe women receiving adjuvant chemotherapy should not try to have reconstruction when they are actually being given anticancer drugs. There is too much risk of developing an infection, and most of these drugs weaken the body's defense (immune) system. Since reconstructive mammoplasty carries the routine risks of any surgical procedure, infection could be a major complication. Therefore, it is usually recommended that reconstruction be postponed until chemotherapy is completed.

Afterward, however, there is no reason why reconstruction cannot be done.

WOULD AN IMPLANT HIDE A NEW CANCER?

Plastic surgeons and radiologists have studied the problem of examining a woman after breast reconstruction, and their conclusions are that there should be no difficulty in detecting an early recurrence beneath or around the implant, using manual examination or mammography (X-rays of the breast). However, for some women, it may be necessary to vary the usual positions for a thorough examination. According to data collected so far by ASPRS and the American College of Radiology (ACR), there have been no known cases of undetected recurrences after reconstructive mammoplasty. Women must be reminded, however, that reconstructive mammoplasty is still too new to have accumulated large numbers of statistics. There is always the chance that future data will be different.

CAN AN IMPLANT BE INSERTED IF THE CANCER HAS ALREADY SPREAD?

At this time, there are dozens of documented cases where women have wanted to have their lost breasts replaced, even though they knew the disease had metastasized (spread) to other parts of the body. This is a personal choice women must make themselves; there is no medical or surgical reason to rule out reconstructive mammoplasty in such instances.

SUPPOSE THE REMAINING BREAST IS TOO LARGE TO BE "MATCHED"?

The amount of skin lost during a mastectomy limits the size of the implant, and the remaining breast may require "reduction mammoplasty"—removal of some of its tissue—to make them as equal as possible in size and shape. In some cases, the skin over the breast-mound can be stretched gradually to accommodate a larger implant. This is usually done in several stages simply by increasing the size of the implant as the chest skin loosens around it. This "expansion" procedure involves reopening the incision for each stage, and so adds some risk. Nonetheless, it is often feasible for those women who do not want to reduce the size of their remaining breast and whose skin is elastic enough to permit such gradual expansion.

CAN THE REMAINING BREAST BE ENLARGED TO MATCH THE MOUND?

If a woman's skin can accommodate an implant that is larger than her remaining breast, a smaller implant can be inserted beneath its tissue. This is routine augmentation mammoplasty and has been used since the 1950s for breast enlargement. However, because women who have had one breast removed for cancer are at higher risk for developing another malignancy in the remaining one, many surgeons would recommend a subcutaneous mastectomy in such cases.

WHAT IS SUBCUTANEOUS MASTECTOMY?

A subcutaneous mastectomy is a surgical procedure in which all of the breast tissue is removed without the loss of any skin, underlying tissue, or the areola and nipple. A curved incision is made at the crease where the breast meets the body. The skin (including the areola and nipple) is lifted, and the breast tissue and fat are removed. An implant is then inserted, and the skin (areola and nipple intact) is replaced. The incision is almost invisible.

Considerable controversy has grown about its routine use to prevent breast cancer in women who are at high risk because of family history or chronic benign cystic disease.

WHAT ABOUT PLASTIC SURGERY TO PREVENT BREAST CANCER?

Plastic surgery is now often being recommended by some doctors to try to prevent breast cancer. Known as a "prophylactic subcutaneous mastectomy," this operation usually involves removing healthy breast tissue through the same kind of semicircular incision just described. This procedure is generally offered to women who are considered to be at "high risk" of developing breast cancer, and many insurance companies are paying for it.

Women who are thought to have such high risks are:

1. Women who have already lost one breast to cancer;
2. Daughters and sisters of these women;
3. Women who have chronic benign breast problems—lumps, cysts, fibroadenomas, etc.—and have had several biopsies.

In addition, some physicians recommend a prophylactic subcutaneous mastectomy for psychological reasons, even if a woman has none of these factors. The problem is being called "breast cancerphobia."

The question "Who is at high risk?" is controversial. No doctor wants to remove a healthy organ simply because it might develop cancer, and most breast-cancer experts oppose prophylactic mastectomies under any circumstances. For this reason, women should be aware of the arguments.

There is no question that a woman who has had cancer in one breast has a higher probability of developing another in the other breast. However, there is evidence that about half of these spots of malignancy never grow large enough to become a threat to life. For this reason, many physicians do not believe surgery of any kind should be done unless a change is actually seen or felt in the second breast.

There is also agreement that breast cancer "runs in the family" and that sisters and daughters of women who had breast cancer are at higher risk of developing it as well. However, no statistical study has been done to put precise values on how high individual women's risks are if they do have such family histories. All that is known is that they are *not* at as high a risk if their relatives developed breast cancer after menopause—the "change of life." Nor is their risk as high if their relatives' cancers are found only in one breast and not in both.

Breast-cancer experts also worry that prophylactic mastectomies may result in a false sense of security. For example, if occult—hidden—cancer cells are already in the breast, they may grow behind or alongside the implant and not be easily detected. The same fear applies to any cells that may be left behind in the nipple. For these reasons, a prophylactic mastectomy is *not* a 100 percent guarantee against developing breast cancer.

Finally, this procedure carries with it all of the possible complications of ordinary surgery plus those of reconstruction. Prophylactic mastectomy should not be undertaken without serious and careful consideration of all its possible problems.

DOES RECONSTRUCTION REQUIRE A LONG HOSPITAL STAY?

The length of time a woman must spend in the hospital depends on the amount of surgery performed. A simple procedure involving no grafts and no complications can be done in less than one hour, followed by an overnight stay. Multiple-stage reconstructions may mean a series of several short hospitalizations, adding up to a total of ten days to two weeks, unless there are unexpected complications. Only the plastic surgeon can predict individual requirements.

IS RECONSTRUCTION PAINFUL?

Like any surgical procedure, breast reconstruction causes some pain. In most cases, it lasts a short time and is easily relieved by medication.

IS RECOVERY DIFFICULT?

Most women can resume all activities within two weeks.

IS RECONSTRUCTION EXPENSIVE?

Plastic surgeons' fees vary with the complexity of the case. For example, simple insertion of an implant costs less than a procedure that requires grafts of any kind; creating a nipple increases the price. Fees also vary considerably in different parts of the United States. In general, the range begins at about $1,200 for the surgeon and may be as high as $5,000. Hospital costs are additional, of course, and depend on the length of the stay.

Most medical/surgical insurance plans in the country are now covering part of the costs of reconstructive mammoplasty as postmastectomy rehabilitation—*not* as cosmetic plastic surgery. Usually, an insurance company will pay for reconstruction only if the woman was a policyholder at the time of her mastectomy. But there are some insurance companies that do not cover rehabilitation of any kind, for anyone. Women who are considering reconstruction should study their policies carefully and discuss the matter with a representative of their insurance company to learn precisely what their coverage is.*

IS THE RECONSTRUCTED BREAST SENSITIVE?

If the nerves of the skin over the removed breast were sensitive after the mastectomy, these feelings will usually remain after reconstruction. There have been reports to plastic surgeons that sexual sensations, lost since the mastectomy, did return to the breast nerves after the reconstructive operation.

WHAT KIND OF COMPLICATIONS ARE MOST COMMON?

Most complications that can occur after breast reconstruction are identical to those that may occur after a mastectomy. One is infection, and antibiotics are usually given routinely to prevent it. Bloody fluid may accumulate to form a hematoma or blood clot around the implant. But a vacuum drain, inserted during surgery, can remove these fluids and prevent this problem.

*California now requires that all insurance companies who pay for mastectomies must also cover reconstructive surgery, as well.

The two complications specific to reconstructive mammoplasty have been described earlier on page 288: contracture and sloughing. According to available statistics, most reconstructions where the implant is made entirely of silicone-gel result in some degree of contracture; the incidence when saline-filled implants were used was small. On the other hand, implants using salt water have a valve, and the fluid leaked out while the silicone-gel is securely sealed and cannot deflate under ordinary circumstances. Manufacturers and plastic surgeons have found a way to combine the two materials so the benefits of each are retained while their disadvantages are eliminated. It is too soon to know whether or not these newer "bi-lumen" implants will be successful.

At this time, it is impossible to predict which women will develop contractures and which will not. However, sloughing can usually be anticipated, because the problem almost always results from an inadequate quantity of skin. As described earlier, putting grafts of healthy skin on the area before the implant is inserted may prevent this from happening.

All implants can be punctured, although the Silastic™ coverings are sturdy enough to withstand even painful bumps and blows. Leaking saline implants must be removed and replaced by reopening the incision. While there is some evidence that microscopic molecules of silicone may migrate into the body from gel-filled implants, there are no indications that they cause any harm. It must be remembered that silicone has been safely used to replace heart valves, bone joints, vocal cords, and other vital parts of the body for decades with no reports of ill effects.

Nonetheless, the Breast Cancer Task Force of the NCI has asked the Food and Drug Administration to continue its investigation of breast implants. Their study began in 1978, and no report has yet been issued, but preliminary findings show that silicone is inert and, therefore, safe.

IF RECONSTRUCTION CAN HAVE SO MANY PROBLEMS, WHY DO WOMEN WANT IT?

As explained earlier, there are about 1,000,000 women in this country who have had mastectomies and fewer than 15,000 reconstructions had been performed by the end of 1978. Therefore, most women do not want it.

But, there are women whose mastectomies left them with feelings of feminine inadequacy, lost body-image and sexuality, and other emotional problems. Athletes, entertainers, models, and women in other professions may have financial reasons for having their breasts reconstructed. And many women want breast reconstruction just for the convenience of being freed from an external prosthesis. It is a personal decision that only the woman herself can make, after consulting her physician, because only she knows how the loss of a breast has affected her life.

14

After Treatment: Physical

"I didn't have five minutes' worth of pain. My years of periodontia hurt me a helluva lot more than the mastectomy did, that's for sure."

The booming, hearty voice coming over the telephone sounded as if it were coming from a large, athletic woman. I guessed right on the sports.

"Three weeks after the stitches were out, I was knocking buckets of golf balls all over the driving range. Nobody could believe it." She laughed, a deep, jolly belly laugh. "And, believe me, everybody was looking at me too. I think they were all trying to decide which one had been cut off, but I fooled 'em. Nobody could tell a thing, even with the skimpy golf shirt on."

"How long ago did you have your mastectomy?" I asked. Quickly I grabbed the notebook I kept ready on the corner of my desk to record the answers to a questionnaire I was circulating to women who had had mastectomies.

"Seventeen years ago next July," she told me happily. "That pretty much puts me in the clear. I hope the same for you."

Seventeen years. No wonder she could not remember the postmastectomy "discomfort" as accurately as I could, after less than a year.

I had been warned about this so-called telescoping phenomenon. "The longer after the mastectomy," several surgeons told me, "the less traumatic it was. For the first year or so, the operation is remembered as excruciating. Then it diminishes to very painful. Somewhere along the line, the 'very' disappears, and ultimately a mastectomy is remembered only as uncomfortable or even altogether pain-free."

"Telescoping" had indeed affected this ebullient woman's

memory. "Did you know ahead of time that you would lose your breast?"

"Hell, no!" she yelled. "Knocked the Captain for a loop too. It was done in a navy hospital," she explained. "My husband was in the service then, stationed out in California. The Captain told me afterward he could have sworn he'd be done and finished in half an hour." She laughed at the memory. "He was madder than a hornet, he was. He was a tennis nut and had a big match scheduled that morning. Had to miss it on account of me."

"How did you feel when you woke up and discovered one of your breasts was missing?"

"Well, being in the service, and being a navy brat to begin with," she told me, "you sort of get used to being knocked around. When my husband came in to see me, he grinned and said something about getting brassieres at a discount from then on, because I wouldn't be needing half. I guess that pretty well sums up what both our attitudes toward the operation were—a bad break. The main thing was to be finished with the cancer, and that took a long time to know."

After seventeen years, telescoping had worked with this woman physically and mentally. I had not yet passed seventeen months, at that time, and the memory was still clearly in focus.

On awakening in the recovery room, the first thing I remember feeling was an intense burning in my throat and in the area of the incision. The throat problem did not last long; it was a local irritation from a tube inserted in my windpipe during surgery. The burning in the incision was caused by two vacuum drains that had been left there to draw out serous fluid, which would otherwise accumulate and cause pain and swelling. The drains were attached to a pouch called a Hemo-Vac, an ingenious gadget that exerted just enough reverse pressure to prevent the unwanted build-up of fluid—important in preventing postoperative swelling and pain. I had been warned that I might have a lot of mucus and that a bubble-blowing machine would be used to clear my pipes. As it turned out, it was not necessary. However, it is common to need to blow some bubbles after such anesthesia.

Except for my throat and the spots where the drains were, I was totally numb in the left side of my chest and in most of the upper left arm. My first thought was that I had become paralyzed. Then I realized that most of the nerves had been cut during the surgery and would need time to reknit. Naturally, I would be numb in the meantime.

"Your sensation will gradually return. Don't worry," Dr. Dao assured me.

What he did not explain was that when the sensation came

back, it would come as pain. But that happened several months later for me, and I have learned that both the time and amount of pain vary considerably from woman to woman. Some women never stop hurting somewhere; some never have pain at all; most women return to normal as I did—gradually.

For the moment, the drains were my only problem, and they were removed on the third or fourth day. My chest did not hurt, but I felt as if a huge, tight rubber band were squeezing me from the armpit to below the rib cage. There were slight pins and needles, tingles, and occasionally a short, sharp, darting sensation, which came unexpectedly and disappeared just as quickly. The area involved was not only that part of me around the incision and the armpit, but also the shoulder, the adjacent part of the back, and the inside of the arm. These are not painful now, but women differ in their responses. My weirdest sensation—or, rather, lack of sensation—was trying to shave under my left arm. Normally, this cosmetic job can be done without even looking; the nerve endings guide the razor to the proper spot. After a mastectomy, these nerves are temporarily deadened, and for a while I had to look to be sure I got all the stubby patches.

These sensations, I later discovered, are common to all women immediately after a mastectomy. But the length of time needed for the nerves to be restored varies with the kind of surgery, (e.g., the number of nodes removed, if any) the surgeon's skill, and the woman's speed of healing.

A mastectomy is major surgery, and it involves a good bit of cutting, regardless of what kind it is. The breast is exceedingly vascular—chock-full of blood vessels—so there is usually a considerable loss of blood. Some surgeons give routine transfusions afterward; others, like Dr. Dao, do not if it can be avoided. Also, surgeons have preferred anesthetics.

Depending on the speed of the scalpel, the operation can take from three to as long as seven hours. I found no mention of duration of surgery as a factor affecting recurrence or survival rates, unless the surgeon worked so quickly that he missed excising cancerous tissue.

Most surgeons make a horizontal incision, with the idea that it is more easily hidden by a conventional bra and will make later reconstruction easier. Some make diagonal incisons. Mine is vertical, beginning about five inches below the shoulder and ending just where the bottom edge of my bra can hide it.

"I like a vertical incison," Dr. Dao told me, "because I like to think of a woman being able to wear a plunging neckline. But it is purely a matter of personal preference with the modified radical. It makes no difference medically."

I had not given a moment's though to any kind of incision. Who had ever though of mastectomy at all, much less how the breast would be cut off? Most women still know little, unless they are personally affected.

Most of what women have learned is the result of numerous magazine and newspaper articles and TV and radio programs that appeared after Betty Ford's and Happy Rockefeller's operations. These courageous women brought breast cancer "out of the closet." Unfortunately, once the spate of publicity about their surgeries was over, breast cancer was banished from the front pages and exiled again to the women's sections. But while the first and second ladies were still newsworthy, women all over the world were able to get some good information from the general media. Even when both were back in the social swim of official Washington—giving out Halloween candy, appearing at luncheons, parties, hearings, and congressional sessions—their mastectomies were still triggering educational materials about breast cancer—among them, my first book.

For example, Mrs. Ford wrote an article in February 1975 and told her readers that she tired more easily and that she rested her arm on pillows whenever possible. In addition, she was getting adjuvant chemotherapy, and so the reasons for this continuing treatment were explained to the public. When Happy Rockefeller had a simple (or total) mastectomy only a few weeks after having a modified-radical, the media informed women about the three different kinds of surgeries in great detail. Betty Ford had had a Halsted radical; Happy Rockefeller had a modified and then a simple. But while the surgical procedures were explained, their physical aftereffects were hardly mentioned.

Pain? Swelling? Not a word. The only problems either woman would admit to were some fatigue and discomfort. As far as the psychological aspects of losing their breasts were concerned, neither woman admitted having any emotional problems whatsoever. Mrs. Ford was quoted to have said that the mastectomy involved only a "little foam rubber," and both she and her husband picked up the pieces of their lives—as far as we knew then. The public was told that Mrs. Ford had given up skiing, and subsequently, we all learned about her addiction to alcohol and Valium. (Of course, this may have been completely unrelated to the loss of her breast. No one will ever know.) Happy Rockefeller wrote an article about her experiences for the *Readers Digest* and said she was putting "breast cancer behind her." As far as I know, she has stuck to that pledge.

I had the feeling, at the time, that their public statements could not be true. Having had excellent surgery by skilled hands, I had still felt pain that was more than "discomfort." Psychologically, I thought I was in good shape (although I learned differently two years later). Letters and telephone calls I had been receiving since writing an article for the *Washington Post* indicated that most women had even more pain and other problems than I experienced. Moreover, I was getting strong hints that women's psyches were also severely traumatized by mastectomies: especially if they did not have the diagnostic biopsy separated from the mastectomy. With all the severe physical and psychological problems there were no real data about women's responses to mastectomy.

To get a broad picture—I somehow had to find a way to reach many women of different ages, marital status, and socioeconomics situations. I called a friend at the National Cancer Institute's breast clinic for advice and, I hoped, help.

"You know," she said, "no matter what you do, you're going to get a very biased sample."

"I don't want to know their names or anything."

"That doesn't make any difference," she said. "Women who are having troubles, either physically or psychologically, will not have anything to do with you, your book, or anything else. They want to block out the whole business and forget it."

I thought for a moment. Of course she was right. A woman would have to be well adjusted to her mastectomy to be willing to talk about it to a total stranger, anonymously or not. Maladjusted women, naturally, would refuse.

"How about talking to psychiatrists?" I asked.

"They would give you an opposite bias," she countered. "You'd be hearing about women so badly adjusted they needed psychiatric help. You would get the two extremes. There's no way I can imagine to get at the women who can't accept the loss of a breast but aren't in bad enough shape—or good enough financial condition—to get help from a shrink. There's no way I can think of to get around this."

I thanked her and put down the receiver. The problem was unexpected, but, after thinking it over, I realized I should have anticipated it. Certainly, women who had never been able to accept the loss of a breast would be unwilling to talk to me or to answer a written questionnaire.

Reach to Recovery! That was the organization to help me. An important branch of the American Cancer Society, the program enlists volunteers who try to visit every mastectomy patient in the country, right after her surgery, to give advice about where to buy prostheses, bathing suits, and clothing; answer general questions, and lift her morale. Once again I was disappointed.

"We didn't want Reach to Recovery to become a crutch," a representative of the program told me, when I called the office of the Washington ACS chapter. "After all, the whole point of Reach to Recovery is to convince women they do not have a disabling handicap. We talked about having a mastectomy club, like the various ostomy clubs and laryngectomy clubs. But that would have defeated our whole purpose. Having a mastectomy is *not* a permanent handicap, and even the worst of scars can be hidden by a well-fitting prosthesis and the right clothes. So we decided we would help the patient for just a few weeks, and then leave her to her own psychological recovery."

This may have made good sense to some people, not to me—not then and not now. What good was a "recovery" program that left women stranded after a hospital visit and a few weeks of telephone service? That was not the time, however, for me to be arguing with the American Cancer Society. That would come later.

In 1974, I had to have data, and I wanted to talk to women who were not immediately "postop," women who were far enough beyond the surgery itself to have some perspective on what they had gone through. ACS rules require Reach to Recovery volunteers to be one or two years beyond surgery but they also guarded the names of the volunteers. So though this group would have been ideal for my needs, I couldn't get to first base with them.

The logical people to help—surgeons—were not likely to cooperate with me. In a *Washington Post* article, I had made it crystal clear that I did not think general surgeons should be doing mastectomies, if there was a breast-cancer expert available. That had not endeared me to members of the American College of Surgeons.

I was still in a deep quandary when a department-store ad appeared in the *Post* announcing a week-long visit by the representative of a prosthesis manufacturer, the Airway Surgical Company. That might be the answer. Immediately I called the representative, explained my problem, and asked if she would mind giving my name and telephone number to the women who came to her to be fitted this week. The representative, Mrs. Loretta Marsh Crowell, agreed without hesitation. On the first day, one woman called; the second day, none; the third day, none. The fourth day I went to the store myself, to be sure she hadn't forgotten me.

"No, I haven't," she said. "I'm really surprised that only one woman called you, because there were about fourteen who wrote your name down and said they would."

As long as I was in the store, I asked it I might park myself in one of the fitting rooms for the afternoon, so that her customers could come in to talk if they wanted to. Of the number who were fitted during those few hours (I do not know how many there were), only three came in to be interviewed. As I had expected, all three had made good adjustments, were open, requested no anonymity, and were positive in their attitudes about the surgery. Two of them were grandmothers and had been postmenopausal when their tumors were discovered. The third was younger, but very down-to-earth and sensible.

After they left, I talked with Mrs. Crowell. She agreed that I would get a distorted picture going this route. "For one thing," she said, "a lot of women don't ever get adjusted enough to buy a prosthesis in the first place. The little bit of confidence or whatever it takes to face me or any other fitter just isn't there. Even to come to this department, she has to first admit she needs an artificial breast, and that is more than some women can do. There are women, I am sure, who live all the rest of their lives with cotton batting or even tissues stuffed into the cups of their bras." (And, judging by the response of those who *did* make it to the fitting room that week, only a few were willing to be interviewed.)

Before Mrs. Crowell left the Washington area, she said she and her firm would do anything they could to help me reach mastectomees in other cities. Thanks to their help, the questionnaire I had devised was circulated via the lingerie departments of stores around the country.

CONFIDENTIAL

1. Age when mastectomy was performed?
2. How long since the surgery occurred?
3. What kind of mastectomy, e.g., Halsted, modified radical, simple, etc., if information is known?
4. What was foremost in your mind when the suggestion of cancer was told to you?
5. Were you aware before the actual mastectomy that your breast would be removed?
6. If the diagnosis was made in a separate procedure, what was this technique?
7. Was the physician a male or a female?
8. Were you visited by Reach to Recovery volunteers of the American Cancer Society? Did these women help?
9. What were the attitudes toward you by other patients?
10. What were the attitudes toward you by hospital personnel?
11. What were the attitudes toward you by relatives and friends?
12. How did you deal with your immediate family? Children, if any?

13. What was husband's attitude or boyfriend's response? This is a critical question, of course, and I would like as much information as possible, especially anecdotes, if any. Unfortunately, I must also pry into the bedroom and ask if there were any differences after your mastectomy. Forgive me!

14. Did you consider having a so-called lumpectomy or other lesser operations in order to save your breast?

15. Did you require postoperative irradiation, chemotherapy, or other treatment?

16. What kind of follow-up care are you being given?

17. Has your physician warned you not to take oral contraceptives?

18. Has the mastectomy made any difference in your life? If so, kindly detail. I am especially interested in your own feelings of womanliness and femininity, male attitudes toward you, and any economic problems you might have encountered. An important aspect is also whether you feel it is a matter you keep privately to yourself or whether you have no qualms about having others know about the surgery.

Any additions that you may think pertinent, based on your own experiences and not covered in this questionnaire, will be appreciated.

At the other end of the spectrum, I asked several psychiatrists with postmastectomy patients if they would have these women call me, and all said they would recommend it. One cautioned that such a sample would represent patients who had serious problems and might slant the results.

"That's what I expect," I replied. "I can't seem to strike a happy medium, so I'm using psychiatric patients to illustrate poor adjustment—if that's the way it is—and, at the other end, women who voluntarily answer questions and seem to have no problem." I described my questionnaire and told him how well adjusted all my respondents had been so far. "These women are slanted in the opposite direction," I said. "I don't know how to get to the ones in the middle—women too adjusted or too poor to see psychiatrists, but not adjusted enough to go to a store to buy an artificial breast."

I never did find a way to reach this group. But I know they exist.

One other group got into my survey—about thirty-five women, some of whom I had known for years, who phoned after my article appeared to ask questions or simply to welcome me into "the club." And, of course, I received dozens of calls and letters from women who had read my article and wanted more information.

Mrs. Crowell told me she had distributed 5,000 questionnaires, but altogether, I received responses from only 130 women as of the time *Breast Cancer* was completed in February 1975. Answers to the questionnaire, by the way, are still arriving in 1981, because many readers of the first and second editions are contributing information about themselves. And, in addition to the data from the questionnaires, I now have a good-sized collection of books and articles by mastectomees written after my book was published. To my surprise, my original data from the 130 responses are holding up.

These women were young, middle-aged, and older. Most were married, but some were divorced, some widowed, and some had never been married. Of those who telephoned, most seemed well adjusted, based on their conversations with me. None of the telephone interviewees asked for anonymity. Several of the women I knew personally asked me not to tell anyone else, just as they had never told me anything before the story about my mastectomy was published. Of the mailed questionnaires, less than half had no name or address; the rest of the women were candid and said I could communicate with them if I needed more information.

Of the women who were referred by the psychiatrists, most said their problems had nothing to do with the mastectomy but had simply been aggravated by it. Several said they had been in treatment when the cancer was discovered, and I verified this with the psychiatrists. Incidentally, as it had been with the questionnaires, more women had been asked to call me than actually did.

In keeping with surgical practice in the United States, most of the women had had Halsted radicals and had not known in advance they would have a mastectomy (although many said the possibility had been mentioned "in passing").

The questionnaire did not ask about education or the kind of work a woman did, and I was sorry later it did not. As a matter of fact, if I knew then what I know now, the questions would have been much different. Luckily, most women volunteered more than I asked. In telephone conversations, both subjects came up, and most of these women had gone to college for a year or two. While I do not think education or a job has anything to do with making the kind of adjustment I was interested in, I do think it indicates (1) the kind of woman who reads the editorial section of the *Washington Post*'s Sunday edition; (2) the kind of woman who seeks psychiatric counseling; (3) the women who are financially able to afford an expensive, lifelike prosthesis and special brassiere, if needed. Therefore, my random and unscientific poll was less random and more unscientific than I thought. However, it gave me a good idea of the physical and psychological problems encountered after mastectomy. As I have said elsewhere in *Why Me?* my conclusions have since been supported by a scientific survey commissioned by the NCI. I also learned how women accept the knowledge of having a potentially fatal disease. In the flurry of articles that followed the first and second ladies' mastectomies, this grim side of the breast-cancer story was somehow understated. The media seemed to concentrate only on the cosmetics of breast cancer. Jacqueline Susann's death after a secret and silent fourteen-year battle, coming as it did during that period, did not help dispel the aura of sexuality and fetishism surrounding the mammary glands.

The surgery that can stop the disease *is* disfiguring, but breast cancer kills. Except in selected cases, mastectomy of some kind was (and still is) considered to be the only treatment that gives women a good chance to live in spite of it. As I just said, if I were composing the questionnaire today, I would include a question about how it feels to be alive, putting much less emphasis on what doctors call "cosmesis." At the time, however, I myself knew so little about the seriousness of the disease that, once I accepted amputation, I was most concerned with questions of physical and psychological discomfort and disability—not of death.

The amount and intensity of pain immediately after the operation and during the months that follow vary considerably. Some women whose surgeries were fairly recent told me they still felt nothing at all except numbness in most of the affected area. One young mother of two girls, who was only thirty-four years old, was hitting tennis balls at a public court less than six weeks after her stitches were removed—and introduced me to friends who had witnessed the feat! I could never have done that. When I interviewed her (about a year after the mastectomy), she still had no pain. All she felt was tightness across her chest.

I was then just a few months postop and still tender in most places; other places really hurt. Apparently my nerves had healed quickly: otherwise I, too, would not have felt anything as early as I did. But tennis? I doubt it.

A woman's recovery, of course, depends on the kind of surgery that was done. Most of my respondents, who had had the Halsted radical, said it was difficult for them to re-educate auxiliary muscles to take over for the pectorals, which had been removed.

For them, regaining the full use of the arm had top priority; pain and cosmetics were secondary.

Also, many of the post-Halsted women required skin grafts (which are usually taken from the thigh) to patch up the breast area. The grafts caused complications of infection, sloughing—the word used to describe grafted skin that refuses to stay put—and itching. But the last is a problem after any surgery. The nerves in the top layer of skin are not functioning and cannot transmit a helpful scratch to the miserable itch.

The late Marvella Bayh, the wife of Indiana's Senator Birch Bayh, had had a modified radical, and had no trouble with grafts or with her arm muscles. "But that postoperative X-ray therapy made me sick," she told me. "I remember that as being worse than anything about the surgery." I learned that Mrs. Bayh's—and other women who reported similar experiences—case was not typical. After *Breast Cancer* was published, dozens of furious radiation therapists called and wrote to complain that my sample of women who had had "prophylactic" irradiation either lied, misremembered, or received improper radiotherapy. For reasons I cannot understand, this is the only major skew in the data from the questionnaires.

The objectionable sentence was, "Invariably, the weakness, fever, retching and nausea—as well as the burned skin—that usually accompany high-dosage radiotherapy are remembered more clearly than the mastectomy itself." Several women complained they had lost so much hair, they were almost bald. Since prophylactic postmastectomy irradiation was routine in most of the United States during the years before 1974, the majority of the women I surveyed had received it. Could all 130 have lied, misremembered, or gotten improper radiotherapy? I will never know. But I did find out in a hurry that properly done, prophylactic irradiation after mastectomy should *not* cause any of the problems above except some loss of hair in the part of the body receiving the irradiation (for example, under the affected arm). Women may also tire easily. Aside from the misinformation about prophylactic X-ray, however, the data from my small sample were accurate.

There were no complaints, by the way, about the sentence, "X-ray treatments can also cause additional swelling and pain by damaging the lymphatics even more than the radical mastectomy did." I stress this because of the current trend toward breast-saving minimal surgery followed by irradiation of the breast. Being able to pay for a linear accelerator—however excellent and expensive it might be—is no guarantee that the radiation therapist is an expert in giving this particular kind of treatment. Irradiating the breast is an art more than it is a science, and the possible aftereffects of poor radiotherapy must be kept in mind by any woman considering going this route.

Now that my errors about prophylactic X-ray have been straightened out and apologies made, I will continue listing the results from the questionnaire. There were other variations in women's physical recoveries during the first months and years, all seeming to depend largely on age, number of small children, and economic status. For example, all the women who were over sixty at the time of mastectomy complained that they had a hard time bouncing back to their preoperative physical condition and energy level. "If I go to the grocery store or to the library," one of them told me, "I am finished for the day." At the time she was eight months postop; I was four. I attribute the difference between us simply to the fact that older women in general do not bounce back as easily as younger ones do.

Having children still in diapers, who must be carried or who crawl all over their mothers, is also something I did not have to cope with. I learned from younger patients that, as happy as they were to be able to look after their babies or toddlers, they had serious physical problems if they had to care for them alone. That is where economic status came into the picture. Those with higher incomes could hire help, and the convalescing mothers had more comfortable recoveries.

Another postoperative problem, which in some women is temporary and in others permanent, is milk arm, or lymphedema. As I have said, the surgeon's skill in dissecting the axilla is probably the most important factor in the development of this complication, and irradiation can contribute even further to its severity. Three of my respondents had had simple (or total) mastectomies. Since their nodes and lymphatic vessels were not removed or cut, they, of course, had no swelling at all. Some women have such mild lymphedema that it cannot even be seen; they feel only a tightness in the upper arm. Others must wear elastic bandages occasionally; some are sentenced to a lifetime of wearing a post-mastectomy sleeve.

This helpful medical accessory is a long elasticized glove minus the fingers, which comes in different sizes. It extends from the upper part of the hand to the shoulder and resembles the long opera gloves that were fashionable for prom wear when I was a teen-ager—gloves with fingered mitts that could be removed without taking the whole glove off. The sleeves are made of the same flesh-colored material as support stockings for varicose veins and act the same way the hosiery does—they squeeze the arm to stimulate circulation.

Many women had some limitation of shoulder motion, and the formation of keloid scar tissue, I learned later from calls to the BCAC, is a further complication many women encounter. Keloids frequently form in black women, and I've gotten lots of calls from them about it. Otherwise, because of variations in surgery, postoperative treatment, age, and possibly the stage of the disease, the women I interviewed had only three common physical problems: (1) the very tight, binding feeling across the chest, a constriction that lasted for months for almost everyone, but with different degrees of discomfort; (2) the strange, eerie business of having to crane the neck to shave under the arm; (3) the refusal of an itch to go away after being scratched. Everything else seemed to differ considerably from one patient to another.

After hearing from more than 3,000 mastectomees since 1974, this is still true. There is no way to predict exactly how a woman will be affected. So I will describe my own postoperative physical experience which may or may not be typical of women my age (forty-five) after a modified radical mastectomy.

The site immediately around the incision was numb for about five months. Once, I developed a small infection in the incision, and Dr. Dao told me, via long-distance telephone, to use hot compresses. The temperature that was comfortable to my fingers was hot enough to print a neat red square on the skin of my chest, although I could not feel anything there. I remember staring in horror as the color appeared—I had not realized that the water was too hot for newly grown skin. My shoulder and arm were extremely sensitive if touched. It was not a constant pain, but even a light brush with a feather felt like a hot iron was branding me. To bump the shoulder or put any pressure on the upper arm was agony.

For anyone interested in my sex life, I must point out that fondling from the waist up was out of the question. I was not one to whip off my bra as soon as I got my husband into the bedroom alone, but even if I had been, it would have been strictly no touch anywhere near the left arm. Some sexual problems that have crossed my telephone wire and desk through the BCAC will be described later in this chapter.

As for swelling, I still have occasional tightness, but nothing that can be seen or measured. It was not poor surgery or X-ray damage that caused the problem, though. I had not followed orders to stay away from 18-hour stretches at my typewriter. I discovered that anything that had made me puffy before the mastectomy still did. For example, I habitually retained fluid before and during the first few days of my menstrual period, and this pattern is persisting. If I eat too many salty or highly seasoned foods, I feel the salt in my upper arm the next morning. Maryland's hot humidity has always made me swell and continues to do so now. (The humidity is one of the reasons a Washington-area job is considered a "hardship post.") Effects of weather on my new incision were the same as they had been after my appendix was removed. For me, pulling or twisting in the incisional site was a better barometer than the weather bureau's. Like the appendectomy scar's improvement, this stopped after about two years.

Because I had my operation away from home, I was hospitalized for more than two weeks. Dr. Dao wanted to be certain the incision was healing well and there were no complications before I left Buffalo. For this reason, all my stitches had been removed by the time I was discharged. The normal practice, however, is to stay in the hospital about a week. The stitches (sutures) in the parts of the chest subject to the least stress are removed first, usually in the hospital. Then, a few days or a week later, the rest are taken out in the doctor's office.

Arm exercises were begun as soon as I recovered from the anesthesia, and this is not routine in most hospitals. Roswell Park has a physical therapy department, and I was taken there the morning after my surgery. It is vital, especially after a Halsted radical mastectomy, to begin exercising immediately to strengthen the auxiliary muscles of the arm that take over for the removed pectorals. It is also important after a modified radical, even though the chest muscles are intact. As I have said, the "radical" part of a mastectomy is the removal of the nodes and some lymphatic vessels and the cutting of other vessels. Exercises help get the blood and lymph circulating through the damaged area. If the arm is pampered or is "sedentary," like mine was, the temporary blockage can become permanent, resulting in ugly and painful milk arm. I was lucky that my stubborn stupidity in refusing to do the exercises religiously did not result in this postmastectomy complication. This clearly is a case of "Do as I say, not as I did."

The most useful and universal exercise is the spider walk. The healthy arm is stretched as high up a wall as it will go and a spot is marked at the tip of the longest finger. The trick is to walk the index and middle fingers of the affected arm up the wall, a little farther each time, until they can touch the same spot. Spider walking is done in two positions: facing the wall and at a right angle to it.

Another helpful exercise is to pull a rope about four feet long back and forth across a high horizontal bar. The shower rod is high enough for a short woman, but a tall one might have to install something different. Women who have had Halsteds also find that squeezing a rubber ball in the palm of the hand strengthens the auxiliary muscles.

A rope, a ball, and a "lounger"—a temporary prosthesis—are given to mastectomy patients shortly after their surgery by Reach to Recovery. At the surgeon's request, and with the patient's approval, a volunteer comes to the hospital the second or third day after the operation to present the kit, a manual of exercises, and a list of dos and don'ts, and to give general moral and psychological support. Naturally, Reach to Recovery volunteers themselves should have made a good adjustment in order to qualify. I did not have the visit, but those patients I interviewed who did were full of praise for the help they got from these volunteers.

Unfortunately, not all volunteers have made good adjustments and some, are not always adequately screened or trained to handle the delicate job they are mandated to do: visit women who have been freshly wounded and permanently scarred. Doing this well is psychotherapy and requires a certain personality plus skilled training. Where such ACS volunteers are early visitors, they are enormously helpful; where the volunteers are not the right women, they do more harm than good. There are more than 50 divisions and units of the ACS in this country, and although I have been impressed with the screening and training of R to R volunteers in many divisions and units, I have also been dismayed by the lack of both in others.

"It only takes one rotten apple to spoil a barrel," I have been told again and again by surgeons who refuse to ask for this service, even when patients specifically request it. (If a surgeon, for various reasons, does not permit R to R to come, women can easily get their own length of rope and rubber ball to squeeze while reading or watching TV.) Unfortunately, this surgical prejudice has prevented many women from being helped. I would like to see all women benefit from this program. I also fervently wish the ACS would expand Reach to Recovery to permit screened and trained volunteers to give presurgical counseling beforehand and to extend posttreatment support for as long a time afterward as women need it. However, the Society's national guidelines for local R to R groups still restrict their activities to giving only nonmedical information.

Another exercise is hairbrushing, a job that is not only good for the hair, but good for the shoulder and arm as well. At the beginning, a mirror is essential, because the affected arm is sore and a woman's reflex is to bring her head down to the brush, instead of vice versa. However, a few sessions before a mirror quickly train the head to stay erect. Swimming is also an excellent exercise after mastectomy, especially the backstroke.

After any radical mastectomy, women are warned—or should be warned—that *never again* must the affected arm be used for taking blood-pressure readings or for innoculations, vaccinations, or injections of any kind. Some surgeons even ban manicures and underarm shaving on that side.

It is also a good idea to avoid exposing the arm to too much sun, although this problem probably varies greatly from one person to another. In my own case, I found out the hard way. Dr. Dao had told me when I got my final instructions to be careful of sunburn, but the warning somehow did not sink in adequately. After I spent a day basking on a Caribbean beach, his words emerged from my subconscious as my left arm began to develop strange swollen curves and to twist and grind.

"I didn't remember," I wailed to Harvey, my arm propped up on three pillows. "I remembered no blood pressure, vaccinations, shots, or inoculations, but I forgot all about the sunburn warning."

"So now you've had a good lesson," he comforted. "You won't do it any more."

When the arm is injured, by either infection, trauma, or sunburn, the underlying tissue generally fills with lymphatic fluid carrying components of the immune system to heal the injury. If the lymphatic vessels have been cut, the fluid cannot circulate normally and sometimes it backs up in the arm. The result is lymphedema and pain. Of course, the fluid did filter back into my system, and my arm was fine after a day on the pillows and far from the beach. But the rest of my sunbathing was done wearing long sleeves. The problem may not bother some women at all; it is also possible that the blockage would not have happened to me if my tanning had been gradual, in small doses, rather than in a full day under the blazing Caribbean sun.

Another curious physical aftereffect of that trip was a reaction to altitude. The cabin of the airplane we flew down in was pressurized to about 6,000 feet at a cruising altitude of 32,000 feet. As we ascended, I noted a gradual tightening in my chest and arm, a sensation that disappeared within an hour or so after we landed. The same thing happened on the way home.

An airplane pilot I questioned said he could not understand

why a higher altitude should have an effect on only one part of the body, regardless of its condition. But a physicist thought this was possible. "It's like having some leaking tin cans of water," he explained. "You change the air pressure on the outside, reduce it the way you do up at 6,000 feet, and you'll have more force pushing from the inside outward than you would at sea level." According to him, even a minor blockage of a few lymph channels would be enough to turn them into "leaking tin cans," which would be more sensitive to changes of external pressure than normal vessels would be.

But that was months after the mastectomy. Immediately afterward, when I first returned home, my main physical reaction was exhaustion. In the hospital, I had been in great condition in comparison with most of the other patients, and of course I had had nothing much to do but brush my hair. My meals were served to me, I enjoyed daily naps, and physical therapy was the only activity that called for any energy. Back home, it was different. Just clearing the breakfast dishes was fatiguing. What had happened to all the vim and vigor I had had in Buffalo?

The vim and vigor were the same. It was only that my home life was taking more of them than my life in the hospital. This is perfectly normal after a mastectomy, especially if no blood transfusions have been given. The operation costs a lot of blood, and that may leave a woman weak, though not necessarily anemic. The important thing to know is that it takes time to get back to a normal energy level, and she must be careful not to overdo at the beginning. This does not mean she has to be pampered though. Mastectomy is not a disabling operation. A woman should get back into her old routine as soon as possible, judging how soon by how she feels.

In addition to the hairbrushing, the spider walk, swimming, squeezing a rubber ball, and pulling a rope, certain household jobs are excellent therapy. For example, the movements of washing windows and walls are helpful—and leave the house shining in the bargain. Anything that requires reaching or stretching is good. There really are no household chores that have to be avoided altogether, but during the first month, the important rule is moderation. While all women have different problems and all surgeons give different instructions, in my case the only restriction was not to lift anything heavy and not to pull or push anything with a lot of weight attached—like an upright vacuum cleaner through a thick shag rug. Other than this, I was encouraged to do anything I wanted to, as long as it did not overtire me.

I have already said that as soon as the bandages were removed I put on a loose-fitting bra and stuffed the empty cup with absorbent cotton. Later, I called my local Reach to Recovery office and was given one of their loungers to wear temporarily.

A surgeon usually does not want his patient to have a permanent prosthesis until her incision is well healed and beyond any possibility of complications. For this reason, most reputable firms require a prescription for the permanent form. That is one case, by the way, where needing a doctor's prescription can help the budget. Medical insurance usually pays for prescribed surgical appliances.

There are many permanent prostheses on the market, ranging from inexpensive Dacron-filled ones to specially weighted, latex-covered, silicone-gel shapes that feel as natural to the touch as a real breast. My strong opinion is that economy should be thrown out the window at this time (especially if the insurance will pay most of the bill). From my interviews with other mastectomees as well as my own experience, I firmly believe that nothing is more important than knowing both breasts look alike, are symmetrical, and "only her corsetière knows for sure."

The silicone-gel prosthesis costs more than a hundred dollars, depending on its size, but mine was worth every penny the insurance company paid. The latex cover made it adhere to the skin, so that it did not shift out of position but stayed where it belonged. The slick, silky coverings of other prostheses I tried often moved when I moved; occasionally I would discover the "breast" up near my shoulder or somewhere under my arm, instead of on the left side of my chest.

The reason for the weighting is simple physics. The smallest breast—even my A cup—does weigh something, and when the weight is removed, that shoulder will ride high. A bra stuffed with cotton is not heavy enough to pull the shoulder back to its normal position. Until I got my permanent form, I had sudden and strange neckaches, backaches, and headaches. All of these problems disappeared as soon as I was fitted with the weighted prosthesis. I had been walking around for more than a month with my shoulders askew, and the resulting stress had brought on the nagging pains. So a weighted form was a medical necessity for me.

Women with large breasts may have to have special brassieres as well. There are also different shapes to accommodate different kinds of surgery. Women who have had the modified radical or simple (total) mastectomy will be uncomfortable wearing the shape designed for the Halsted. It has a short "tail" intended to fill any cleft left in the axilla. If the surgery was less extensive and no such cleft is present, the tail feels lumpy.

Because the Halsted was by far the most common mastectomy

in 1974, my biggest problem was finding the shape manufactured for the modified radical in my size. Most surgeons do not get involved in advising patients about prostheses. Once they write a prescription, they count on Reach to Recovery volunteers or on expert fitters in lingerie departments of stores to take care of it.

Many large cities now have "mastectomy boutiques" that specialize in selling prostheses, lingerie, and other clothing needed by breast-cancer patients. These shops have well-trained fitters and dressing rooms with solid doors that close tightly—not with flimsy curtains. Women who are well-adjusted enough to go shopping for underwear may not mind being seminude and exposed in ordinary dressing rooms, but saleswomen and other customers who walk by are often startled and embarrassed by the sight of a single-breasted or no-breasted woman. For this reason, I suggest checking the yellow pages of the telephone directory to see if there are any such specialty stores nearby. As a rule, they are listed in the category of "Intimate Apparel."

When I had to go prosthesis shopping, there was no such store in my area, and I did not even think of calling a general department store or of looking in the Sears or Montgomery Ward catalogues. Instead, I went through the depressing experience of going from one "surgical appliance" store to another. The salespeople were wonderful, but the atmosphere sent my morale plummeting. These stores, much as they are needed, house wheelchairs, hospital beds, braces, and artificial limbs for "real" amputees. If this kind of store should be the only place a prosthesis is available, there is no choice. But my experience was unpleasant enough that I urge women to look for a place that is less threatening and grim. This is especially important at the beginning—right after surgery—when standing before a triple-viewed mirror can be devastating. By the time a second or third replacement is needed, mastectomy scars are faded and women have become accustomed to their flat half-chest.

Most of the countries I have visited, by the way, do not have a Reach to Recovery program at all. In 1976, I met Mrs. Fumi Morioka, a mastectomee who modeled an R to R program in Japan after ours. Mrs. Betty Westgate started a similar organization in England—the Mastectomy Association. But in other countries, nurses are usually the only sources of information women have.

Silicone-gel forms are relatively new: they have only been available for about fifteen years. At the end of 1974, I interviewed several women who had had their mastectomies more than ten years earlier, and I was told again and again what a blessing these forms are.

"I fought many a battle with a bulge," one fourteen-year (at that time) veteran said, laughing. "These new jobs are marvelous! You don't know what you missed."

Another women, who was only thirty-two (and four feet, ten inches tall) when she lost her breast eleven years before, complained bitterly about the ugly surgical-support brassiere she had worn for years. Even the golfing navy wife, who was neither young nor tiny—she weighed 176 pounds when we talked—waxed eloquent over not needing a "garment" anymore.

"It's made all the difference in the world to me," she boomed. "Now I can wear see-through blouses without worrying that the ugly old thing with five hooks and two inch straps will look like hell underneath."

Loretta Crowell told me that before the end of 1974, prostheses, like breast cancer itself, were "unmentionable."

"Until Mrs. Ford and Mrs. Rockefeller," she said, "I could never have put the kind of ad in a family newspaper like the one you saw in the *Post*. Talking about mastectomy forms and bras was strictly taboo."

So women who are unlucky enough to need mastectomies nowadays are nevertheless lucky to have so many postoperative services and products available. All of these are important aids in physical and psychological rehabilitation, aids that were not available in decades past when women had to make their own prostheses using cloth bags filled with birdseed. Reconstructive mammoplasty—plastic surgery to rebuild a lost breast—is probably the most important service/product in this category, and the previous chapter is devoted to that topic. But women who are unable or who do not want to have breast reconstruction, for one reason or another, have unlimited choices now. Manufacturers have designed special lingerie, bathing suits, and ingenious ways to simulate lost breasts for difficult-to-fit clothing.

One of these is simply called a "puff," a short cylinder of lightweight fabric stuffed with as much polyester fiber-fill necessary to match the remaining breast. Puffs are sewn into nightgowns, housecoats, bathrobes, and other clothing where a missing breast would be noticed if a bra and prosthesis were not worn. Before I had breast reconstruction (and before I learned about professionally made puffs), I invented my own for clothing too revealing for a bra-filled with a prosthesis. Fiber-fill is sold in most slipcover and upholstery stores, and I packed this stuff into the feet of discarded stockings. Although I did not think of putting my homemade falsies into nightgowns, I did sew the padding into the empty cups of my bathing suits and sundresses. Then I stitched the nylon covering of the falsie about a quarter of an inch from the edge of the built-in bra cup. To notice it someone would literally have to lean over and peek inside my cleavage to see. When I was afraid the tan of the stocking might show, I simply covered the "prosthesis" with a patch of fabric the same color as the dress. Using such devious disguises, I am able to wear my premastectomy bikini and a dramatic dress with one bare (naturally, the left!) shoulder, which I had bought a week before I found the lump. I can also wear plunging necklines.

Unfortunately, all this may not be helpful to those who have had a Halsted radical mastectomy. I know of no clever, ingenious ways to camouflage the scars left by that operation except sleeves and high necklines.

Aside from the cosmetic aspects, the physical problems of a mastectomy are very like those following any kind of major surgery. Everyone heals and recovers at a different speed and experiences different reactions. Because the woman around the corner was playing tennis six weeks after her surgery does not mean that anything is wrong with a woman who, like me, could not. As long as her doctor is satisfied, there is no cause for worry. The aftereffects of the surgery will not last forever, and inevitably the mastectomy will stop being a good excuse for getting out of club or committee work. Enjoy it while it lasts.

An unfortunate aftereffect of mastectomy, which is not cosmetic, is job and credit discrimination. Since I had worked on my own for years as a free-lance writer, it had never occurred to me that having had a mastectomy could hurt a woman's ability to get a job. Then, in the *New York Times*, on November 28, 1974, it was reported that Mrs. Joyce Arkhurst, a New Yorker, had been denied a job at the United Nations because she had had a mastectomy in April 1973.

Her cancer was cured, according to her doctor, but the personnel office at the UN, where she had applied for a job would not hire her. Although everyone who had interviewed Mrs. Arkhurst thought she was qualified, she could not get the necessary medical clearance. The United Nations, she was told, does not hire cancer patients until five years have passed since their last treatment.

Mrs. Arkhurst came to the National Conference on Cancer Management, held in New York, to demonstrate to the physicians attending that the problems of a cancer patient are more than medical. Dr. Robert McKenna, a cancer surgeon, who was also at the meeting, reported on fifty other cases of employment discrimination against cancer patients he knew of in California alone, and said that most government agencies and many private companies have employed practices identical to the United Nations'.

Certainly it is hard to think of any major surgery less handicapping than a mastectomy. Except for a job as a go-go girl, a striptease dancer, or possibly a lingerie model, I cannot imagine why any employer would argue against hiring a mastectomy patient. I called the personnel offices of several firms in my area, as well as the United States Civil Service Commission, to ask about it.

"There's no way to know if a cancer patient is cured for five years," I was told. "Suppose we invest a lot of time and money in training the person, and they get sick with cancer again. All that goes down the drain."

"Suppose you invest all that time and money in training someone, and the person walks into the street and is hit by a car!" I responded in disbelief. "Anything can happen. If you hire a young secretary, how do you know she won't get married and leave because her husband is transferred? What about getting pregnant?"

Later, I found out that it was illegal for the federal government or any of its contractors to have discriminated against a cancer patient. That person in the Civil Service Commission should have been fired himself for not knowing about Section 503 of the Rehabilitation Act of 1973. According to this Act, "the term 'handicapped individual' means any person with a physical or mental disability which constitute or results in a substantial barrier to employment . . . " The entire Rehabilitation Act explains what Affirmative Action is and what the penalties are if any federal agency or one of the government's contractors discriminates against a handicapped person. Few cancer patients consider themselves to be "handicapped" in the general sense of the word. However, Congress made it clear that all cancer patients are considered handicapped, as far as the law is concerned.

Because there are few schools, colleges, universities, hospitals, and large business firms that do not have a federal contract, Section 503 covers a large proportion of the twelve million handicapped people in the United States. However, there are thousands of firms and factories that are neither unionized (labor-management agreements usually forbid discrimination) nor have government contracts. So discrimination is a fact of life.

Discrimination against cancer patients seems to make no sense at all, but hiring someone who has had this disease does, apparently, present some real problems. First of all, many places have insurance and pension plans that will not cover employees with preexisting chronic diseases of any kind. Even though a separate policy could be written for these people, they do not want to take the bookkeeping trouble to do so. There is still a ridiculous, but persistent superstition that cancer is contagious, and many businesses are afraid of losing employees who have this fear.

Another, often legitimate, reason is worry about absenteeism. Now that adjuvant therapy of some kind has become routine whenever a woman has positive nodes, absenteeism may be a problem, even if the woman does not develop a recurrence. Most adjuvant therapies must be given by injection during the doctor's office hours, and time must be taken off from work.

In addition, many women have unpleasant side effects immediately after taking the medication and may not be able to work as well or at all. While this should not be a problem in a company with dozens or hundreds of employees, it obviously is a serious one for owners of small businesses with only one or two. It could be a hardship for such firms to have to hire an extra employee to cover for the necessary, frequent absences. This last category is the only one where refusing to hire a cancer patient is at all acceptable. As far as large firms not covered by Section 503 are concerned, it is outrageous that there is any such discrimination.

At the National Conference on Cancer Management, Dr. McKenna pointed out that cancer of the breast is considered curable today and that, whether the personnel director knows it or not, one of every thousand job applicants is a "closet" cancer patient. He also calculated that such discrimination against cancer victims means about a $500 million annual cost to the United States economy in taxes, welfare, and other financial assistance. In October 1974, the American Cancer Society had formed a study group on the problem of job discrimination, with Dr. McKenna as its chairman.

One way to get around the persecution, of course, is for the former patients not to tell their employers. However, they would then have to pay their own medical bills, in most cases, since they could not collect anything under a firm's group plan. This would be an enormous—and obviously unfair—hardship. Another suggestion is to initiate a mass-education program aimed at personnel officials with the goal of convincing them that a former cancer patient is no higher risk than any other employee. Still another approach being considered is to give special tax benefits to employers who hire the handicapped—cancer patients and all others. So far, it is mostly talk.

Coincidentally, shortly after I learned of Mrs. Arkhurst's problem with the United Nations, I was invited to a party given by someone in my husband's company. One of the other guests, a senior employee—a very sharp, highly trained, competent woman of perhaps fifty—took me aside and told me she envied my being free to talk about my cancer openly without fear of a penalty.

"What do you mean?" I asked.

"Exactly what I said," she whispered. "I had a mastectomy last April and went back to work half days after only two weeks, just to be sure my supervisor didn't suspect I had anything serious."

I stared at her in disbelief. This was, after all, the same place where Harvey worked—presumably a sophisticated, enlightened, well-educated bunch of people. "They couldn't possibly have refused to give you back your job, you know," I told her. "There are laws now—"

"I wasn't worried so much about this job," she told me quietly. "I do know my rights, and if I had been fired I would have gone to the EEOC (Equal Employment Opportunity Commission) before they could have blinked. No, I was worried about my prospects of getting another job. Who knows? Something might happen here, and I'd be out of work. Where would I get a new job with a fresh mastectomy printed on my personnel record? That's the big problem I face—getting a new job. We don't have to worry about hanging on to the old ones. We're protected there. But getting a new one is different."

"But don't you think you could accomplish more by going public and fighting?" I asked.

She shook her head sadly. "I've got three kids in college and a lot of expenses. I'm afraid I'm just not in a financial position to do any fighting for the cause." She smiled and patted me on the shoulder. "But right on to you, for anything you can do."

She got up and looked around to see if anyone had overheard us. "Please keep my secret. I really have to go on working."

Since then, I have read and heard more such stories. Dr. McKenna's committee tried to get employment policies changed for former cancer patients and the NCI has staff in the Division of Community Activities working on the problem now. Other organizations are working to change the climate for all handicapped people. Undoubtedly, there are many jobs that victims of certain handicaps cannot manage. But having one breast instead of two? I doubt it would handicap even a prostitute.

I had not mentioned credit discrimination in *Breast Cancer* or in the first edition of *Why Me?*, because I did not even know it existed. After all, no one I have ever done business with ever asked me to fill out a health form when I applied for a charge account. But in 1976, a writer called me to tell me she had been turned down by a famous New York store because her breast cancer put her "at high risk at not being able to pay the bill." Not married, she held a well-paid job at a major newspaper, and she was earning about $28,000 per year. In spite of her high salary, being unmarried meant she had no one legally liable for her debts. She was a savvy woman, knew this was patently and blatantly illegal and was able to straighten it out with no help from me.

But I could not help but wonder how this store knew she had had breast cancer. It was only then that I learned there are no laws prohibiting insurance companies from "leaking" medical information to both employment and credit agencies!

When anyone is admitted to a hospital for anything, he or she signs a form permitting the hospital to give all the relevant information to the patient's medical insurance company. Of course, all of the health professionals involved in the case are sworn to confidentiality, except for the office that handles insurance forms. The information must be given to the third-party-carrier (as medical insurance companies are known), and then the information is up for grabs.

Sen. William Proxmire of Wisconsin has repeatedly tried to get the Senate Banking Committee he chairs to propose legislation to prevent this leakage, but the insurance lobby argues that it is essential for them to be able to exchange data. Otherwise, they claim, epileptics and diabetics, who are not being controlled by medication, would be able to get driver's licenses.

No one can question the need for insurance companies to have these kinds of interchanges to protect the rest of us folk on the roads. Yet there must be a way to prohibit them from leaking personal medical information to employment and credit agencies.

Since I first became aware of this dirty business, I have collected a file of muckraking investigative articles about such schemes from all over the country. In some, indictments were handed down, and the people are in jail. But most of these cases involved the small-fry racketeers who were caught in hospital records rooms while posing as legitimate insurance investigators. Their employers at the top, as far as I have been able to learn, have never been touched by a policeman's glove. In my state, Maryland, Charles Docter, a member of the legislature, pushed through (against massive pressure from the insurance lobby) a state law forbidding these practices. Obviously, though, a single law in a small state can do nothing to help the millions of people who are being hurt in the rest of the country.

Remember—this affects not only cancer patients but people who have had heart attacks, tuberculosis, and other diseases that could put them at "high risk" for leaving unpaid debts behind. (It also, by the way, permits abortions, VD, hemorrhoids, psychiatric care, and other private problems to get to prying eyes.) This is clearly a scourge that needs to be cleaned up by Congress. Anyone interested in helping Sen. Proxmire can contact him at his Washington, D.C. address: Room 5241, Dirkson Senate Office Building, Washington, D.C. 20510.

In both *Breast Cancer* and *Why Me?*, I listed the follow-up examinations I was having at Roswell Park, so women would know what they and their doctors should be doing to detect a recurrence as early as possible. Since then, I wrote a short leaflet about this for the National Cancer Institute, which I have inserted here. It is called "If you've had breast cancer . . ." and copies are available by calling (toll-free) 800-638-6694 or by writing: Office of Cancer Communications: National Cancer Institute: Bethesda, Md. 20205. These are free; everyone's tax dollars pay for them.

IF YOU'VE HAD BREAST CANCER . . .

Surgery—removal of a breast containing a malignant tumor—is usually enough treatment to cure the majority of cases of early breast cancer. However, women who have had a mastectomy should realize the disease may return (or recur) in spite of the surgery. Most women worry that such a recurrence will develop in their second breast. If this should happen, the recurrence is probably a new cancer and not a sign that the original disease has spread. The reason is that breast cancer is often a "multicentric" disease, that is, if one malignancy should develop, there may be other cancerous spots in both breasts. For this reason, a new tumor in the opposite breast is usually completely independent from the first and is known as a "second primary." This is why it is important for women to continue to practice breast self-examination (BSE) after surgery. If a new growth appears, it will be found at an early stage of development when it is most likely to be curable.

Women who have had one breast cancer should also be aware of some of the early warning signals of recurrence elsewhere in the body. For example, a symptom might develop in the incision itself or in the area around it. It sometimes happens that lymph nodes not treated by surgery or X-ray may become malignant. The disease may also spread, or metastasize, to another part of the body, such as the bone, lung, liver, or—infrequently—to the brain.

According to the American College of Surgeons, 60 percent of all recurrences appear within the first three years after surgery, 20 percent within the next two years, and 20 percent in later years. Because of these statistics, women who have been treated for breast cancer should be checked frequently during the first five postoperative years and should continue to be checked by their doctors as often as is recommended in the years afterward.

It has been generally accepted for decades that early detection and treatment of primary breast cancer will save thousands of women's lives. However, there was little that could be offered if the disease returned. Now, the development of potent anticancer agents has given hopeful evidence that early detection and treatment of a recurrence may succeed in lengthening the lives of— and perhaps even curing—those women whose disease returns.

WHAT WOMEN CAN DO

Regular visits to a physician are important, and every woman and her surgeon should decide who will be responsible for her follow-up care. Many surgeons monitor their patients themselves. Others may refer them to medical oncologists, to internists, to a radiotherapist (especially if the breast had been preserved and irradiated instead of being removed by mastectomy), or to a family practitioner. Between professional examinations, women should also be on guard for symptoms that they themselves may find:

1. Monthly self-examination of the remaining breast (BSE) and of both underarm areas to detect any changes. Report any difference in skin texture, color, size or shape; dimpling, lumps, thickenings, rashes, nipple discharge, or tenderness (not associated with the menstrual period);
2. Report any bone pain;
3. Report persistent coughing or hoarseness;
4. Report digestive problems—nausea, vomiting, heartburn, diarrhea—not present earlier, but which persist for several days;
5. Report unexplained losses or gains of weight;
6. Report any changes in menstrual patterns such as the length of time the flow lasts, time between periods, the differences in type of flow, etc.
7. Report any persistent dizziness, blurred vision, severe and frequent headaches, unusual difficulties in walking, balancing, etc.

While women should be careful to observe and report these possible symptoms of recurrent disease, especially during the first three postoperative years, they must always keep in mind that problems like arthritis, influenza, the menopause, and even the common cold are usually the cause—*not* a recurrence of the cancer.

WHAT MAY BE EXPECTED FROM THE DOCTOR

During the first three postoperative years, women treated for breast cancer should have professional examinations approximately every three to six months. During some, examination of the neck and previously treated area and palpation of the remaining breast may be done, simply because nothing else is necessary. Other visits, however, may include all or some of the following procedures:

1. Examination of the incision, nearby chestwall, both axillas, the base of the neck, and the second breast;
2. A *mammogram* of the remaining breast. While an annual X-ray is usually recommended, the intervals may vary depending on individual characteristics such as size and density. Under no circumstances should women who have had breast cancer refuse to have a mammogram because of fears of the radiation. The controversy about possible dangers of breast X-rays does *not* apply to them. The debate about mammography concerns only the routine examination of women, under age 50, who have no symptoms of breast cancer;
3. Manual examination of the abdominal area; blood tests for liver function and/or liver scans, if indicated;
4. Other blood and urine analyses, including the alkaline phosphatase test. Many breast-cancer experts are doing certain experimental studies of blood and urine specimens, and permitting such research to be performed can do no harm and may do a great deal of good;
5. X-rays and/or scans of the chest, spine, and pelvis, at irregular intervals. These are usually "scattered," so the patient's exposure to radiation during a single visit is reduced. Some doctors may take a baseline X-ray or scan of the skull for future comparison;
6. Annual pelvic examinations, including a cervical or "Pap" smear.

For the fourth and fifth postoperative year, the above examinations may be done every six to nine months, but there may be reasons for a physician to see a patient more frequently.

HAND AND ARM CARE AFTER REMOVAL OF THE AXILLARY NODES OR RADIATION THERAPY

A potential problem that may arise after surgery is swelling of the affected arm, a condition known as *lymphedema*. Not all women develop this postoperative complication, because most primary treatments being used result in the removal of fewer axillary lymph nodes, and routine postoperative radiation of the axilla is rarely done now. Lymphedema is caused by the loss (by surgery) or damage (by X-ray) of underarm nodes and their connecting vessels, a problem that slows the passage of circulating lymph fluid from the affected arm. If swelling should occur, it may be disfiguring, and sometimes painful. At this time, lymphedema cannot be cured but can be helped by elevation and massage, the use of an elastic sleeve, or by pneumatic compression.

Women who have had axillary nodes removed or who have been treated by X-ray should follow these simple rules to prevent infection that could worsen the swelling:

1. Avoid cuts, scratches, pin pricks, hangnails, insect bites, or the use of strong detergents on the affected arm and hand;
2. If the affected arm or hand is injured, treat the cut or scratch with antibacterial medication and cover it with a dressing.

The National Cancer Institute has prepared a list of recommendations for women to follow to avoid lymphedema and to prevent its complications even if mild swelling has already occurred. These are:

Don't carry anything heavy with the affected arm.
Don't suspend anything heavy on this shoulder.
Don't wear jewelry that might scratch or squeeze the arm.
Don't cut or pick at the cuticle on this hand.
Don't do any gardening without wearing heavy protective gloves.
Don't use the affected arm to check a hot oven.
Don't let anyone give injections or draw blood from the arm.
Don't let anyone use the arm to measure blood pressure.

Some other precautions:
Wear rubber gloves when washing dishes.

Use a thimble when sewing.

Order an identification tag engraved with:

"LYMPHEDEMA ARM—NO TESTS—NO HYPOS"

Use an elastic sleeve, if necessary, and be sure to have it remeasured periodically so adjustments can be made.

Ask the doctor about pneumomassage if the swelling persists.

These recommendations apply to all women who have had axillary nodes removed or who have received X-ray therapy, even if they have not experienced any swelling. But they are especially important to any breast-cancer patients who have noticed signs of lymphedema.

Women may wish to show this leaflet to their physicians for their comments or additional suggestions about hand and arm care after breast surgery.

Breast cancer is a chronic disease, just as diabetes is a chronic disease. Like diabetics, women with breast cancer must always be on guard for symptoms. That may be a cruel and heartless thing to say to a woman who has gone five years or even more without trouble and thinks she can stop worrying forever. But to lie would be more cruel and heartless, because it could result in unnecessary deaths. The years without recurrence or metastasis are called disease-free years; cancer specialists do not speak of cure rates but of survival. Women who have had breast cancer must face the facts.

We can relax and breathe easier after two years—the period when more than half of the recurrences and metastases first show up. And we can breathe even more deeply after five years. But the definitive time for measuring breast-cancer survival is now ten years. The five-year period formerly applied to all cancers is under no circumstances valid for mammary carcinoma. We must be on guard, although not as intensively, for ten years.

I hope that by the time I am ten years postop, "mastectomy" will come right after "leeches" in the medical-encyclopedia listings of quaint old surgical practices that have been abandoned.

15

After Treatment: Psychological

"Do you still feel attractive and appealing?" the young host of the TV talk show asked.

I squinted at him angrily. The subject of sex, I thought, had been laid to rest during an earlier off-camera break for a commercial.

"I don't feel any different from the way I did before," my fellow guest began to explain. "I've always thought too much of myself to think that everything I am, my personality, my intelligence, had anything to do with whether I had one breast or two." A sensible explanation, but a totally unnecessary one.

We had been invited to appear on a local daytime show to talk about the problems of mastectomy after Betty Ford and Happy Rockefeller had their operations. My partner was attractive, in her late forties, fourteen years postop, and she seemed to have been subjected to that kind of question before. She also had had enough mutilation from her surgery for me to be able to see a dip in her upper chest, even though she was wearing a high neckline.

Our host was a young blade-about-town with a reputation for smart-alecky wit and an ability to get to the heart of a panel's subject quickly. To him, the heart of breast-cancer problems is sex.

"Now, I'd like you to talk about the differences in your relationships with your husbands after the operation," he had earlier instructed us during a commercial. "This is what our viewers are interested in, you know—the changes it has made in your marital situation."

"That's ridiculous!" I had snapped. "Women watching this show have more sense than to be curious about our sex lives when we've had operations for cancer."

Then the light flashed, signaling our return to the air. From his first question, it was obvious that he either had not heard or had not paid any attention to my comment. Even after my partner did her best to close the subject politely, he could not let it pass.

"If you've seen Coke ads since the age of eight as I have," he continued, "you obviously have to dwell on the fact that having breasts is part of our culture."

I stared at him, through what I hoped were narrowed, angry slits, and did not answer. My partner, however, tried womanfully to mollify him without prostituting the principle that sex has no place in any intelligent discussion of breast cancer.

"It really has nothing to do with—" she began.

I thought he was about to break in with a more pointed question, and, television or no, I could not hold back any longer. I remember leaning so far toward him that the microphone hanging from the cord around my neck jerked to one side.

"Just a minute!" I interrupted. "The thing you're forgetting is that we're discussing a fatal disease, and the important thing is that the doctor get rid of the cancer, and are you going to live? Unless a woman is unbalanced, the first thing she worries about is her life."

He didn't seem to understand. "But once she wakes up, and she doesn't have her breast, but she has her life—" he broke in.

"The first thing she says is 'Did you get it all out'? " I completed his sentence.

It must have seemed incredible to him. "It is?" he asked softly.

"You better believe it," I snapped.

I don't think he believed me.

Earlier, when I discussed the physical aftereffects of breast surgery—specifically, of a radical mastectomy of some kind—I listed the items in the questionnaire I had used to get information and I had reluctantly included one about sex, because I knew this was an area readers would be interested in. I use the word "reluctantly," because it seemed wrong to pry, and I felt like a Peeping Thomasina.

When I evaluated the replies, I decided my response to the TV host had really reflected the attitude of most women, because—as I wrote—"To almost all the women who wrote or telephoned, sexiness and being appealing and attractive to men *were* unimportant. They had more significant things to worry about."

How wrong I was! I have already described my statistical incompetence elsewhere and it was this enormous gap in my educational repertoire that led me astray. About 5,000 questionnaires had been distributed by Mrs. Crowell throughout the

United States and Canada, but only 130 women were comfortable enough about themselves to send them back or call me to answer the questions by telephone. Even a freshman student in statistics would know that the data I used to reach my conclusions might not be representative: if N = 5,000, then N–130 = 4,870. When that many women do not respond to a questionnaire, the results are undoubtedly skewed.

By pure luck, however, my small sample did accurately reflect women's attitudes as well as later "well-designed" statistical studies did, but my data had not probed into sexuality, femininity, self-esteem, and body image. (I did not learn about these problems until the next year when thousands of letters and telephone calls from women—and men—began to pass across the desk and telephone line of the Breast Cancer Advisory Center.) So to write the postsurgical chapter for *Breast Cancer,* I blithely took it for granted that all 5,000 women who received my questionnaire had picked up where they had left off when they found their symptom of breast cancer. (Just as I thought *I* had picked up where I left off . . . until the Jacksonville fire showed me how wrong I was.)

So I went ahead and began my analysis of the "data."

Making some rhyme and reason out of the questionnaires turned out to be complicated, even with a 130-women sample, I quickly learned.

"All you have," Dr. William Granatir, a Washington, D.C. therapist explained, "are women whose emotional lives were not seriously damaged by losing their breasts."

He was the first person to point out the "telescoping phenomenon" I described earlier.

"The farther away in time a traumatic emotional experience is," he said, "the better it may seem to have been. It would be interesting to know what these women would have told you right away—or if they would have told you anything right away."

Another psychiatrist friend told me his experiences with patients showed that the most severe psychological problems occurred before a diagnosis of breast cancer was confirmed.

"That's what you've got to look into to get a real picture of what breast cancer does to a woman," he said. "Maybe you ought to make that your next project."

And I did exactly that later, after I had that enormous sample of responses statisticians demand. But in 1974, I could not do more than I did. As I have said, it is amazing that the 130 women who "felt good enough about themselves" to share their attitudes with me did represent views that have been described in surveys since then.

On the other hand, it is possible that the women who responded to these more scientific and valid questionnaires were the same kind who responded to mine.

From my nonscientific, small, skewed, and biased sample, I discovered there were several variables that affected women differently. These were: extent of disease; the woman's age; her marital and family status; the condition of the marriage; whether she has young children or older ones still living at home; and unrelated premastectomy psychological problems. For example, unmarried women under forty-five seemed to be in better psychological health than the postmenopausal unmarrieds. But only eight women in the younger group responded, and only three of these were under thirty-five—a sample that is out of proportion with the overall incidence statistics. Many such young women, I suspect, did not call me or return their questionnaires. After all, most of the current clamor here for lumpectomies and reconstructive mammoplasties seems to be coming from women in this category. In both Stockholm and Moscow, I was told, young women were the ones who wanted to be involved in the trials of lesser surgeries; in those countries, too, the young unmarrieds apparently thought two breasts are essential for finding husbands.

Immediately I discovered a dramatic dichotomy between the attitudes of women who had already gone five or ten years with no recurrence or mestastasis and those who knew their cancers had not been stopped by the mastectomy. The difference was so stunning that the two groups seemed almost to represent completely separate diseases.

Women whose doctors "did not get it all out" or who were too advanced for a mastectomy to help at the time of diagnosis had little interest in discussing the kind of surgery they had had. They usually couldn't even recall the details. Their worry about the spreading cancer overshadowed such relatively minor woes as ugly scars, lymphedema, disability, and all the other things we have been led to believe are the major problems after mastectomy. This applied to all ages. The youngest woman in this group had her surgery when she was thirty-three, only six months after her youngest child was born. The oldest, sixty-seven when I interviewed her, has since died. None of these patients cared much about skin grafts or Halsted versus modified versus lumpectomy. They had left these concerns behind them long ago.

"What I couldn't understand," the youngest of them told me, "is why everyone in the media—including you—thought it was so important that Betty Ford had a Halsted instead of something else. What the hell's the difference if the surgery cures her?"

Then forty-two and a practicing architect, this woman had survived nine years of flare-ups and hospitalizations. She was adjusted to living with recurrences and metastases and to the knowledge that she would always have cancer. "But nobody even
hinted at the time of my surgery that it was going to be a chronic
disease," she said. "All my lymph nodes were fine. I was cured,
they told me."

Her first metastasis, to the lung, was not discovered until her
chest was X-rayed for pneumonia almost three years after the
mastectomy. "I *have* gotten better examinations since I had that
first metastasis," she said ruefully. "Before that, it was just a
quick examination of my other breast. I'm getting much more
attention now." She paused. "But not as much as I think I should
have. Sometimes I have to insist that I *know* something is wrong
before anything is done."

Nine years after surgery, mastectomy itself was as buried in her
memory as her own birth. She died in 1979, but her attitude when
I interviewed her in 1974 was typical of the women not cured by
mastectomy. Again and again, over and over, I heard the same
lament from them. Doctors did not examine carefully or often
enough to find the recurrence or metastasis early, when they
might have been able to stop the cancer from spreading farther.

When I pointed out that treatments being used so effectively
then—especially drugs—had not been available even five years
earlier, most long-term survivors seemed to feel better. But nothing assuaged the bitter, sometimes violent, rage of women like
Ann Scott whose metastases, if they had been found early, could
have been helped by drugs already on the shelves of cancer-
hospital pharmacies.

"What kind of checkup do you get at Roswell Park?" I was
asked repeatedly. As I described the procedure there, I could
often hear a pencil or pen taking quick notes. Several women
even asked me to slow down a bit. Only one of those I talked with
had been scanned before her metastasis was finally found—and
then only after she complained of chronic backaches. Some had
never had a postoperative mammogram; some had had chest
X-rays, but only as a part of routine physical examinations by
their family doctors. Several of the women, however, had been
X-rayed periodically to see if their spines, ribs, and skulls were
free of disease. In general, the architect's experience was typical:
the women got more thorough examinations *after* their metastases appeared.

Without question, the women who knew their disease had not
been stopped by their mastectomies had totally different emo-

tional problems from those who were either "waiting" or who were breathing more freely after ten or more years.

"I wish all I had to worry about was whether my scar shows in a bathing suit or if I can pick up a ten-pound bag of sugar," one woman told me. "It depends where you sit how you stand, I guess." She roared with laughter when I told her about the questions I had been asked on the television program. "Now, that has got to be the epitome of insanity," she finally spluttered. "Who in her right mind would be worried about being appealing when she finds out she's got cancer?"

From my nonscientific, biased, and miniscule sample, I concluded that unless a woman is so insecure or neurotic that having two real breasts means more to her than staying alive, her main concern after a mastectomy was, "Does the surgeon think it was caught in time?" and not "What will my husband think when he sees me naked?"

Who cares what he thinks? If he loves her, his first concern will also be for the cancer, not for the imbalance in that part of her under the shoulders. A man who throws away a woman because of a mastectomy, or even two, is not worth having.

Television talk shows and the worry about being appealing notwithstanding, the single biggest psychological adjustment a woman must make after breast surgery is to the sudden knowledge that she has a chronic, potentially fatal disease and that removing the breast is only the first step in trying to stop its malignant spread.

Her family and friends know it, too, but are helpless to do much about it. In order to keep them from falling apart, the woman tries to keep her chin up and have a smile plastered on her face—at a time when she herself is most defenseless and in need of support.

Being in another city, I had no friends visiting me at all, but it was supportive for me to be in a hospital devoted exclusively to the treatment of cancer, as Roswell Park is. My first roommate was a retired librarian, Betty Butterfield, who had had miscellaneous skin cancers for thirty years. When I arrived, shaken and trembling, almost a week before the mastectomy, she was just waking up from her latest bout of skin grafts. Her grogginess lasted only a short time, and then she was bouncing around cheerfully, bandages swathing her face.

"You're in the best place there is in the world," she assured me. "I found my first cancer thirty years ago, and now I'm seventy-four and still going strong. It's because I have Roswell Park to come to. If anybody can keep us going, they'll do it here."

With that kind of person around, I couldn't wail and whine.

"If you've got to have cancer"—she grinned weirdly through her bandages—"the best kind to have is what I've had all these years—skin. But the second best is your kind, the breast. If it's caught in time, it's the easiest to cure. So what if you lose a breast? There are a lot of patients in this hospital that would change places with you in a second." She looked at her watch. "It's almost time for dinner. I'll introduce you to some of them afterward."

Next to Betty, (who is now learning the hustle and who led a senior citizens' tour to Alaska), Larry Bohne, who died early in December 1974, did more to help me adjust to living with cancer than anyone else. When I met Larry, he had already been declared terminal three times, and many of the drugs that had pulled him through had had their first human trials on him.

"I guess I'm the first person after the gorillas," he quipped. "It's been fifteen months now since I should have gone, and I'm still here. Every day is worthwhile. It's not the quantity of life that counts, it's the quality. Remember that."

With so much courage from a thirty-year-old whose first child was born just before he discovered he had cancer, how could I complain about losing a breast? And there were others whose first cancers had been diagnosed years before and who came regularly to Roswell Park for checkups or treatment.

It was difficult at times. I had to tread delicately with patients who were seriously ill and not rub salt in their considerable wounds by appearing to be so hearty and healthy. The first few hours were hard too. It was painful to look around at people with amputated organs, skin grafts, missing hair, and miscellaneous pipes and drains, and to accept the knowledge that I belonged here, that it was not just a ghastly mistake. On the other hand, it was enormously helpful in more important ways.

Cancer had always been a scare word to me, an automatic signal to order a cemetery plot and a tombstone. Meeting people who had lived for years with as many as fourteen tumors made it much easier for me to hear that I now had a chronic disease to take care of for the rest of my life. The only long-term survivor of breast cancer I had ever heard of was Theodore Roosevelt's daughter, Alice Longworth, Washington's *grande dame*. While there was no breast cancer in my own family, as far as I knew, I kept remembering the close relatives on Harvey's side of the family who had had breast cancer, none of whom had survived.

These first days at Roswell Park made me realize that the kind of surgery performed, how ugly the scar would be, whether I could wear low necklines and bikinis—everything that had concerned me earlier—were frivolous worries. After talking to Betty, Larry, and others on my floor, I was glad I would be cared for by a breast-cancer specialist in a cancer hospital. But for a far more significant reason than the one that took me to Buffalo in the first place. Never mind the beauty of a modified radical mastectomy. Suddenly, quite suddenly, I was surrounded with proof that being cared for (or treated) by an oncologist could save my life.

Once, on her morning television show Barbara Walters asked the late Marvella Bayh why she had been so public about having a mastectomy and not secretive, as the novelist Jacqueline Susann had been.

"I really had no choice in the matter," Mrs. Bayh replied. "Birch had already declared himself to be a candidate for the presidency in 1972, people had already begun working on his behalf, and money had been collected. He could not have dropped his plans without explaining the urgent reason for withdrawing."

She said that afterward she had been happy there was no choice. She had discovered how much good she could do by telling about it and letting people see that she was well enough to lead the busy, active—often frantic—life of a senator's wife. Mrs. Bayh, who looked radiant, said she hoped her example, like Shirley Temple Black's, Betty Ford's, and Happy Rockefeller's, would help get rid of some of the fears that keep women away from early-detection clinics and doctors' offices.

In my case, there was no urgent reason to tell the world. I simply discovered that I, like most writers—especially those of us in and around Washington—abhor secrets. To us, a secret is something to dig out and tell to the public. It never occurred to me to keep my mastectomy quiet. In fact, I began keeping notes the night I found the lump. It may seem macabre, but that's the way it is with people whose job is communicating—we have to communicate. With these notes, jotted down as I went along, I have been able to reconstruct accurately the changes in my attitudes throughout the whole dreadful business. Without them, I am certain I would have suppressed a great deal.

Everything—the first panicky terror at finding the lump, the confusion and conflicting points of view about what to do, the inaccuracy of the diagnostic techniques available, the ignorance of the average doctor, and, finally, the subtle but sudden switch in my thinking during that first bull session in my room at Roswell Park—is not only in my memory but also on paper.

Since then, I have found out that writing about the experience

is a catharsis for many women, not only for "communicators." I
have files of poems, short stories, documentary-type essays ("I
Came In With Two . . . ") and even book manuscripts written by
patients who simply had to put something on paper. Betty Rollin,
a television reporter for NBC, wrote about her mastectomy, and
her attitude represented the typical premenopausal woman with a
rocky marriage. Jean Zalon's fight for breast reconstruction is
also detailed in her book *I Am Whole Again*. The plight of women
who develop recurrent disease has been described in many eloquent articles by Natalie Spingarn, a Washington writer who is
now writing a book about "hanging in there." This may well be its
title when it reaches the shelves of stores and libraries.

The list can go on for pages. Many of the articles I received
were published in local community newspapers and magazines;
some were in college or club newsletters. Most were never published at all and stayed in manuscript form to be sent around to
other patients. One of these was "published" by a woman who
called me about her "crippling arthritis" after reading *Breast
Cancer*. Unfortunately, Yvonne Burkart's disease was already so
advanced that she could not even be helped much at Roswell
Park. But while she lived, she circulated a round-robin newsletter
for women receiving chemotherapy and included witty recommendations for coping with drugs' side effects, patterns for
unique turbans, and other hints for breast-cancer patients whose
surgeries were not enough.

Professionals often wrote scientific papers, did studies and
surveys, and many switched from whatever interest they had had
before to work with the many problems surrounding breast
cancer.

Most of the material, however—especially the unpublished
works—were bitter accounts of having been railroaded into a
Halsted radical mastectomy, of having no choice in the decision-
making or of nontreatment and/or mistreatment by general physicians and surgeons. Many of the women with artistic ability drew
illustrations reminiscent of the kinds that came from concentra-
tion-camp memories to accompany their stories.

In rereading *Breast Cancer* for its first revision, I noticed
flashes of anger and outrage in parts of my own chronicle. This
may seem strange, because I was lucky enough to get excellent
treatment. But I vividly remember feeling furious, for my own
sake and for the sake of other women, that I had to battle so hard
and have "connections" to get good treatment. Suppose I did not
live near the National Cancer Institute? Suppose I had not had
friends to steer me to the right place? What would have happened

to me? So I too was outraged by the medical/surgical establishment. Many times I still am.

Overall, however, my description of what happened to me is, I think, objective and free of diatribe.

The two days after my admission were busy with preoperative tests and X-rays to let Dr. Dao know if I was an eligible candidate for mastectomy. Everyone was rooting for me, and when the good word finally came, Betty, Larry, some of the other patients and I had a wild evening over a pint of Scotch (permission requested and granted). Who would have thought, just a few days earlier, that I would be celebrating the prospect of losing my breast?

There were moments though, that were not spent in jolly celebration. Frequently I would realize I was cuddling my left breast as if to say a last good-bye. On the weekend prior to the surgery, I was given permission to leave the hospital, and Harvey and I drove to Niagara Falls, which neither of us had ever seen. The gaudy, honky-tonk Wonder of the World was filled with people old and young who had come to see the spectacle, and often I found myself looking at some particularly ugly, grotesque, or obnoxious woman and thinking bitterly, enviously, "Why me and not her?" It was not a nice thought to have.

I was so ashamed of myself for having it that I am sure my mind would have blanked it out if it had not been written down at least a dozen times, in different notes. Later, when I began interviewing postmastectomy patients, I found this jealousy was not unique to me; everyone had felt it at one time or another. And everyone had been ashamed too and had never mentioned it, even to husbands, friends, or closer relatives.

The questionnaires and telephone conversations taught me how wrong my ideas had been about other aspects of breast cancer. For example, I had automatically assumed younger women—especially unmarried ones—would be hardest hit psychologically by the loss of a breast. My poll said this was a false assumption. On the other hand, only eight younger women responded, while about thirty older ones did. According to the responses I got, older women who are widowed or divorced suffer far more, and even the older married ones have greater problems adjusting—particularly those whose husbands are going elsewhere for sexual solace.

Of the eight premenopausal unmarried women I interviewed (please remember, a biased sample of well-adjusted women), *none* spoke of any problems with sex after mastectomy. One wrote that—while she was already engaged before the surgery, and her fiancé had not been disturbed by it—she did not believe him and was afraid that he had the "wounded bird syndrome."

"He's the kind who takes in stray kittens and nurses birds with broken wings back to health," she told me. "I thought he was just saying it didn't matter not to hurt me."

She also told me she wondered whether she could get a new man. To test her appeal, she invited an "admirer" to her apartment. Apparently, he was not at all fazed by her single-breasted-ness, and her self-confidence was completely restored.

My first encounter with the special difficulties of a postmeno-pausal widowed or divorced woman came the night of that televi-sion program. "It's easy for you to sit up there in front of a television camera and tell everybody the important thing is that cancer is fatal, and that losing a breast and sex come second," an anonymous caller reprimanded me over the telephone. "You're married, you said the 'baby' of your family was almost sixteen and you had more than a week between the biopsy and the operation to get adjusted to the idea. You're really nobody to talk."

My caller was very angry and was, of course, right. It was easy for me to say what I said five months after the shock of the mastectomy was behind me. But she had more on her mind than the television program.

"I'm sorry if it got you upset—" I tried to apologize.

"I'm not upset. I'm just mad. Are you old enough to remember the movie *King's Row*?"

"I even read the book."

"Do you remember that scene when Ronald Reagan woke up and began screaming to Ann Sheridan, "Where's the rest of me?""

"Well, that's exactly how I felt and exactly what I yelled when I woke up in the recovery room and found myself wrapped tight in bandages," she said. "The doctor had told me all I would have was a Band-Aid and that I didn't even have to cancel a dinner party I had planned for that night."

"He never told you he might have to do a mastectomy?"

"No, absolutely no. Never! The word cancer was never men-tioned. He said it was a cyst and that it ought to come out—that's all."

Poor woman. "What kind of surgery did you have?" I asked her.

"What else? The bad one—the kind that cut all the way into my armpit and left my rib bones sticking through the skin like spikes. That didn't happen to you."

"Are you having trouble with your husband because of it?" I asked gently.

"That bastard!" she spat. "We were separated almost a year before the operation. I called him afterward and asked if he would mail some checks for me and go up to Bowdoin to tell our boy, so he wouldn't have to hear about if first over the telephone. He told me that when the judge gave me custody, he gave me custody, and I'd have to take care of everything myself. He's remarried now, and his new wife is pregnant. Imagine!" She almost moaned with pain. "A fifty-eight-year-old man able to get a twenty-six-year-old wife and starting a whole new family. If the situation was reversed . . . but it wouldn't ever happen."

"I'm sure you'll be able to find somebody—"

"Oh, sure, I'll be able to get somebody else, with a chest like this," she cried. "Who would want to look at me now? If I had it to do over again, I would do what you did—sign the paper only for the biopsy. But if the verdict came back and it was cancer," she said angrily, "I would take my chances."

What could I say? I had had so many advantages. I could not imagine going through the long ordeal without a loving, reassuring husband to hang on to, to have at my side all the time, and, in addition to his emotional support, to do chores like filling out hospital admission forms, getting airplane tickets, and managing general logistics. How had she managed? Now, apparently, she felt alienated from everyone because of the mastectomy. "It really isn't that important how you look if someone loves you, is it?" I said.

Her voice became harder. "Sweetheart," she said evenly, "it's different if you already have someone who loves you. Then it probably doesn't matter. But I'm fifty-five years old and have no one in sight. Getting someone new to love me at my age would have been hard enough." She laughed, almost a cackle. "Look at my ex-husband, getting a woman less than half his age. Have you ever heard of that happening with a woman, unless she's rich or something? I've never been a beauty. Now I'm completely shot." She began to sob and could not finish the conversation. I heard the receiver quietly put back into its cradle.

I cannot adequately convey the psychological trauma mastectomy must be to these women. I could think of little to say to those I spoke with, except that men need a lot of educating about the unimportance of a missing breast. I can only record the problems of these women, so that they will know they are not alone. For—extrapolating from my unscientific sample of the luckier, well-adjusted woman—there must be thousands in this cruel situation.

Young unmarried women were also upset and shaken, but, according to my poll, were third from the top in the degree of severity. However, I did receive only eight responses; such a small number can hardly be typical. There is more trouble smoldering quietly than these examples indicate. With the eight I interviewed, the major complaint was the extent of the surgery and the fact that they were not offered any choice. (All were free of disease, as far as they knew.)

"I probably would not have taken any chances with my life," one twenty-nine-year-old secretary told me. "I'm positive I would have agreed to the mastectomy. I'm not so up-tight about having two breasts that I would have risked dying of cancer." A sharp edge came into her voice. "But I feel I was duped. The surgeon didn't mention even the remote possibility of needing a mastectomy before the biopsy. He told me later that the odds were so much against it, because I was under thirty, he was surprised at the diagnosis himself. But he did a Halsted," she continued, "and never mentioned any other operation. I didn't know there was another kind until the publicity in the newspapers after Betty Ford's mastectomy. The s.o.b. never said he could have saved my muscles." Now she sounded very angry. "Athletics have always been the big thing in my life, ever since I was a little kid," she explained. "And tennis has been sport number one for me. It took me months to get that arm back, and it still isn't as good as it was."

She paused. "After I read about the modified radical Happy Rockefeller had, I called the surgeon and gave him hell. He tricked me, pure and simple. There are no two ways about it."

As I have said, I was surprised to discover that younger married women were not as horrified by the loss of a breast as postmenopausal married women, whose youth and sexual attractiveness have begun to fade (or so they thought). These women are far more vulnerable to psychological problems, because they tend to have emotional troubles at this time of life even without the loss of a breast. Their children may no longer be living at home; husbands may show little concern for their wives. Then the pain and strain of breast cancer and mastectomy are added.

The emotional condition of the older married women seemed to depend on the status of their marriages. If their relationships with their husbands had been rocky—if he had been adventuring around or was a "workaholic" who was never home—losing a breast was a more severe psychological jolt than for women who had good marriages.

"It's just one more thing to keep him away from me," a wealthy fifty-eight-year-old woman told me. While she had no financial worries and was still covered by the security blanket of her husband's name, social status, and reputation, she did not have him. "He's always traveling or working overtime," she complained. "And when he is home, he's upstairs in his office with that briefcase. This awful scar is just another reason for him to want his own bedroom."

Psychiatrists assured me that the mastectomy was not the problem here and seldom is when divorce follows soon after the surgery. "Those marriages were on the skids long before," they agreed. "The mastectomy was only an excuse to get out of a situation that was already bad." Without exception, none of the psychiatrists or other physicians I talked to knew of a sound marriage that had been destroyed because the wife had a mastectomy. Other problems, especially work and other women, had probably already shaken the marriage. To these older wives, losing the breast meant losing any chance they might otherwise have had to reattract their errant husbands.

An interesting sidelight is that none of the young married women I heard from had any worries about their husbands running around with other women. "They're secure in the inherent sexuality of youth itself," a psychiatrist explained. "They have enough sexuality not to fear their men will go away because a piece of themselves had to be removed."

Young women with good marriages seemed to have few problems adapting to the silicone gel in their future. They were primarily worried about having cancer and being incapacitated.

"Who would take care of the kids if I had to go in and out of the hospital for treatments?" one thirty-four-year-old mother of seven asked. "My mother is dead, and my husband's mother can't manage even two of 'em, much less the whole brood. That's my main worry, the kids and dying, not losing a breast."

None of the young married women I interviewed had considered removing only the lump, even for a moment. "I've got four kids to worry about," one explained realistically. "They need a mother, not a second breast."

One young married woman had to have a second mastectomy the year after her first. She told me—though I did not believe her until she explained—that she had been delighted!

"My real ones were so enormous." She laughed. "Before my first mastectomy, I could never wear a store-bought dress from the racks. The top of me was size 44, and the bottom a size 10. I spent my whole adult life in skirts and blouses, except for a couple of things I had custom-tailored."

She grimaced. "I even had to have the blouses altered, because the shoulders of the size 44 reached my elbows. My own sewing ability stops at buttons, and I had to pay a dressmaker to take darts in the shoulders of everything I owned. When I had to buy my first prosthesis, I had trouble finding one big enough to match my right breast. And I had to wear a horrible surgical brassiere, with thick straps that dug into my shoulders.

"Now," she continued, "I'm a perfect 34B—just what I've always wanted to be."

Older women who had never been married seemed to have the least emotional trouble getting used to having only one breast. Their major concern, like that of the young married women, was having a possibly fatal disease. They usually had a large circle of friends, who rallied around to give aid and comfort, and had also maintained close ties with relatives. But all the responses I had, written or telephoned, showed they were terrified that the cancer might not have been stopped.

"Taking the breast off didn't bother me at all," a retired schoolteacher told me. "But I'm sixty-seven, and I've had so many friends, now, go through with the mastectomy and die anyhow. So many of my friends over the years. That's what I am really most frightened of."

Such women have long ago made their adjustments to living alone, and the mastectomy seemed to have little effect on their attitudes, except for the fear of cancer itself. The schoolteacher explained her feelings. "Maybe I'd think differently if I were thirty, or even forty, but at my age the fuss they're calling the breast-cancer controversy makes no sense at all."

Wise woman.

It was very different with the women who were still hoping to find someone to occupy the empty side of their double beds. Suddenly, with the sharp precision of a surgeon's scalpel, they saw their hopes for catching another man slashed away.

All the women who had not known they would have mastectomies complained about the absence of information before they were wheeled into the operating room, although most seemed to have rationalized it by the time I talked to them.

"I was furious with the doctor then and there," one woman told me. "But it would have had to happen anyhow. This way, I got it over with in one operation instead of going through it twice. Now I'm glad I didn't have all that worry and aggravation in advance."

Everyone who had had the Halsted radical mastectomy said she would have chosen the modified radical had she been asked. "I'm just sorry it wasn't invented fourteen years ago," one woman said, smiling. "But I guess that's true with everything in medicine, isn't it?"

Actually, the modified radical mastectomy was "invented" as long ago as 1900, when Cleveland's Dr. George Crile, Sr. and some courageous colleagues challenged Halsted's routine removal of the pectoral muscles. Thirty years later, in England, Mr. David Patey introduced a similar operation. In most countries, the Halsted had virtually been abolished in favor of some kind of modified radical mastectomy by 1974.

As I said earlier, all the women who complained about disfigurement or the loss of a breast were those who had not suffered recurrences or metastases. Such women made up about three-fourths of my poll, and the biopsy, mastectomy, and associated psychological shocks were the main themes of their conversations. The one-fourth who had developed new cancers did not mention the original surgery at all unless I brought it up, and then they were usually vague about the details.

So, in terms of age and marital status, the women who took the mastectomy hardest, were according to my poll, in their fifties or older and were either widowed or divorced. Their desire to ignore the tumor completely, to have only the tumor removed, to have a lumpectomy or partial mastectomy, or to investigate plastic-surgery procedures was greater than I found in any other group I interviewed. But I must repeat that this may be bias of the responses I received.

Second on the list of badly adjusted postmastectomy respondents were the older women whose husbands paid little attention to them, for various reasons (usually the suspected reason was another woman). All but one of these had passed the menopause or were going through it at the time, and all had grown children who no longer needed a mother's care and attention. Most of the children were gone from home entirely; five women still had children at home, commuting to college or working. For this group, finding a cancer in their breasts had been an additional emotional shock at a time when their womanliness and motherliness were at an end.

The third most affected group, my sample indicated, were premenopausal unmarried women. None of the eight responses I received reported any differences in "self-esteem," "self-worth," or "inherent sexuality"—to use the psychiatric jargon. While I would like to believe this is universal, I'm afraid the statistical odds are against it.

Premenopausal married women (most in my poll had young children) were most concerned over dying and leaving their children motherless. As far as their marriages and their husbands' attitudes toward the mastectomy, all replied that the experience had brought them closer together than they had been before. Older women who had never been married were similarly most affected by their fears of the cancer itself, the pain and possible imminent death.

In 1975 I complained about the one-stage biopsy + mastectomy procedure, blaming this terrible surgical habit for much of the psychological damage done to women. Happily, this barbarous custom is being abandoned in favor of the more humane two-stage procedure, and there is no longer any need for me to beat a dying horse to death.

Obviously a major trauma is waking up from the anesthesia and finding the breast gone. While I knew in advance this was going to happen, the utter and absolute totality of the amputation was still a chilling shock. It was (and still is now, I must add) impossible for me even to try to imagine what it must be like for women with no advance knowledge.

In addition to the more widespread use of the two-stage procedure now, the availability of breast reconstruction has helped avoid much of the postsurgical psychological traumas of having a mastectomy. Most medical insurance plans are now covering reconstructive mammoplasty as rehabilitation, and this has probably been the most important factor in its popularity.

Another reason women are having fewer emotional problems is the knowledge that there are options to mastectomy, and those having confirmed diagnoses of breast cancer can usually find a clinical trial or else a private physician who will do less surgery. Doctors are now willing to come out and say, "I don't really know what is the best treatment."

That is quite a change!

None of these were common in 1974, however. Even though women who discover they have breast cancer now and in the future will benefit from the changes, there are still tens of thousands of women in the United States today who are suffering from the emotional damage done in past years. My poll cannot and must not be taken as an accurate summary of the psychological troubles that followed a mastectomy prior to 1979, when the NIH officially endorsed the two-stage procedure. While few of the poorly adjusted women responded, I did receive some replies. One, for example, admitted changing her life style drastically because of the mastectomy. "If these are my last five years," she wisecracked, "I'm entitled to live it up." She had gone on a wild shopping spree and, along with an expensive wardrobe, had bought a fur coat—none of which her family could afford. She had also gone alone on a Caribbean cruise.

"I don't care if I do leave debts behind me," she insisted. "He'll be alive, after I'm in the ground, to work and pay them off. I don't want another woman spending my money later when I'm doing without now."

But she was an exception in her bitterness about her husband and her worries about a possible successor. She was, by the way, referred to me by a psychiatrist, and had already been in treatment when the cancer was discovered.

The major symptoms of disturbance I found in my poll were relatively minor from a psychiatric point of view. Primarily, these were intense bitterness that it had happened at all ("Why me?"), a deep jealousy of women with two healthy breasts, rage at the surgeon for mutilation later found to be unnecessary, and fury about poor follow-up care that resulted in not finding recurrences and metastases until these were far advanced. If these can legitimately be called "disturbances."

By and large, even these were muted, however. Except, of course, for the women with metastatic disease, almost all my respondents had accepted their mastectomies—multilating or not—and had found that the surgery made little difference in their lives. Their main problem was worry about the future. But even here there were rationalization, resignation, and reconciliation. The general philosophy (my own, too, I should add) seemed to be: "You never know when your number's up. I could walk out and get hit by a car in front of my house."

Because I was an insider and had changed many of my own ways, I knew some of the right questions to ask about what changes others had made. (These, by the way, were not on the written questionnaire. I was afraid too many answers to write might mean no response at all from many women.)

"Haven't you found that you have reordered your priorities?" I began. "Isn't it less important now whether the beds are made every day than it was before?"

"Well, when you put it that way, I guess I have changed," one mother of five told me. "I was always after the kids to do this and that, or not do this and that, and now I sort of let it all pass me by. In the end, what difference does it make if they spill juice on the floor or get fingerprints on the wall? The house will be here long after I'm gone."

"Do you feel as if you want to go places and see things now that you might have postponed, even if it means borrowing money?" The answers to this question seemed to be related to the family's standard of living.

"Well, my husband and I did talk about going to Scandinavia someday," one thirty-two-year-old told me. "But we were going to wait till the kids were old enough to really appreciate traveling. Then, after the mastectomy, we decided what the hell. So we packed them up and went last summer. The doctor told me I had six positive nodes, and there is a very good chance I might develop another cancer within the next few years." She laughed. "But we didn't really borrow. We did the whole trip with credit cards."

Women who had no yearning to travel to other countries did admit they were visiting relatives or taking holidays and vacations more frequently.

To my surprise, I discovered that the United States is not the only breast-conscious country in the world. On the basis of my tour abroad, I think Sweden outranks us, and even in the Soviet Union women are very reluctant to lose their breasts, although perhaps for a different reason. The Intourist guides for my group, for example, were young women, and I asked them how they would feel about having a mastectomy. They said their reactions would be not so much sexual as maternal.

"When I was growing up," one told me, "a woman's breasts were a symbol of fertility and motherliness. This is not important in big cities like Moscow and Leningrad, but if I return to my hometown, it would be a real reason for hiding such an operation." She explained that centuries of superstition, folklore, and mythology might tag single-breasted women as freaks in rural areas. Also, she added, cancer itself is highly feared in the countryside as something unnatural, as a disease that might be "catching."

In the oncology institutes of Moscow and Leningrad, I learned that *no* cancer patients were ever told the disease for which they are being treated. The oncologists deleted the word cancer even in our discussions; it was always mammary carcinoma.

"But what do you tell a woman when she has her breast removed nowadays?" I asked. "Even in the country, women must know that breasts are removed only for cancer."

"I do not know what they think," Professor Melnikov, in Leningrad, said. "I know only that in the Soviet Union the word cancer is never mentioned, by doctor, patient, or family. If a woman suspects it is a mammary carcinoma, she will not speak of it."

Since the plaque on the wall of the hospital clearly said INSTITUTE OF ONCOLOGY, I wondered what the patients thought they were there for. On the other hand, I also know how people can block, suppress, repress, and lie to themselves. At Roswell Park,

I had spoken with several patients who hastened to tell me they were not being treated for cancer, that their presence in the hospital was a dreadful mistake. This trick of the human mind may well be the reason the word cancer can so easily be avoided in the Soviet Union.

In Sweden's Karolinska Institute, Dr. Westerberg told me the Breast Clinic had once conducted a psychological experiment to ascertain how Swedish women felt about mastectomy. Dr. Jerzy Einhorn, the chief of the Breast Section, had agreed to the survey, although he was confident it would show sensible Swedish women to be more concerned about the disease than about preserving the organ.

"Dr. Einhorn was shocked," Dr. Westerberg said, "and he said so repeatedly. He was shocked to discover that almost all the women were very much afraid of losing the breast and wished to do whatever possible to preserve it." She laughed. "He was indeed very, very surprised."

Dr. Westerberg explained the procedure. As women came into the clinic, they were asked if they could spare the time to meet with a psychologist and several other women for about an hour a week to discuss their attitudes about the loss of a breast. But the sample, planned to be random and consecutive (the first hundred women who came into the clinic, regardless of age, marital status, and other factors), could not be done as planned. Many worked, had large families, or for other reasons could not participate. So all the women involved in the survey were those who were relatively free of other cares. Nonetheless, Dr. Westerberg feels it was a good enough sampling to give the psychologist an idea of how Swedish women felt about mastectomy.

"As I said, Dr. Einhorn was shocked to learn that almost all the women would do anything to avoid it." A lovely example of Swedish womanhood herself, Dr. Westerberg chuckled again at Dr. Einhorn's astonishment. "As a matter of fact, one of the most difficult cases I can recall was persuading a very attractive woman of about fifty-five or sixty that she should not risk a simple removal of the lump. She was divorced and had a fiancé who would, she was quite certain, leave her if she underwent a mastectomy. Ultimately, I was able to persuade her that life was more important than her breast or the man, but it was very, very difficult to do so." Again, as in my sample, an older unmarried woman was most resistant.

At the Royal Marsden Cancer Hospital in London and the Royal Infirmary in Edinburgh, there was no language barrier, and I was able to talk directly to patients. Four women I interviewed were still bandaged, carrying their drains in little knitting bags. All had known in advance they had cancer, and all were primarily worried about whether the disease had been stopped by the surgery. None was concerned about the lost breast, and all said their husbands had been more tender and attentive since they became ill than they had ever been before in their years of married life.

And that brings us to sex. Apologetically on the written questionnaire, and even more apologetically over the telephone, I had asked if there were any before-and-after differences. Women who had good marriages said the surgery had brought them and their husbands even closer. "It's a subtle change that I can't put into words," one woman explained. "But the difference is for the better. We have never enjoyed each other so much."

One caller confided over the telephone that she was a member of the rare breed whose nipples are so generously endowed with erotic nerve endings that kissing and caressing them can produce an orgasm. "I've gotten so used to that," she laughed, "I'm not sure I'd be able to enjoy sex without it."

"Well, you still have one," I reminded her.

"I know, and as long as I've got it, I'm okay," she said. "But what in the world will I do if I have to have another mastectomy? I think I'd lose my mind."

As for my own psychological feelings after the mastectomy, I seemed to be typical of premenopausal married women with older children. While the idea of leaving them motherless was not as poignant in our case as it was where young children were involved, none of us wants to die without seeing our children into full adulthood, and happy. Many women, including me, would like to be around to baby-sit with their grandchildren.

I confess that I did not let Harvey see the incision immediately. Because I'm a small person and did not have much skin to spare, Dr. Dao had pulled the edges of the cut area very tightly together so that I would not need a skin graft. The immediate postoperative appearance of the incision was a puckered, ugly slit—like a fiery red shirred seam. Even I had trouble looking at it without flinching. In a few months, though, new skin grew, and the repelling wrinkles disappeared. I stopped being shy. But there was no blare of trumpets, like Salomé shedding her seventh wisp of cloth. I was in the tub, and Harvey came in to get something from the medicine cabinet. That was that.

He probably misses my left breast just as I sometimes miss his once thick head of curly hair. When we were first married, I wore a 36D bra, and he broke a comb in his thatch every week. Neither of us is the same as we were thirty years ago.

One woman described her husband's attitude beautifully and eloquently on the questionnaire. "My husband is now, if possible, more tender and loving than he ever was before," she wrote. "Our love life has a brand-new dimension that wasn't there until I had the mastectomy. It's as if he suddenly realized that I was something very precious that he almost—and could still—lose. This feeling of being 'cherished' like something very valuable, a treasure, is what has been added to our love."

Immediately after surgery, I had other problems, although these pale to insignificance in comparison with some I have been told about. Nonetheless, they were (some still are) serious to me. The first one I encountered after coming home, was enduring the doom and gloom of friends and relatives. Many came through the door and immediately burst into tears. Men treated me as if I were a fragile, very delicate piece of rare Meissen porcelain or a vase from the Ming dynasty to be handled with great care. I could not reach for a tissue without having six people jump to get it for me. At first it was funny, then tedious, and finally oppressive.

During the spring, my daughter Lesley (who planned to work every summer after that one) had persuaded me to rent a beach apartment for her, one of her friends, and me for this last free vacation. When I became ill, I called the landlord and explained my predicament. "If you can rent it at this late date, I'd appreciate it," I said. "If you can't, I'll honor the contract." The week after returning from Buffalo, I was finished with the tea and sympathy. Luckily, the apartment had not been rented yet. I called my daughter's friend's mother, extended the invitation to include her, and we packed off for two weeks on an ocean beach. Between sessions of the House Judiciary Committee's impeachment hearings, I began to assemble my notes.

The surgery had had an immediate impact, by the way, on Lesley. A few days after the operation, the same friend's mother had called me in Buffalo. "Lesley doesn't think you're telling her the truth," she said. "She's scared about your having cancer and is sure the reason Harvey hasn't brought her to Buffalo to see you is that things are worse than you and he are saying."

The reason no one except Harvey had come to Buffalo was just money, but as soon as I put down the telephone we decided Lesley had to fly up. We also brought our son Todd from Cambridge (where he had a summer job in a chemistry lab). I had called our older son, Gantt, a rock-and-roll musician then playing in a Denver club, to assure him that the only difference was a little more flat-chestedness. He was twenty-two then, did not frighten easily, and seemed to take it well. Once Lesley and Todd came to

Buffalo, went with us to Niagara Falls, and we had a little time together, both were confident nothing was being withheld from them. They were also reassured by Dr. Dao's explanation of what had been done to their mother and why.

Remembering to include older children in parents' problems at such a time, I found, is important for *their* psychological well-being. Having lost both my parents when I was young, I had sometimes worried that my children would have secret fears of my dying early too. What could I do to reassure them? The only route I could see was to be open and candid and answer every question.

After a week or so at the beach, Lesley got so used to protecting my left arm from bumps and flying Frisbees that it became an automatic reflex. Later, after I had begun the research for this book, I heard her tell Harvey that she was "sick and tired of hearing about breast cancer night and day. I wish she'd finish and get on another subject." What had been a horror word just a few months before had become a subject, like manic-depression, Tay-Sachs disease, and some of my other total-immersion projects.

Both boys were and are, at least outwardly, adjusted to having a mother with breast cancer. Todd called with the latest immunological data on the disease from MIT labs. Gantt, back from Denver, was very matter-of-fact about it. As he put it once, "So when did I ever have a well-balanced mother?"

As for my feelings about still being attractive to other men, it had not occurred to me to wonder about my appeal to anyone other than Harvey. I am not sure if this was because I was sedately married and older, or because I was too busy after my surgery to think about other men. To find out, I would have had to experiment with an admirer, and the idea did not and still does not appeal to me or to Harvey—even for the sake of science. But I have had a couple of experiences since my mastectomy that shook me into thinking my attitude about my desirability might have changed. When I was in Moscow in December 1974, an American businessman, quite attractive and much younger than I, invited me to dinner. I had already eaten with the group I was traveling with, and so I told him no. He tried to change my mind, arguing that our dinner had been meager (it was not) and that I would be hungry again in a few hours. But it had been a long day, and I still had work to do before I could crawl into my fluffy featherbed and go to sleep. "No, thanks," I smiled gratefully. "I've got too much to do."

Then we met again in the elevator and discovered we were both on the seventeenth floor, only two rooms apart. He had told me he had been away from his wife for almost two months, and remarked about the convenience of our locations, but I pretended not to hear. Suddenly, fleetingly, a picture flashed into my mind. What would his reaction be, I giggled inwardly, if I invited him in, whipped off my bra, and confronted him with the still blazing scar where he expected a breast? It was only a momentary thought, leaving as quickly as it came. But it may be significant to a psychiatrist.

One change that I know would be tagged as significant was a strange feeling of being "protected" by the mastectomy.

In Stockholm, I was fast asleep one night when there was a knock on my door. "Who is it?" I asked, completely unafraid.

"Jeemee." I could hear him trying to jiggle the lock to open the door.

"Jimmy who?" I called, still totally unpanicked.

"Italian Jeemee," he said, in heavily accented English.

"I don't know any Italian Jimmy," I answered.

He went away.

In my travels as a free-lance writer I have had a number of similar nocturnal visitors. Apparently it is customary for Jimmys to watch hotel lobbies for single women and call on them later in the night. Always before I had been petrified, but not this time! Again, the same thought had flown across my mind. Suppose I had opened the door and pulled off my long, baggy thermal nightgown? What would his reaction have been? Would he have fainted? Would he have screamed with shock and run away?

Back in those early postmastectomy years I worried that all this meant I no longer considered myself worthy of seduction. Quite honestly, I didn't know. I only knew there was some difference in the way I reacted. None of the women I interviewed mentioned similar feelings of being "protected" from unsolicited ardor, by the way. On the other hand, I didn't ask.

I hasten to add that I no longer feel at all "protected" from lecherous lobby-lurking Jimmys and am just as fearful of being raped as most women are. Thinking back, I do not remember when the change began; it probably happened gradually. But suddenly, the lost breast just stopped mattering. If I had not written *Breast Cancer* and become a "professional patient," I would hardly ever think of the disease anymore, except for continuing to have frequent examinations in Buffalo. As it is, I deal with breast cancer every day as the director of the Advisory Center, so it is impossible to imagine what life would be like otherwise.

More than the healing of emotional wounds by time, I think the reconstructive surgery that put a breast on my bony ribs had the most profound impact on my forgetting I even had a mastectomy. True, it is only a mound under the left pectoral muscle, a mound with no nipple, a mound that does not look like my other breast at all. But at my age and stage of life, I spend little time in the nude, and the differences between the two are not visible even in a brief bra. To me, the most important result was the return of my cleavage (such as it ever was), although Dr. Teunis, the plastic surgeon who did the operation, still wants to top the mound off with a nipple made by splitting the remaining one.

"I feel like I've fixed a car and left off one of the headlights," he jokes.

"I just don't want to be cut again," I tell him, "unless I absolutely have to."

So far my feeling is still that it does not seem important enough to send me back to a surgeon's scalpel.

It is difficult for a staid, married and middle-aged woman to know whether or not she is still attractive to other men. It was a shock to learn, years ago, that when I walk along a street with Lesley, men's eyes turn for her, not for me. This phenomenon began (although I did not really accept it) when she was in her early teens and has continued onto this very day. Obviously, the men with the turning eyes do not know I have only a paltry mound where a high, firm breast once rested.

When Lesley is not around, however, I feel just as attractive and appealing to men as any woman old enough to be a grandmother is entitled to feel. When the Center finally moved from my house into a real office on May 4, 1981, a mastectomee volunteer, Mattie Boker, and I flirted shamelessly with the building's handsome agent to get extra parking spaces for her and Dorothy Johnston, the Center's staff director since 1975. After batting our eyes and using every other feminine wile we could muster to wheedle the precious bumper-stickers from him, we stopped and laughed.

"Do you think anybody would believe this," I asked, "two women with missing breasts trying to flirt parking places out of a man?"

Neither of us had even thought about our "lost sexuality." Neither did Glen Gaskins, apparently. We got the parking stickers.

Of course, I know that thousands of women do not feel as Mattie and I did. As a matter of fact, from my 130 initial interviews, I discovered that my experience was not typical from the very beginning. For example, because I have been a medical writer for a long time, I can understand doctors' jargon and can read "the literature" without its being simplified in the popular press. Also, I had the advantage of being ten minutes away from two of the finest medical libraries in the country—the National Library of Medicine and the library of the National Institutes of Health. Most women do not have either piece of good luck. They must rely on their doctors to explain. The word most of my respondents used to describe their feeling was "helpless." One said she "suddenly became a shivering bit of jello who followed my surgeon like a toddler following mommy on the first day of nursery school." And, of course, I knew in advance that I would have a mastectomy. Only one of the women in my poll was prepared for the shock in advance.

The most important result of my "poll," in my opinion, was the pitifully few women who bothered to respond to it at all. A report published in April 1975 by the NCI said there were then about 677,000 women living in the United States with a known history of one or two mastectomies. Yet the only documented number of cases I could find at the time I was writing *Breast Cancer* was 300,000 to 350,000. Where were the missing statistics? Were they suffering out there—secretly and silently? More current NCI data show that the number is now about 1,000,000, but there is no way to know for sure. Most of them may be hiding in closets.

In 1974, no one seemed to care much about such women. In a paper published in the January 1975 issue of the *American Journal of Psychiatry,* Michael J. Asken wrote about the "Psychoemotional Aspects of Mastectomy." At the end, there were only twenty-two references in his bibliography. Asken's report gave a brief glimmer of what went on in the minds of the "unreachable" women I just described. According to his research, only a few thought in terms of having a potentially fatal disease. "While mastectomy performs a gratifying service by saving a woman's life," he wrote, "her appreciation is muted by the price she must pay for that service—the loss of a breast and permanent disfigurement. Within the value system of American society, that price is a considerable one."

Asken referred to "mastectomized women" and called their anxiety and depression "psychological morbidity." On his anxiety scale, their fear of death ranked below "concern over sexual desirability, interpersonal and sexual relations. And, if the woman was married, "dangers to her marriage." She felt herself to be "untouchable," Asken said, and "fears she herself did something at some time in her life to cause the cancer to develop."

Looking for someone or something to blame is not confined to women in psychiatric journals. I have spent many an hour wondering what I did or took or was exposed to that might have caused my cancer. Before I finally settled on diethylstilbestrol, the suspects ranged from a breast abscess to our microwave oven to the color television set. One of the psychiatrists I interviewed told me his patients usually blamed people, *not* things. Most often, they blamed themselves and felt the cancer was some kind of divine retribution for past sins—especially sexual sins like masturbation, promiscuity, extramarital affairs, or abortions. Other disturbed patients blamed their husband, children, or their parents. All things considered, I guess I am in relatively good mental health for blaming DES.

Times have changed.

As I said in Chapter 9, where I discussed the psychological problems women endure before breast cancer is diagnosed, I think health professionals may now be paying too much attention to the problems of "coping" with a lost breast. The two-stage procedure and breast reconstruction, combined with a more enlightened public attitude about single- or no-breasted women, have changed the climate from the one that prevailed before the mid-1970s. All of these factors together have considerably reduced the emotional trauma of having a mastectomy.

There are, however, post-treatment psychological problems today that did not exist before. For example, many women are now being treated by some kind of segmental surgery, with or without irradiation of the breast, and they have completely different worries from those encountered in the past. They know they opted for a form of treatment not yet "proven" to be as good as amputation. True, they have the comfort of hearing that data showing the effectiveness of these procedures are being gathered by both clinical trials and by doctors who do them routinely outside of randomized studies. But still, the dread that they may have played "Russian Roulette" frequently lurks in the backs of these patients' minds.

There are other worries that plague women who chose to have less than a mastectomy. Those who rejected radiation because they feared exposure to a potential carcinogen, nonetheless wonder if there were other foci hidden in the breast, foci the X-rays would have destroyed . . . if only they had "listened to the doctor." At the other end of this spectrum, patients who received the prescribed five or six weeks of high-dose radiation after partial surgery often suffer whenever the media play up a radiation disaster of some kind.

"When Three Mile Island was all over the newspapers and

television," one woman told me, "and reporters kept talking about the dangers of 'low dose leaks,' I was scared to death. All I could think about was the damage those X-ray treatments might have done to me."

At the time TMI was banner-headlined, she was about to reach the magic five-year mark and was planning to celebrate the occasion by wearing a dress with a neckline that plunged almost to her navel.

"I wore something with a high collar instead," she said sadly. "My mother and sister have both had mastectomies and always kept telling me I was committing suicide because of vanity. With all that stuff in the news about radiation, the last thing I wanted to do was call attention to having both of my breasts."

She told me her sister acted as if her mastectomy scar was a "red badge of courage."

"Much as I love her, I can't stand having her act so brave and heroic—as if having her breast cut off had automatically turned her into some kind of saint," she explained. "Sometimes I think women who had bad radicals are doing a lot to keep doctors from changing. How can a surgeon who cut a woman's muscles out last week explain that he doesn't have to do that anymore?"

So many women who had limited surgery decades ago have sworn me to secrecy that I often think counting these long-term survivors would probably affect the "statistically significant" data scientists are looking for. But these women, like those represented in Michael Asken's paper, are also hiding in closets—but for a different reason.

"I just got so damned sick and tired of having people tell me how stupid and vain I was," a friend whose cancer was treated only by lumpectomy in 1959 told me, "that I stopped telling anyone about it." She paused. "I've really forgotten all about that operation by now; it's been so long ago. Maybe I was just lucky."

Of course, she will never know, just as I (and hundreds of thousands of other mastectomees) will never know if another cancer would have grown in the breast that was removed.

But the problem now is "coping with cancer"—all aspects of living many years with a potentially fatal disease—not coping with the loss of a breast. In the past, breast-cancer experts were primarily concerned with simply prolonging life, somehow or another. They have come a long way since this was their only concern. Women are living longer—thanks to anticancer agents that keep the disease under control *without* cure. And cancer experts now accept the fact that "quality of life" is almost as important as "quantity of life."

In addition to the unique emotional problems of women who

had partial surgery of one kind or another (with or without irradiation of the preserved breast), women who must receive some kind of adjuvant therapy after surgery, because the disease was found in their axillary lymph nodes, have others. Of course, they suffer from knowing they have cancer and are at higher risk of dying from it, and they may also have lost a breast. (Women having partial surgery must also be given adjuvant therapy of some kind if positive nodes are found after an axillary sampling or complete dissection.) But now they may have to face the various side effects of cytotoxic drugs.

The problems of adjuvant therapy's side-effects could just as easily have been included in Chapter 14, where I discuss coping with the physical aspects of breast-cancer treatment. However, calls and letters to the BCAC have convinced me that these particular problems are more serious because of their traumatic emotional impact than because of any physical suffering they may cause. Alopecia (jargon for hair-loss) is such an example. Besides their primary concern with damage to the immune system, oncologists are now more and more interested in helping women (indeed, all cancer patients receiving chemotherapy) to avoid or to lessen side effects that are not actually life-threatening.

"As doctors," one explained to me, "we've got to be concerned with the whole patient—not just with his or her platelets and white-cell counts. If a breast-cancer patient's morale drops to zero because she's bald and won't go out of the house, that's as important a medical problem as immune suppression is."

One result of oncologists' concern with quality of life has been research into ways to prevent drugs from affecting hair follicles. At the Tuscon Cancer Center, studies proved that chilling the scalp with ice for about twenty minutes before giving chemotherapy often prevents hair loss entirely. Many patients do lose some hair but not enough to need wigs (with the help of clever hairdressers). Several commercial "chemocaps" are now on the market, but, before investing in one, it is probably a good idea to find out whether or not the scalp-chilling will help. This can be done easily by improvising a turban made from plastic bags, then filling it with ice.

However, stunning wigs are available nowadays, and (with the help of good toupée adhesive) only a women's oncologist needs to know. In some cities, I have been told, groups like the ACS' Reach to Recovery, the YWCA's Encore, and informal self-help groups formed by breast-cancer patients have set up "wig banks." This permits women to change their coiffeurs just as easily and often as if they were visiting their favorite beauty shops again.

Another common side effect of adjuvant therapy is nausea and vomiting, a problem that may be helped by prochlorperazine (the most popular product is trade-named Compazine). Women should know, however, that this is primarily a drug used for disorders of the central nervous system, and the Physicians' Desk Reference lists dozens of possible side effects that may be worse than the nausea and vomiting. Above all, the PDR stresses that the substance not be used if there is evidence of immune suppression. Of course, oncologists would be aware of these contraindications when prescribing this drug. I know of many cases, however, where women share useful ideas about this, that or the other—including drugs—without even telling their oncologists. For this reason, I want to stress the possibility that what may be harmless and helpful for one woman could very well be dangerous to another. As it is with any medications, drugs involved in cancer treatment should not be swapped.

In early 1981, marijuana (also known as "grass" or "pot") was approved by the Food & Drug Administration for use by cancer patients whose nausea and vomiting are not stopped by any other means. The approval finally ended years of battling between the NCI and the FDA for legalization of THC (tetrahydrocannabinol—the component of marijuana that prevents these problems) in tablet form for cancer patients. No, the marijuana ingredient is not available from the corner drugstore; it must be dispensed only by oncologists administering chemotherapy. Curiously, older patients, conditioned to thinking of marijuana as evil as well as illegal, are often not helped by the pills. But, according to reports, young people are. As experienced (and unconditioned) pot-smokers grow older and reach the ages when adult cancers strike, this situation will probably change, and more patients will be helped.

To return to my discussion of only breast cancer, every woman reacts differently to the drugs, estrogens, anti-estrogens, and other hormones used to treat this disease—either as adjuvant or for a recurrence. I have, by now, spoken to and received letters from thousands of women being given various regimens. Most do complain of varying degrees of baldness, nausea, vomiting, diarrhea, and stomatitis (soreness of the membranes in the mouth), often even if only two substances are used. And if one of them is vincristine, it can also make it difficult for women to walk normally; they may have tremors, dizziness, double vision, or other neurological problems. Most premenopausal women stop having their menstrual periods, and often they do not return when the therapy is ended.

On the other hand, I have also heard from many women who

have been zapped with five, six, or even seven cytotoxic agents yet have neither missed one period, lost a single hair, nor been nauseous for a moment. Oncologists may be interested in knowing that such women receiving the drugs as adjuvant therapy—where there are no symptoms that can be seen or measured by current technologies—suffer from a chronic fear that the absence of any side effects means the drugs are not working.

One woman who falls into this category lives only a local telephone call away from me, and I hear from her often.

"Damn it!" she once cried, after her visit to the Bethesda Naval Hospital where she was being treated. "Everyone else in that clinic was wearing a wig or a turban and kept telling me how much weight she had lost because she had been so sick. And there I sat, fat and hairy, listening to them. I'm sure this stuff isn't doing me any good. Otherwise I'd be bald and vomiting too."

She had had twenty-three positive axillary nodes and was fifty-six years old at the time of her mastectomy in late 1979. Her doctors at Bethesda Naval had not wanted to give her any adjuvant chemotherapy at all, because they accepted the data that showed it was of little or no benefit for postmenopausal women.

"I raised all kinds of hell," she told me, "because I thought they were taking away any chance I had to beat this thing. I'm no dummy. I knew that having so much cancer in my nodes meant the odds that I'd live five years were zilch."

The Navy doctors had told her about the side effects she would encounter, side effects that would probably make her suffer for nothing.

"Can you imagine the nerve of those guys? Just saying no and not even wanting to let me try to see if I did 'suffer'," she asked. "I just insisted that I wanted everything they had, and I got my way. After all, my husband's not an admiral for nothing."

So her doctors had relented and prescribed Cytoxan, Methotrexate, 5-Flourourocil, vincristine, and prednisone. Because her tumor was strongly estrogen-dependent, they added tamoxifen as well.

Eighteen months later, they stopped the treatment. She was still free of disease—the only way to "test" any adjuvant regimen—and throughout the entire time, she had not experienced even one of the drugs' usual toxicities.

"That's why I'm still so scared," she told me frequently. "I'd feel a heck of a lot more confident about my future if I had been a little sick."

As I explained in Chapter 11, where I discussed adjuvant therapy, data from many trials have been published since 1979.

These studies show that older women do benefit from cytotoxic drugs after all—if enough agents are given, if the doses are high enough and if the treatment is given long enough. At the annual meeting of the American Society of Clinical Oncology (ASCO) held in Washington, D.C. in May 1981, however, it was clear that the matter was still controversial.

What does knowing this do to the emotions of the majority of women who *do* suffer from the drugs' many toxicities? When this meeting was held, the media reported the differences of opinion in detail, and I was deluged with calls and letters from women whose quality-of-life was being wrecked by cytotoxic chemotherapy. Certainly, the data regarding drugs' effectiveness for premenopausal women was consistently dramatic enough so I could honestly recommend they continue the prescribed therapy, in spite of the many side effects.

But the data were not so clear-cut for postmenopausal women, especially for those whose cancers had been strongly estrogen-dependent. Nor was there agreement about what to do for younger women who were estrogen-dependent.

A few days after the Breast Cancer Advisory Center opened its doors in Rockville, Maryland, a 46-year-old woman in this situation called for help.

"I had both breasts taken off three years ago, and the surgeon told me I was Stage IV, that it was already in my bones, and I couldn't live for more than two years. But he took out my ovaries and put me on Cytoxan, 5-FU and tamoxifen anyhow, because he felt like he couldn't just let me die without doing something."

She told me she had had "every side effect in the book," but had managed to go through eighteen months of treatment, "vomiting all the way."

"But I was alive after the two years they gave me," she said, "so I figured it had been worth it. The cancer in my bones never went away, but it never got worse either."

The reason for her call was that a liver scan done that morning had shown metastatic spots, and her oncologist wanted to put her on five drugs plus the anti-estrogen, tamoxifen.

"I had read all the stuff in the papers about the arguments the experts are having," she told me, "and I told him I knew. I reminded him he had told me I was very estrogen-dependent and that maybe it had been taking out my ovaries and the tamoxifen that put me into remission, and not the chemo. He came right out and told me those miserable drugs might not have anything to do with keeping me alive. But he said he wasn't sure and didn't want to take any chances."

Having gone through so much hell from only a two-drug regimen plus tamoxifen, my caller did not want to go through it again, especially with three more added, if she did not have to.

"Isn't there some way to know what helped me without all this trial-and-error business?" she pleaded.

Unfortunately, there is no other way. Breast-cancer experts are struggling with the same problems in chemotherapy as they are with those in learning how much surgery is "enough."

Hundreds of clinical trials are going on now all over the world. Different combinations of anticancer agents, in different dosages, using different schedules (including day vs. night) and different methods of administration are being tried. Just as one example of the current confusion, I will point out that Dr. James Holland believes in a five-drug combination; Dr. Gianni Bonadonna believes three are sufficient; Dr. Bernard Fisher, in two. I might mention that Dr. Thomas Dao believes *no* cytotoxic drugs are necessary, if the woman's tumor was estrogen-dependent.

All are experts; all have different opinions. Until those clinical trials are completed so that ten years of survival rates can be analyzed, no one will know. Until then, we women will have to make decisions based on faith.

Having to make these vital decisions with only faith as a guide is, as far as I am concerned, one of the most stressful emotional traumas women must endure after any surgical treatment for breast cancer. Certainly, they put worries about body-image, femininity, and sexuality into their proper perspective.

Stress.

Will my caller's cancer be worsened by the emotional stress she is undergoing because she must make a potentially lifesaving (or lifelosing) decision about her future treatment?

This is another one of the great unknowns. As I explained in Chapters 2 and 5, the hypothalamus is the part of the brain that masterminds emotions like anger, fear, and sexual drive. It also controls the production of the hormones linked with the development of breast cancer.

In Leningrad in 1974, I had interviewed Professor V. M. Dilman, an endocrinologist, who had used L-Dopa (L-3, 4 dihydroxyphenylalanine)—a medication used to control Parkinson's disease—to treat advanced breast cancer. He had also used an anti-epileptic medication, Dilantin. Although there had been no remissions as a result of using these drugs, they had relieved pain and reduced the size of the tumors. The professor told me he thought the reason was the drugs' effects in inhibiting the secretion of prolactin, the female hormone that is to a cancer cell what gasoline is to a fire, if estrogens are also present.

If neurological drugs should be effective agents against breast cancer, perhaps there is a psycho-physiological link somewhere, a link that is yet another factor in the development of this disease.

There has been much publicity about the possible role of the emotions—especially of stress—in not only the cause, but also in the prevention and even the cure of breast cancer. There are even some epidemiological surveys showing that women with various psychiatric problems appear to have higher incidences of the disease than other women do. (Of course, it can be argued that this "high-risk factor" is more related to having enough money to consult psychiatrists than it is to being clinically neurotic or psychotic.)

Until recently, however, epidemiological studies have been the only way to search for a possible link between emotional factors and breast cancer, because the technological know-how was not available to do anything else. Now there are some techniques for evaluating "stress" and "psychiatric disorders" objectively. Certain hormones have been discovered within the central nervous system, and these can be measured to see if an excess or deficiency may be indicators or "markers" of breast cancer, as well as of emotional problems. But such tests are still too preliminary and still too difficult and expensive to even consider for routine use. It is part of The Future.

In the meantime, there are health professionals of one discipline or another who are advocating various "stress reducing" programs for cancer patients. Certainly, anything—yoga, transcendental meditation, hypnosis, biofeedback, imaging, visualization, etc.—that can help a cancer patient cope with the problems caused by the disease itself is valuable. There may also be some benefit in programs designed to prevent a recurrence of the disease . . . so long as the stress-reduction is done in addition to and *not instead of* prescribed therapy. The problem that often arises is that patients are convinced they should substitute some kind of psychotherapy for recommended surgical, radiation, or medical treatment.

Like prayer, any emotional therapy may help cancer patients overcome some of the psychological problems of breast cancer. But any woman who relies on any of them for cure is risking her life.

16

Male Chauvinism, Sex, and Breast-Cancer Politics

There is a patron saint of breasts. She is Saint Agatha, an early Christian martyr. Born in third-century Italy, when the Christians were still being persecuted by the Romans, she was so beautiful, according to legend, that Quintianus, the pagan governor of Sicily, fell madly in love with her. The only way he could manage to meet the young beauty was to have her arrested and brought to him for trial. The charge was her religious beliefs.

Quintianus made it quite clear that the case would be dropped if Agatha let him make love to her. However, she had no use for a man who felt the way Quintianus did about her God. She refused. Unable to get Agatha to submit, the governor found her guilty and sentenced her to a brothel. A term in the House of Aphrodisia (named for a "wicked woman of unsavory fame and wanton reputation") was supposed to convince the young virgin that she should mend her ways and give up not only her church but also her chastity. Somehow, Agatha was able to keep both, even after a month at Aphrodisia, and when Quintianus called back to see if she had changed her mind, he found her still "pure and undefiled."

Hell hath no fury like a man scorned. Agatha was tortured mercilessly, and several harrowing versions exist of how Quintianus took his revenge for her rejection of him. According to some records, he ordered that she "be bound to a pillar and her breasts be torn off with iron shears." Another description tells how Agatha was stretched on a rack and red-hot iron plates were put on her body. Then her breasts were ripped off.

Breasts were so important that Agatha's reward for her martyrdom was their miraculous restoration. Saint Agatha's ordeal has been immortalized by artists, Anthony Van Dyke among them, through the centuries since, and poems have been written about her suffering. Even in Sicily, over a millennium ago, breasts were a very important part of the female anatomy, and having them hacked off as the price necessary to keep one's faith was a good reason for sainthood and divine intervention. Agatha's story floated as far north as Scandinavia, where February 5 is Saint Agatha's Day, as it is in the calendar of the Book of Common Prayer. Hundreds of thousands of women pray to her if their breasts are too small, too large, or too pendulous, do not produce milk or develop disease.

Breast consciousness is a universal obsession, which probably began with Adam and Eve in Eden. But why? Why did Atossa hide her breast tumor from her husband 700 long years before Saint Agatha? Could she have been afraid that King Darius would find himself another wife? A mistress? When a modern woman discovers a lump, does she delay in seeing a doctor for the same reason?

Whether we liberated women admit it or not, fear of not catching a man or fear of losing one probably is the main reason we are so "obsessed" with keeping our breasts, even when doing so could be fatal.

In his book *Early Detection,* Dr. Philip Strax wrote:

> We live in a breast-oriented society. To the average woman, her breast is the badge of femininity, an important part of her allurement to charm her male. To the man, the breast is a source of excitement and erotic stimulation. It has become a bridge between male and female and is used as a reward to be flaunted before the eyes of the male in the female's attempt to attract him. This emphasis on the breast as a sex symbol begins in adolescence and apparently persists throughout life.

Dr. Strax supports this opinion with some "typical incidents" he encountered in the course of a day as a physician.

> "I'm a school teacher," said an attractive 45-year-old woman. "I first noticed this lump in my left breast 2½ years ago. At first, I thought it would just go away. It didn't hurt or bother me in any way. Then as I watched it get bigger and produce changes in the skin, I thought it was probably serious. I felt strongly about breast surgery and the fear of losing my breast. I simply couldn't bring myself to see a physician. I even wear a bra at night to hide the condition from my husband."

A twentieth-century Atossa. Another conversation between doctor and patient:

Mrs. K. lowered her eyes, clasped her hands, and began shyly. "My husband likes to manipulate my breasts as part of our love-making. Sometimes he's rather vigorous and once my breast was black and blue. I've heard that an injury can lead to cancer. Is that true? I've been worrying about our relationship."

Dr. Strax says that the "common thread in all these episodes is the tremendous preoccupation with the female breast that has been developing in the past 30 years. . . . Billboards, movie marquees, newspaper ads, and magazine photos all stress the female breast as the sex symbol of our age."

A successful movie must show a close-up of a woman's breast with the hero looking at it admiringly. Topless waitresses, dancers, and actresses have become a hallmark of our society. The younger female is being stampeded into a bra-less generation. Designers vie with each other in attempting to emphasize the bosom with low-cut or transparent blouses. . . .

This elevation of the female breast as an important sex attribute has brought with it a greater apprehension and anxiety about breast conditions . . . and the totally erroneous idea that has been spreading among many women that the loss of a breast is equivalent to loss of sexual attraction or prowess or both.

But, Dr. Strax, who is creating all this apprehension over being sexy and alluring?

Men. Entrepreneurs of machismo like Hugh Hefner and Bob Guccione, that's who!

When I discussed my opinion with a young man, he sneered. "What are you talking about, Rose? The girls do it to us. From the time I was in seventh grade, when only a couple of the girls in my class had anything, they were always sticking them out and practically shoving them in our faces. You've got it all wrong," this budding MCP insisted. "It's not the males who do it to the females. It's the girls who make breasts a sex symbol, not the boys."

"I bet you were sneaking *Playboy* centerfolds into your room long before you were in seventh grade," I said.

"Well, maybe I was," he admitted. "But the girls were the ones who started it."

"How many girls have anything before they're twelve?" I snapped.

He looked down at his hands, as if he were trying to count the number of chesty girls in his elementary-school class. Sheepishly, he conceded there were none. "I guess I didn't know any."

Having two boys and a girl and having watched their progress through early childhood, adolescence, and now young adulthood, I feel qualified to say that by the time a girl is old enough to have anything to put into a training bra, little boys have had two or three years to teach her the importance of those small eruptions on her chest.

It does not take much time or effort; it almost seems to be instinctive. But learning experts know that breast consciousness is definitely nurture, not nature. Either way, our culture certainly considers breast loss a sexual deficiency of some dire kind.

Several years ago, one of the mathematicians who works with Harvey lost the tip of one of her middle fingers in a garbage disposal. For months afterward, she worked tirelessly to retrain her other fingers to punch the buttons of the calculating machine she used all day on her job.

"I'm not having as much trouble after my surgery as you did after you lost that little piece of your finger," I quipped, when she offered her condolences at an office picnic. "I'd be in the same bad shape as you were if I had lost a part of my finger instead of a breast." We both laughed.

"Yeah," she said. "I never thought of that. You can't hardly do much typing with a breast."

Even though her loss was actually more handicapping than mine, no one ever asked her if she still felt "attractive and appealing"; nor did anyone ever wonder whether she might lose her husband because a piece of her body had been lost.

Dr. Strax made much ado about the influence of the media—magazines, book jackets, movie billboards, et cetera, *ad nauseam*. I agreed. He set the time frame of such media influence within the past thirty years, only dating back to the time when the "boyish" figure went out of style. I do not know about this. I doubt the obsession is so recent. What about the buxom ladies who graced the *Police Gazette* in the 1890s, Lillian Russell, or those cruel girdles designed to pull in the stomachs and push out the chests of our great-grandmothers?

Men dominated the media then and still dominate them today. Obviously, they believed then and as they do now that emphasizing the breast is good for business.

Even now, with the Equal Rights Amendment, the Equal Employment Opportunities Commission, women's liberation, and the urgent rush to hire women, there is still only a handful of them in the policy-making echelons of all the media. The National

Broadcasting Company, for example, was brought before the
EEOC because it had no women in the top executive levels. In
advertising, where most of the sexy-breasted brouhaha is born
and nourished, only a faint sprinkling of women is found in the
major jobs; when a Mary Wells Lawrence reaches the top, it is so
noteworthy that the achievement merits stories in national magazines.

But merely having a woman in a top advertising job or putting
one in charge of a national magazine does not necessarily make
the difference it should. Look at the exploitation of breastiness in
the advertisements in *Cosmopolitan,* edited by Helen Gurley
Brown, a major source of journalistic wisdom on how women can
win in a world of men.

Dr. Strax is right. The media have made breasts into the ultimate erotic symbol, to men and to women too. The media were
responsible for the long hours my sons spent discussing who was
32A or 34B and—wonder of wonders!—the fifteen-year-old who
had a 40D. The media are also the main reason my daughter and
her girl friends, at the age of twelve or thirteen, stood before their
mirrors trying to make the bumps in their training bras larger with
the help of cotton balls, Kleenex, or ripped nylons (those worked
best, by the way).

Yes, Dr. Strax, you are absolutely right. You men have done an
appalling thing to us with *your* billboards, *your* marquees, *your*
centerfolds, *your* advertisements. Every time a man leaves an
extra-large tip to a topless waitress or pays to see a Blaze Starr or
a Racquel Welch, a woman is made to believe she must have two,
preferably large, breasts, no matter what the cost—even death.

Girls and women do not want breasts so they can show them off
to other girls and women.

Male influence has likewise affected the search for treatments
and cures of breast cancer. It is curious that those early Egyptian
medical papyri gave instructions for treating breast tumors only
in men. Today, only about one percent of all breast cancer attacks
males, and many of its victims are older men who develop it from
taking estrogens for prostatic cancer. Is it possible that breast
cancer was a more masculine disease in the days of the pharaohs?
Or is it more probable that not as much medical effort was spent
on treating women's ailments?

Although a lot of money and attention is now devoted to breast
cancer, its treatment is still influenced by male opinions and
masculine attitudes. In the United States, the American College
of Surgeons had—until the past few years—a female membership

of only three percent. In the past, all medical schools had strict quotas governing the admission of women, and those who did succeed in overcoming the discriminatory obstacles, often became physicians who could easily be "slapped down" by their male colleagues. In breast-cancer treatment, for example, the pioneering work done in Canada and the United States to preserve women's breasts by using irradiation instead of the knife was done by two women, Drs. Vera Peters of the Princess Margaret Hospital in Toronto and Eleanor Montague in Houston. In spite of their successful data, being females in a male-dominated profession resulted in having their work overshadowed by men who are getting the credit they deserve. It will be interesting to see if this kind of "inferiority complex" will affect today's generation of women M.D.s.

I should not be using the past tense here. Although anti-discrimination laws have banned admission quotas, most medical schools and hospitals still have rigid and inflexible rules demanding that women students, interns, and residents be "on call" at all hours of the day and night, rules that do not permit maternity leaves and make no exceptions for women to care for sick children or absent babysitters. Such rules, while not legally discriminatory, are nonetheless, obstacles that keep many capable women out of medicine.

What does the small number of women doctors have to do with breast cancer? I think the number of women involved in treating the disease in the United States—especially in the surgical treatment—makes an enormous difference in what is being done.

Of course, there is no way to prove a negative, no way to prove that the small number of women in medicine here is related to the small amount of progress made over the last century. But I can not help but compare Professor Sviatukhina's work in Moscow, where she has been doing partial mastectomies, with the work of Professor Melnikov in Leningrad, who swears by the Halsted radical mastectomy. Breast-cancer staffs that include many women are generally more interested in and sympathetic to saving as much of the breast as possible. Men just do not understand the importance of that. A search through the medical literature shows that many more women scientists are involved in looking for alternatives to mastectomy than would be expected from the small number of them in the medical profession. Many dedicated male doctors would also like to do away with mastectomies of all kinds, of course, but where there are more women, there invariably seems to be a greater effort to do less chopping and more preserving.

No, I cannot prove that the absence of women doctors has caused the lag in progress in the surgical treatment of breast cancer in the United States. But I cannot accept it as mere coincidence either.

And nowhere are women doctors as sorely missed as in the presurgical period. Premastectomy sympathy and understanding from a woman surgeon are seldom available. Afterward, under the care of male surgeons, women were left almost entirely on their own until Terese Lasser, a mastectomee herself, began the Reach to Recovery program in 1952, a program which is now under the aegis of the American Cancer Society.

When *Breast Cancer* was written at the end of 1974, I wrote that in spite of its sponsorship of Reach to Recovery, the ACS was dominated by men. By the time the first edition of *Why Me?* was published in 1977, I was able to add more women to the Society's top-level professional roster. Now, I am delighted to write that Dr. Diane J. Fink was named to be the vice president of the ACS' Division of Service and Rehabilitation, effective June 15, 1981. The first director of the NCI's Division of Cancer Control and Rehabilitation (DCCR), Dr. Fink subsequently was appointed to be the NCI's representative on the NIH's OMAR Committee. This acronym refers to the Office for the Medical Applications of Research, and she was responsible for helping deliver new procedures and technologies from the NCI out to the public as quickly as they were proven to be safe and effective.

Having known Dr. Fink's interests during the years since my involvement with the NCI, I am confident she will be influential in initiating new and valuable programs and in abolishing archaic ACS traditions. I am particularly anxious to see the American Cancer Society begin to move with the times and abandon its longstanding philosophy that all medical information must reach patients directly from their physicians and not through organizations like the Breast Cancer Advisory Center or other health groups. This would be of particular importance to women concerned about breast cancer, because no busy doctor has the time (or, sometimes, the inclination) to explain all the options and alternatives available to treat this disease.

I have also heard a rumor that Dr. Jimmie Holland, a woman oncological psychiatrist especially interested in pretreatment counseling, may also be working with the American Cancer Society. Until now, the ACS has not considered it appropriate to help women cope with breast-cancer problems until surgery (a mastectomy, as a rule) has already been performed. Then, and only if the surgeon grants permission, a Reach to Recovery volunteer visits a patient in the hospital to give her a temporary prosthesis, teach her arm-building exercises, and give her lists of stores where lingerie, bathing suits, and other suitable clothing may be bought. With Drs. Fink and Holland involved in ACS business, I believe this anachronism will not be allowed to continue.

I use the word anachronism, because the letters M.D. no longer stand for Mystical Deity in the minds of most women today. It is ridiculous for the Society to continue to act as if we are living in a vacuum surrounded only with information doctors dispense as they see fit. Newspapers, magazines, television, and radio have educated us about breast-cancer treatments and the unknowns and controversies surrounding them. While menfolk may still be timid and trusting about their medical/surgical problems, we women want to know. What's more, we want to have at least a tip of our fingers in deciding our own destinies. Current ACS standards prohibit giving women (or anyone for that matter) anything other than predigested information that has been approved by a board of physicians. Giving referrals to breast-cancer specialists is an absolute no-no. (Some divisions, chapters, and units around the country "cheat" and do not adhere to this national policy. These are more liberal in giving any assistance they can—including referrals to breast-cancer specialists.)

On the home front, husbands and/or lovers can and should give their women maximum emotional support in the critical weeks after surgery.

While some women may be eager to resume love-making, most of those who have had some kind of radical mastectomy will be too sore even to think about it for weeks. It may seem too obvious to say, but husbands and lovers must be understanding about this, and often they are not. Also, a mastectomy has traumatic psychological components not present in other surgical procedures. A woman may be reluctant to be seen nude for a while, as I was, for a variety of reasons. In such cases, her husband or lover may finally have to rely on his/her instincts and take some kind of positive action to help her get through this phase. (If the shyness and withdrawal go on too long, they could be signs of a severe disturbance.) For all I know, Harvey may have deliberately come into the bathroom to take something from the medicine cabinet just to break my pattern of reticence. The strategy was enough for me, and something like it may be enough for other women. But please, for a month or so—patience. The woman must have a little time to get used to the idea.

By all means, a man must go out of his way to be loving and

tender to show that, whatever physical difference the mastectomy has made, it has not changed his feelings (a warning usually not needed for female lovers). This is difficult for most undemonstrative American males, but they must somehow learn how to show affection without its having any sexual connotations and must try to make the woman feel even more precious than before.

The late Marvella Bayh told me about her anxiety and fear the night before her mastectomy. "I'm only thirty-eight years old," she had cried tearfully, "and I have to live the rest of my life with only one breast."

"Honey," Mrs. Bayh recalled her husband saying, "I'm forty-three years old, and I've lived all my life without any breasts at all."

I mention this here because it is the kind of answer every husband should file away in his memory box to use when and if his wife ever needs it.

Among the women I interviewed, older women—the married and the previously married—were the ones who had the most difficult emotional adjustment to make. Divorced husbands must make a special effort to help their former mates. Few second wives would object if their husbands visited their predecessors in the hospital after surgery, took care of finances and other household problems for a short time or offered to look after the children. Ex-husbands should read, in the chapter on postsurgery psychological problems, about my conversation with a woman whose first husband gave her no help at all. This kind of cruelty is barbaric. A divorced woman in our family subsequently had a mastectomy, and I am very proud of the cousin who was always at his ex-wife's side in the hospital, has chauffeured her for postoperative treatments, and has helped her financially as well. That is the way it ought to be.

Men who are still living with their wives but whose marriages are no longer close need the strongest lecture. It is a difficult enough time for an older woman, even if the marriage is fairly good.

"Let's face it," one fifty-eight-year-old woman told me. "My husband is sixty, very handsome and distinguished-looking. He can and, I've been told, does get women in their thirties to go out with him. He may even have a mistress, for all I know. Why should he bother with me?"

This woman's attitude was more bitter than usual, because she did apparently have some reason for doubting her husband's fidelity. What an awful additional blow the operation must have been for her! But the difference is only in intensity, not detail. It is a bad time.

So, to husbands of women in this very troubled—physically and psychologically—age group, I make this plea: Be with your wife as much as you can throughout the ordeal, and support her with your presence as well as your checkbook. If you have ever had any feeling for her as a human being, a partner, and perhaps the mother of your children, assure her, above all, that it does not make any difference to you whether she has one breast or two. She may not believe you, but she will nonetheless be happy to hear you say it.

Nowhere is male domination more evident than during the short interval in which the decision must be made about the mastectomy—because we patients are usually unconscious! Since most surgeons do not take the time in advance to outline the different surgical alternatives, the patient does not have the knowledge for making a decision even if she is awakened and asked—an argument doctors use to defend the system in the past and still repeat now.

Occasionally, however, surgeons do bring husbands into the decision-making process. This was apparently the case with both Betty Ford and Happy Rockefeller.

I remember very well the night of September 27, 1974, the evening before Mrs. Ford underwent her mastectomy at the Bethesda Naval Hospital. She had entered the hospital earlier and news broadcasts mentioned the event. But they soft-pedaled it by saying she was to have a simple, routine biopsy of a small "nodule" found during her regular gynecological examination. A friend in the White House press corps told me the rumor was that mammograms had already been taken and the diagnosis from them was positive. The Washington news reports indicated that if the biopsy confirmed this diagnosis, a Halsted radical mastectomy would be done immediately.

Having just gone through my own surgery, I knew such speed was unnecessary. Besides, there could not have been enough time between the discovery of the tumor and the scheduled operation for the doctors to have done any preoperative work-ups—the staging examinations of the bones, lungs, skull, spine, and liver—so necessary before a mastectomy. From the news reports, it did not sound as if these tests had been done.

"The poor woman is being railroaded," I told Harvey at dinner. "To the Bethesda Naval Hospital, in the bargain!"*

Wanting to put some of my hard-learned knowledge to use, I

*Later, I asked a veteran cancer specialist who had served many years as a navy doctor what he thought about having a mastectomy in that hospital. "Well," he answered, "I was over there for a long time. Bethesda Naval does a great hernia."

tried to call Ron Nessen, the President's press secretary, whom I had once met briefly at a press conference. He was not available; no one was available. President Ford, Nessen, and everyone else on the White House staff were attending a "mini-summit" on the economy and a reception for the delegates. Finally, at 11:45 P.M., I was able to reach one of the President's speech writers, to whom two mutual friends had referred me.

Introducing myself quickly, I told him why I was calling. "I'm not a kook," I said convincingly, I hope. "I've just had a mastectomy myself, and I want to pass along to the President some of the information I've learned."

"What is it?" he asked.

Briefly, and as simply as I could, I told him that the biopsy should be done and that then, if the diagnosis was cancer, certain tests should be completed before a mastectomy was performed. And, I added, the President should not let a general surgeon do the operation, but should find the best breast-cancer specialist in the country.

"If the President's wife isn't going to get the best," I asked, "who is?"

There was silence.

"Are you still there?"

"Just a minute," he finally replied. "I'll see what I can do."

I held the line, feeling like a toenote to history. But that was not to be. In a few minutes, he returned and transmitted what may well be the most memorable line in feminist history.

"I am sorry, Mrs. Kushner," he told me. "The President has made his decision."

I was speechless. Finally, I blurted out, "The President has made *his* decision? It's not his decision to make. Mrs. Ford should make the decision, don't you think?"

It was his turn to be speechless. Then, in an emotionless monotone, he answered, "I'm sorry, Mrs. Kushner, but that is all I am authorized to say. The President has gone to bed, and he has already made his decision."

The next morning I read the paper, heard the news, and learned that the President's decision indeed had been made. Betty Ford, at 8:30 on the morning of September 28, 1974, had been found to have breast cancer. A naval surgeon, Dr. William Fouty, and a professor of general surgery at George Washington Medical School, Dr. Richard Thistlethwaite, were at that moment performing a Halsted radical mastectomy on the wife of the President of the United States.

Harvey was listening to the radio with me. When the broadcast was over, he turned to me. "Well," he said, "it looks like the wife of Harvey Kushner got a hell of a lot better treatment than the wife of Gerald Ford."

It may seem in questionable taste to recount my conversation with the White House speech writer here and I would prefer to forget it. But even the President of the United States is not free of a lifetime of conditioning in our masculine society. Just as I hope women will learn from reading this book what they have a right to expect and demand, I hope men will understand that their wives should not be denied a conscious voice in their destinies.

Only a few weeks later, the absence of "freedom of choice" again became public knowledge when Happy Rockefeller's second breast was removed for a mirror-image carcinoma.

According to the late Vice President Rockefeller's own statement, broadcast and telecast live, he had been told immediately after the first mastectomy that there was a microscopic tumor in the second breast. (The routine policy at Memorial Sloan-Kettering is to do a biopsy of the same spot in the opposite breast whenever a mastectomy is performed, because about 1 per cent of women with one breast tumor have a mirror-image cancer in the other breast.) However, Vice President Rockefeller told the millions in his radio and TV audience that he had withheld this information from his wife after the first operation because of her emotional state. In the interim, he, her surgeon, Dr. Jerome Urban, and other surgical consultants had pondered what should be done because it was a lobular carcinoma *in situ*. Among them, they had decided that removing the second breast was the safest thing to do. Finally, in the middle of November, Happy Rockefeller was informed of her fate. The second breast was removed, as the men around her had decided.

Of course, that may be exactly what Mrs. Rockefeller herself would have chosen, had she been consulted. She had plenty of time after being told of the decision to say no, and she didn't. But—in her husband's own public words—she had not been told anything for more than a month. The decision about treatment was made by her husband, her surgeon, and whatever other specialists had been asked for advice.

Writing about politicians inevitably leads me into the role of politics in breast cancer. Research is not cheap. A lot of money is needed to develop equipment and to hire top-notch people. It is very expensive, and the major source of such huge sums is government and government means politicians.

Congress, as the world knows, is predominantly male. Nowhere does its masculine orientation show as clearly as in the number of dollars appropriated by that august body to study cancer of the breast.

Cancer of the lung and bronchus has been the top malignant killer since data were first collected. (Although breast-cancer *incidence rates* exceed those of lung cancer, the *death rates* of the latter are higher.) Because men have been smoking cigarettes longer than women, until recently lung cancer has been considered a masculine disease. I could not find an estimate of the millions—perhaps billions—of dollars spent before the tars and nicotines in cigarettes were found to be a major cause of lung cancer, mainly because the money came from so many different sources. Before the early 1960s (when cigarette smoking was officially blamed), the NCI, the National Institute of Heart and Lung and Blood Diseases, the American Cancer Society, the American Medical Association, anti-lung-disease organizations like the Christmas Seal and emphysema societies, the tobacco companies themselves (at least $10 million spent to prove the reverse), and numerous privately supported foundations poured hundreds of millions of dollars into a search for the cause of this (then) masculine cancer. And because so much lung cancer is associated with certain jobs, labor unions, insurance companies, and government agencies concerned with occupational hazards spent additional millions for research.

Even now, the costs of the battle against lung cancer can't be counted. Dollars are still flowing to enact legislation to stop smoking in public buildings, elevators, department stores, theaters, on common carriers, and even in certain areas of motels, hotels, and restaurants. Who knows how expensive it was to drive cigarette commercials off radio and television? In addition, miscellaneous environmental agencies—federal, state, local, and private—are spending money to regulate or prohibit the emission of various carcinogenic pollutants into the air. And I am talking only about funding with American dollars. Other countries have also contributed from their treasuries to get rid of lung cancer. With so many millions—probably billions—flowing into anti-lung-cancer budgets, from so many sources, it was and is impossible to calculate, even roughly, the totals being spent.

It has been a different story with breast cancer. This disease has been the top killer of American women between the ages of forty-four and fifty-five for a long time, and, within the past decade, it has been attacking younger and younger women. Yet Congress did not declare financial war on this specifically female cancer until 1966, several years after cigarettes had been pinpointed as the cause of lung cancer. In that year, Congressman

John E. Fogarty introduced a resolution for the creation of a breast cancer task force with a starting budget of $500,000. By 1970, it had about $2.75 million to spend on all federal research into the causes, treatment, and cure of breast cancer. Tiny cost-of-living raises were given to the Task Force since then, and in 1975 the budget was about $9.75 million. Then the funding began to be reduced (as all nondefense funding was reduced).

Finally, in 1981, NCI director Dr. Vincent T. DeVita decided the Task Force had done such a superb job of "stimulating research into the field" that the time had come to eliminate it. True, the entire NIH was under fire, and the NCI's cut was disproportionate. Money had to come from some source to fund other important work. By that time, I had been appointed by former President Jimmy Carter to the National Cancer Advisory Board and was in a position to do more than write letters to the editor. As the only patient-advocate (also known as "Writer/Consumer") on the NCAB, I argued that it was ridiculous to penalize a successful research program because it had done a good job. To do so, I said, might be interpreted by other programs to do poorly in order to perpetuate their grants and contracts.

Without getting into the intricacies of the federal research bureaucracy, I will only say that the final death sentence (in my opinion) of the Breast Cancer Task Force was averted by women's protests—plain, old-fashioned lobbying, picketing, and agitating. A single telephone call to Anne Kaspar of the Women & Health Roundtable resulted in a protest at a Consensus Development Conference on Caesarian Sections the next day at the NIH. Women who had come from all over the country to attend the C-Section Conference were, without any help from me, alerted into action. From reports I heard, a bulletin had been miraculously (for the Women's Movement) prepared overnight insisting that if breast-cancer research was to be abolished, prostate would have to go as well. Letters, I have been told, poured into Dr. De Vita's office, and he asked to attend a meeting of the Roundtable to explain his position. I did not go to this monthly brown-bagger, but Ruth Segal, an aide to former Secretary of Health and Human Services Patricia Harris, told me that the health professionals and concerned laywomen who packed the room were not convinced by his arguments.

Women showed what could be done by using the political clout we 53.1 per cent of the United States population have—when we decide to use it. The Breast Cancer Task Force (and the Prostate Project) are both alive and as well as they can be, considering the general economic climate of the decade facing us in the 1980s.

Women have been too reticent and timid about exercising female power, but it does work. In Massachusetts, for example, women marched on Springfield (the state capital) demanding that breast reconstruction after mastectomy for cancer be considered "rehabilitation" rather than cosmetic. The State's Blue Cross-Blue Shield plans had refused to cover this plastic surgery procedure, although testicular implants had *always* been paid for (as penile implants have been). The Massachusetts women won, and now almost all medical insurance plans pay for postmastectomy breast reconstruction, if the initial surgery was covered by that carrier.

Massachusetts seems to be the best place to be for fighting against legalized male chauvinism. On May 22, 1979, an act was passed making it illegal for doctors to railroad women through any breast-cancer surgical procedure (read mastectomy) without informing them in advance of other alternatives. Not only did this open the door for women to know about these alternatives, but it guaranteed the two-stage procedure. Obviously, no surgeon will take the time to explain all treatment options and their risks and benefits to all women who develop something that might be a symptom of breast cancer. And informed consent cannot be obtained from a woman who is unconscious on an operating-room table. So, in Massachusetts—and now in California since September 17, 1980—women may not lose their breasts without their specific informed consent. A similar bill is pending in the Connecticut legislature. Violating surgeons may be fined, have their licenses and hospital privileges suspended, or incur all of these penalties. In spite of strong protests by the Massachusetts and California medical societies, the laws fortunately have not been rescinded or repealed.

There are forty-seven more states that need this law.

There are also other arenas where political pressure must be applied. Around Washington, there is a slogan that cancer is "political," and the lobbies for laetrile and interferons (among other special-interest groups) are usually used as examples. But there are uniquely breast-cancer issues that are political because their only resolutions will be in the chambers of Congress.

For example, as discussed previously, except for the developing fetus, the female breast is the most radiosensitive of all human tissues. This means that all diagnostic X-ray equipment used to examine any part of our bodies must be top-quality, well-calibrated, and operated by qualified personnel who know what KVP and MA/S buttons to push. Yet there are *no* federal laws regulating usage of this potentially dangerous equipment.

The Bureau of Radiological Health is our watchdog over ionizing radiation, but it is a toothless watchdog because it has no power over usage. It can and does inspect the components in the manufacturing plant, and it can and does inspect the components after they are assembled in a radiologist's office (radiology apparatus is often put together like stereo equipment—one part from one firm and a second from another). After the complete setup is checked by someone from the BRH, continuation of monitoring is up to the individual states. Some, like New York, Massachusetts (again), California, New Jersey, and New Hampshire have excellent state radiation-control offices which spot-check both public and private diagnostic facilities at random, with no warning. A few states also require that all radiation technologists be certified by the American Registry of Radiological Technologists (ARRT).

But in the other states, regulation is literally catch-as-catch-can. My own state of Maryland, for example, is woefully understaffed and underfunded. Cosmetologists are under tighter control than radiologists are! A handful of people have the job of watching all uses of ionizing radiation—from possible leaks in sludge deposits in the western mountains to the nuclear power plant at Calvert Cliffs on the eastern shore along the Chesapeake. Other states, no doubt, have similar staff and financial problems. We women (and men: their gonads are almost as vulnerable to damage from poorly done X-ray examinations!) must see to it that the Bureau of Radiological Health is given the power to control this outrageous hodgepodge of mismanagement.

The BRH offers a free dosimetry calibration service to any and all radiologists—private or affiliated with institutions—in the United States. At no cost, the Bureau sends them a specially treated square which, when it is exposed by their equipment and mailed back (postage-paid), can be analyzed and any problems are reported back to the radiologists by BRH experts.

Ron Jans, chief of the program since it was born in 1976, however, told me that the voluntary program has still not caught on with most of the radiologists in this country. Moreover, he said that many breast X-rays are still being done in 1981 on so-called "general purpose" equipment.

When the first edition of *Why Me?* was written in 1977, one-third of all mammograms were being done on so-called "general purpose" X-ray equipment—machines used to image broken arms and legs. Another third was being taken with X-ray equipment adapted in some way to image only the breast, and only the remaining third were being done with "special purpose" mammography equipment—designed and built only to X-ray breasts.

The 1981 statistics showed an improvement and the trend will probably continue, but—in the meantime—many women are being X-rayed by equipment that should be in a Smithsonian Museum of Ancient Technology.

Radiation usage is an area so vitally in need of regulation that it can be done only on the federal level. Radiologists must be forced—not urged—to comply with radiation standards and to hire only qualified personnel. A "voluntary" program will not succeed.

Another federal problem is full coverage of all breast-cancer problems for women covered by Medicare. As late as early 1981, Senator Charles Percy was responsible for having *external* prostheses covered by this national senior-citizens' health insurance as a necessary, and not a cosmetic, postsurgical "appliance." Banning drugstore sales of diethylstilbestrol is still another federal problem.

Some breast-cancer problems must, by definition, be fought for on the state level, however. Teaching breast self-examination in the senior year of high school is a local issue, and it should be mandatory. (So should TSE—testicular self-examination for young men.) Victorian thinking has prevented this vital part of health education from being adopted by most school systems in the country.

Another state issue is third-party-payments for nurses. This, again, is available in Massachusetts, but, as far as I have been able to learn, no other state requires Blue Cross-Blue Shield plans to pay the fees for nurses other than enterostomal therapists and, in some cases, midwives. To women, this means that unless a surgeon pays a nurse out of his own pocket to explain options and alternatives in breast-cancer treatment, they will probably not have them explained. This, indeed, is why NURSUPPORT failed: the grant given to the Georgetown University Hospital by the NCI for an oncological nursing program ended, and the nurses who staffed the "hotline" went elsewhere.

It is also the reason why the Breast Cancer Advisory Center has been so sorely needed. If women fought as they did for the Breast Cancer Task Force in October 1981, these issues would probably be resolved.

And these are only a few examples of the political aspects of breast cancer.

A recent political problem affecting breast cancer—indeed, all cancers—is related to the tightening of the federal purse strings for the National Cancer Institute. While the absolute number of the current annual budget sounds more than adequate at about $1 billion, when inflation and the cost of living are taken into account, financial support for the NCI has been drastically reduced since 1979. In comparison with the more recent massive flow of dollars into the Department of Defense, the funds devoted to cancer research seem to be petty cash in the Pentagon.

What does this mean to us?

The obvious result is that the quick pace set during the early years of the Breast Cancer Task Force and of the entire National Cancer Program must inevitably slow down. Many of the projects I will mention in Chapter 17—The Future—will be postponed or rejected entirely, because priorities will require ongoing research to be completed before new studies can be started.

A less visible result of government's parsimony, however, is that scientists are being forced to turn to the private sector for money to do their research. This means that the kinds of data liberally shared in scientific journals and at seminars and symposia become industrial "trade secrets" that are locked in corporate vaults until they can be exploited commercially. While there may be researchers who sell patents and grant licenses for their work so they can become wealthy themselves, these people represent a small minority of those looking for private support. The reason they are selling their ideas to the highest commercial bidder is usually that this is the only way much basic research can be continued. As far as the vast majority of scientists is concerned, a free interchange of ideas and data is the only way progress can be made. Unpublished trade secrets, by definition, result in duplication, overlap and in a waste of time, talent, and resources. Yet this unprecedented situation has begun and is spreading with the speed of light.

At an international meeting of cancer scientists held in Washington, D.C. in the spring of 1981, people, who gladly gave me preliminary results of various studies in the past, were suddenly mysterious and silent.

"I've applied for a patent on that," I was told.

Or, "I've granted a license to a drug company to produce a test kit, and I can't go into detail about that yet."

The situation became so serious in June 1981 that Congressman Albert Gore, Jr. of Tennessee announced plans to hold hearings into the matter. As far as breast cancer is concerned, there is no way to know how many studies once funded by the Breast Cancer Task Force will now become (or already are!) Top Secret, because a pharmaceutical or chemical company has bought the rights.

This political issue, like the one concerning the lack of regulation over radiation, is in no way related to male chauvinism: it is everyone's problem.

However, there are still issues directly related to MCP. For example, there is a grave lack of women legislators in all state and local governments. The U.S. Senate has usually been entirely male, and the House of Representatives has always had few women. The only way to get bills introduced and laws passed is to become politically active ourselves or to work for legislators who will do their best for our needs.

I said it was impossible to prove a negative when I discussed the probable role male chauvinism plays in the problem of saving women's breasts. It is equally impossible to prove a negative here. There is no way to correlate the lack of progress in breast-cancer research with the almost all-male Congress and other male-dominated organizations. It is an historical fact, however, that even the weak push given to breast-cancer financing did not begin until 1966, after a major cause of lung cancer had already been found.

Male chauvinism plays an important role in all aspects of breast cancer, from the moment a sixth-grader's budding chest bumps make her popular with pimply-faced boys. Later, the belief that breasts are vital in getting and keeping a boyfriend, and then a husband is reinforced by the blatant blandishments of our male-dominated media. Next, there is the malevolent influence of a male-dominated medical profession, specifically in surgery, rein-forced by decades or discrimination against women by admis-sions offices in medical schools, policies that have perpetuated medical masculinity. Although entrance statistics indicate that the number of women in schools of medicine in the United States is higher now than ten years ago, those stalwart women who finally receive their M.D. degrees usually go into pediatrics, obstetrics and gynecology, psychiatry, and dermatology—not surgery. Their reason is not schedules, but another kind of dis-crimination.

Americans do not accept the notion that women doctors should be in certain fields of medicine, and one of these is surgery: Americans—men and women—just do not cotton to the idea of female surgeons. Naturally, they would not make worthwhile incomes, and most women doctors do not even try. The result, of course, is the 3-percent-female component in the American Col-lege of Surgeons.

Finally, the money for breast-cancer research is voted by a male-dominated and male-oriented Congress. And, in spite of the cancers that struck Mrs. Ford and Mrs. Rockefeller and in spite of the rising breast-cancer incidence rates, President Ronald Reagan is keeping cancer-research funds low, as a part of his battle of the budget. At the same time, he is insisting that Congress provide money to "rescue" San Salvador. Somehow, men have their priorities scrambled in strange ways.

Not long before I found my lump, I attended a press conference held to protest the so-called Buckley amendment to the Constitution, which, if passed, would have invalidated the Supreme Court decision liberalizing the abortion laws of most states. Several leaders of the women's liberation movement, feminist groups, and the Women's Political Caucus spoke against the amendment. In her remarks, the writer Gloria Steinem lashed out against male doctors who do unnecessary mastectomies, hinting that there is some kind of male-chauvinist conspiracy whose goal is to mutilate women by cutting off their breasts.

In the research I have done and the conversations I have had, I did not find any suggestion whatever of such a sadistic conspiracy in the present situation where amputation of a breast is the best first treatment.

But other kinds of male chauvinism? Plenty!

17

The Future

I am gazing into a "crystal ball" made up of thousands of grant proposals to the National Cancer Institute, proposals submitted from scientists all over the world, and—better than any clairvoyant—I can envision great hope for The Future.

When I wrote *Breast Cancer* in 1974, my research was based on already-published articles and books and on interviews with scientists who were kind enough to take the trouble to talk to me. Most of the time, they were happy to postulate and speculate about their research, and *Breast Cancer* reflected this cooperation.

But since then, I have discovered that any data already printed, even articles in professional journals (forget books altogether!), must be at least six months old. And, usually, they are even more ancient. The only way for anyone to have current, up-to-date information is to either interview researchers about what they are doing or to go to conferences where results of research are announced orally. Much of *Why Me?* came from this kind of first-hand listening. I was lucky, and I have continued to be lucky, because of the geographical accident of living five minutes away from the National Institutes of Health—the world's foremost biomedical research center. Throughout *Why Me?*, I have detailed meetings and international conferences I attended at the NIH; the kind and generous cooperation given to me by scientists there who let me pick their brains for hours about mundane (to them) aspects of their work and who gave me copies of unpublished manuscripts; help from librarians at the NIH library and the National Library of Medicine.

This accident of living near the NIH made it possible for me to do so much first-hand listening that I did not have to rely on published material that was often obsolete before its appearance in a journal or book.

Again, because I was lucky enough to have been appointed to the National Cancer Advisory Board (the NCAB), The Future, in the form of pink summary sheets comes to me regularly (since September 1980), courtesy of the U.S. Postal Service.

These pink-sheets are as top-secret as any scrambled CIA intercept, until the NCAB has voted approval or disapproval of the verdict given by each researcher's peer-review committee. Although I am not permitted to give specific details, I am allowed to pick through the pink and write about general ideas and trends. So my stacks of pink sheets give me more than a glimpse into the future: they actually tell me what research scientists are now doing and—more important—what research they would like to do, if they can get the money to support it.

For example, it is not difficult for anyone reading the past year's proposals to see that the latest rage in the cancer-research community is not recombinant DNA, not genetic engineering, and not interferons. Monoclonal antibodies have all but pushed these competitors out of the scientific race entirely.

"They're the greatest things that have come down the pike," Dr. Jeffrey Schlom had told me, when I asked him to review the section on immunotherapy. "We haven't even begun to learn what they'll be able to do. In the fight against cancer, they will be useful everywhere."

And, indeed, scores of pink-sheets from virtually every corner of the earth seem to be based on this exciting field of new technological know-how.

All cells—including cancer cells—carry certain "fingerprints" that identify that particular kind of cell and none else. Often found on the surface of the cell's membrane, but sometimes inside its body (or cytoplasm), these fingerprints are proteins that scientists usually call (in the case of cancer) "tumor associated antigens," or TAAs. Without understanding the esoteric biochemical complexities involved, I can make the over-simplified statement that for every antigen, there is, somewhere, an antibody. And, just as iron filings cling to magnets, keys fit into locks, and estrogens bind to estrogen-receptors, antibodies are attracted to and latch themselves onto their ordained antigens.

Of course, the basic principle of this magical attraction is not new; it has been known since the days of Edward Jenner and Louis Pasteur. But because each living cell has tens of thousands of individual antigens—each with its own antibody—past attempts to exploit their natural affinity for each other were trial-and-error or educated guesswork. What is creating the almost delirious excitement now is the potential development of a way to identify, isolate, and then to produce, in enormous quantities, pure antibodies that will be able to zoom directly to their antigens—wherever they may be in the body. Once perfected, the implications of such technical know-how for cancer prevention, detection, and treatment are literally limitless. But at this time, the technology is a newborn babe in laboratories all over the world. Scientists still have a great deal of work to do before they can use the child properly.

Like so many babies, monoclonal antibodies were conceived accidentally. In the early 1970s, two British scientists—Drs. Cesar Milstein and George Köhler—were trying to discover how the molecules of an antibody are bound to each other. Curiously, although antibodies have been used for almost a century, little was known about these amazing proteins except that their job was to "inactivate" a foreign invader by either killing it or by preventing it from functioning. Drs. Milstein and Köhler were doing basic research to learn more.

The result of their work was the "hybridoma," a way to take a single antibody and put it into a tub full of the nutrients it needed to grow and multiply. Scientists would then have a steady supply of pure, antibodies always available for their research. Although many had tried to do this in the past, all had failed, because—left to their own devices—antibodies die quickly. To make them live longer, Milstein and Köhler took cells from the spleen of a mouse (cells that manufacture great quantities of antibodies) and fused them to cancerous myeloma cells.

One of cancer's lethal characteristics, of course, is that its cells rarely die but proliferate endlessly, so this fusion "conferred immortality" on the mouse antibodies. According to an interview of Dr. Milstein by *Science News*, he was not able to convince the administrators of Britain's Medical Research Council—supporters of this research—that the procedure had "important enough applications" to be patented. Yet the pioneering studies of Drs. Milstein and Köhler have given the world's scientists a way to keep antibodies alive, perhaps forever: the hybridoma, an incubator for growing pure, cloned generations of antibodies to specific antigens.

The word "clone" achieved some notoriety a few years ago in the book and movie *The Boys from Brazil*. Their author, Ira Levin, invented a bizarre tale about a last-minute attempt by

Hitler's scientific henchmen to immortalize the Fuehrer forever. To do this, Levin's villains manipulated Hitler's sperm cells (they wanted no female chromosomes interfering with Hitler's sons) and planted them into the incubator (hybridoma) of a healthy woman's uterus. Lo and behold! a crop of mini-Hitlers were born and raised in various countries, offspring who were supposed to meet and resurrect the Third Reich a generation later.

Not long after *The Boys from Brazil* was published and filmed, a medical writer hoaxed the world by writing, *In His Own Image*, a "non-fiction" account of an anonymous, wealthy man who wanted a child carrying no genes or chromosomes except his own. To solve this problem, he had himself "cloned," and his child—according to the book—is living in blessed anonymity somewhere. This "true" story caused a brief, but exciting flurry in scientific circles in the late 1970s and earned its author a place on the best-seller list.

While making exact duplicates of humans or even lower mammals is still science-fiction, there is no question that antibodies can and are being cloned, and their potential for the detection and treatment of all cancers seems to be unlimited.

To sum up the frenetic international scene in a few lines, imagine a situation where a harmless antibody, known to be attracted to a known antigen on a breast-cancer cell, is tagged with a miniscule dose of radioactivity—a "label". Every six or twelve months, it is injected into women, as part of their routine physical examinations, to see if a breast cancer is growing. When and if the technology is perfected, the labelled antibody would shine like a Times Square marquee on a photograph taken by a gamma camera, as soon as it made a connection with its tumor-associated antigen—even if there was only a single cancer cell in that breast!

Obviously, mastectomies would not have to be done, because other foci of malignancy would also shine as soon as they made the radioactive antibody-antigen connection. Surgeons would simply remove the cancerous centricles wherever they appear on the photograph. No one could hope for earlier detection. The same mechanism would be used to see if axillary or internal mammary nodes have been invaded; they would no longer have to be removed surgically for pathological examination.

Monoclonal antibodies, when they are perfected, would also indicate which women should receive adjuvant therapy after primary treatment, because the radioactive tracers would target in on micrometastases this treatment is designed to eradicate. If none are seen on the gamma scan, drugs would obviously not be necessary.

Some women, of course, will have invaded lymph nodes at the time of diagnosis and will need to be given some kind of adjuvant treatment. For them, periodic monitoring with radioactive antibodies to see whether or not the chemo- or endocrine therapy is working would be a real blessing. As I've said, the only way anyone can now know if adjuvant treatments are working is simply that no second cancer appears.

Antibodies, I have been told, may also turn out to be the answer for treating existing disease. Once the antibodies to known breast-cancer antigens are identified and cloned, cancer weapons of all kinds would be loaded on them. Like "smart bombs" and homing-torpedoes, the antibodies will carry their lethal cargoes directly to the tumor. Since the cells of healthy tissues *en route* would not have these breast-cancer-specific antigens, none would be affected by cytotoxic drugs or radiation being carried by the antibodies.

These, of course, are the applications of monoclonal antibodies most women are interested in, but there are more basic, laboratory uses as well. Plans and promises can be seen in scientific magazines and journals, already filled with advertisements from various firms producing this or that strain of monoclonal antibodies. Television "breakthrough" programs have triggered letters and telephone calls to the Breast Cancer Advisory Center asking where breast-cancer patients can go to be treated with monoclonal antibodies.

With so much excitement in both the professional and lay media, they must be explained in detail. But since I know there are still enormous obstacles that have to be overcome before monoclonal antibodies can be applied clinically, predicting their possible future value to women is more difficult than walking on eggs with combat boots.

"What shall I say?" I wailed to Dr. Taylor, coordinator of the Breast Cancer Task Force's research programs. "Everybody I talk to tells me something else. Some immunologists I've interviewed insist they're going to be a false alarm. But other people I've talked to—people who usually hedge their bets and never say anything is any good until it wins the Nobel Prize—think they're the answer to everything . . . cause, diagnosis and cure. I just don't know what to write."

"Just tell it the way it is," she said firmly. "Monoclonal antibodies may be a valuable tool some day, but there are just not enough data yet to know their full potential in breast cancer, even though the field looks promising.

"Explain what monoclonal antibodies are, how they're obtained, and why there's so much excitement about them," Dr. Taylor instructed. "But you've also got to explain what today's real problems are, so you don't stir up a lot of false hope. We've had enough of that during the past few years."

With her words in my mind as bright, blinking yellow lights, I am proceeding with caution. Monoclonal antibodies may turn out to be all that their most ardent advocates expect: a way to detect and treat a breast cancer when it is a curable, microscopic cluster of only a few cells. On the other hand, they may only be another piece of technical know-how—like the electron microscope and the computer—that will make it easier for scientists to get answers to some questions.

One of the problems that still needs to be solved, for example, is a way to identify those antigens that are present only or predominantly (thousands of times more frequently) on a malignant cell. As I have said, each cancer cell carries hundreds of thousands of antigens on its membrane and inside its cytoplasm. To find antibodies to any of them, these cancer cells are injected into an experimental animal (rabbits seem to work best), so its immune system begins to manufacture antibodies against the antigens of that tumor cell.

The animal's blood or lymphocytes then become packed with antibodies against all, most, or some of the antigens on those cancer cells. This has been proven, because injecting the serum or strained lymphocytes into other animals with cancer has made their tumors shrink or go away entirely. But which antibody in the injection caused the reaction? No one knows for sure.

So scientists must then do the tedious, laborious, and time-consuming work of plucking out individual antibodies that seem to be likely candidates from the blood or lymph-node cells in order to fuse them with an immortal cancer cell. Hybridomas filled with the precise nutrients these antibodies need must be created. Then once a colony is thriving, researchers must make educated guesses about which clones will actually be useful.

As far as breast cancer is concerned, Dr. Jeffrey Schlom of the NCI has published several papers showing successful reactivity between the monoclonal antibodies produced in his laboratory and the mouse mammary tumor virus, the MMuTV. He has also been successful in demonstrating reactivity with human metastatic breast cancer cells.

As enthusiastic as a miner who has struck a rich vein of gold, he told me plans are already in place to begin Phase I trials, in women with advanced disease, at the Sidney Farber Cancer Center in Boston.

"If we can show that internal mammary nodes can be identified without surgery," he explained, "that will be tremendous progress for women who have primary breast cancer. This trial will have enormous implications for treatment, almost immediately."

The unspoken corollary of course is "if it works."

Dr. Schlom is confident that he has identified (at this time) eleven monoclonal antibodies that react with human breast cancer cells and not with normal tissues. But Dr. William D. Terry, Chief of the Immunology Branch of the NCI also urges caution.

"So far, no one has identified an antigen that is present *only* on breast cancer—or any cancer—cells and not on normal ones," he explained. "We do know of antigens that appear several thousand times more frequently on malignant cells than they do on normal cells, and that could have clinical implications.

"But so far, none is cancer-specific enough to be reliable if potentially harmful substances like radioactivity, cytotoxic drugs or large doses or irradiation are to be used," Dr. Terry continued.

So without precise identification of cancer-specific antigens, there is still no sure way for scientists to know whether an antibody is useful, and so monoclonal antibodies have no immediate application to the detection or treatment of breast cancer.

However, their future potential—as reflected in the pink sheets—seems to have the sky as the ceiling.

Another research area I have mentioned frequently in *Why Me?* is "markers." This word means different things to different people. To children, they may be a rainbow of colorful drawing pens; to gamblers, they are life-and-death IOUs inscribed to a casino boss; to athletes, markers are the goals showing how far they have run in X-number of minutes. But in cancer, markers are indicators to show the extent or progress of disease.

As far as breast cancer is concerned, we women need markers desperately, but little is ever heard about them in the reams of literature we are given to read. We need a safe, easy, quick and reliable marker for: 1) detecting and diagnosing an invasive cancer early; 2) distinguishing between an "atypical" cell that is truly premalignant, a precursor to invasive cancer and one that is merely abnormal and likely to remain abnormal forever; 3) predicting whether an invasive cancer cell is virulent, and likely to metastasize quickly, or one that is sluggish; 4) showing that there is only a single malignancy in a breast or whether there are other foci of cancer; 5) pointing to the presence of cancer in axillary and internal mammary lymph nodes, without the need to cut them out for confirmation; 6) indicating which women with negative axil-

lary nodes are, nonetheless, at high risk of recurrence and shou
receive adjuvant therapy after primary treatment; 7) telling which
women receiving adjuvant therapy are actually being helped and
which should be switched to another combination of agents.

Although it is possible that one technology like monoclonal
antibodies will be able to accomplish all of these miracles, achieving these seven goals will probably require developing several
different kinds of tests.

At this time, dozens of scientists around the world are looking
for unique pathological, biochemical, immunological, and biological substances in the tumor itself, in the lymph nodes, and in the
blood and/or urine of women who have been treated for breast
cancer. This research is not an academic exercise but an attempt
to find these elusive "markers" to answer these unknowns of
breast cancer.

For example, many scientists are looking for a breast-cancer
test that would meet women's criteria of being as accurate, safe,
easy, quick and inexpensive as the Pap test is for cervical cancer.
Dr. Georg Springer, in Evanston, Illinois has been perfecting a
skin scratch-test he has named the T-antigen test (no relation to
T-cells: the name refers to Thomsen-Friedenreich). It is similar to
the well-known tuberculin scratching, and if a woman's skin
reddens or swells, she is examined for breast cancer thoroughly.
To verify the test's reliability, Dr. Springer is following several
hundred high-risk women (because of family or personal histories
of the disease) to see if those developing a strong reaction to the
scratch do, eventually, develop breast cancer. So far, healthy
women have had no reaction, while those with known breast
cancer have had strong ones. The problem is that about ten per
cent of women with benign breast diseases like fibroadenomas,
chronic cystic problems, mastitis, etc., also develop a strong
reaction. The T-antigen test is, therefore, not yet ready to replace
mammography or other early-detection modalities.

A marker to identify precursor cells was not even needed until
the advent of early-detection gadgets that have the capability of
visualizing microscopic clusters of abnormalities. If invisible
cells were indeed precursors of cancer, they made themselves
evident soon enough; if they were destined to remain abnormal
and never become invasive and life-threatening, neither women
nor their doctors ever knew they were in the breast at all.

So until mammography and other super-vision apparatus came
along, women had no choice but to worry and wait for the ax to
fall, if it was going to fall. With the beginning of mass-screening

programs aimed at finding breast cancers long before they could
be felt, an unexpected problem was discovered: some "atypia"
seen by the mammograph were so miniscule that many surgeons
refused to biopsy the women. Then in 1969, two pathologists at
the M.D. Anderson Cancer Center in Houston—Drs. H. Stephen
Gallager and John E. Martin—studied serial sections from amputated breasts after surgery and reported that they had found
multiple precancerous microscopic lesions and even real invasive
carcinomas in as many as fifty per cent of the organs. They also
discovered malignant foci in second breasts that were removed
for various reasons.

The result of their now-classical research was the concept that
the development of breast cancer is a "continuum" with no
precise beginning except variations from what would be considered normal. Earlier, scientists believed there was an exact moment in time when a healthy cell became malignant, that the
disease remained localized to the breast for a certain period of
time, and then—for unknown reasons—it began to spread. The
Gallager-Martin research suggested this long-held belief was
wrong and that healthy cells gradually go through several stages
before they become frankly invasive. Doctors even coined a new
nomenclature for hyperplasia, dysplasia, metaplasia, atypia, and
carcinomas *in situ*: they named them "Stage 0" cancers. As I
explained in Chapter 7, the Breast Cancer Detection Demonstration Projects (BCDDPs) showed that hundreds of women were
treated by extensive surgery, including Halsted radical mastectomies, because of a diagnosis of carcinoma *in situ*. Women began
to be afraid of breast screening because of the possibility of
having unnecessary surgery, in addition to fears of overexposure
to ionizing radiation. A grand debate has, since that time, been
going on in the radiological/surgical/pathological media about
what to do to treat atypical cells that are not yet—and may never
become—real cancer.

To women, the issue is more than an academic problem to be
argued at conferences and in journals. We need a marker that can
distinguish between true precursors of invasive cancer that could
kill us and those cells that simply do not look normal to a pathologist's eye.

Dr. Pietro Gullino, chief of the Pathophysiology Laboratory at
the NCI, is convinced that angiogenesis, the ability of cancer cells
to create a blood supply, is an important marker that can predict
whether or not benign atypical cells are likely to become malignant. Tests for angiogenesis, however, are still far from being
useful in the average U.S. hospital, although Dr. Gullino feels the

vascularization-factor could be isolated tomorrow. So angiogenesis is of no value to us women today.

We also need a marker to settle the issue of multicentricity. If all goes according to immunologists' plans, monoclonal antibodies may provide the answer. In addition, the handful of women who refused any treatment at all during the BCDDPs—in spite of grim mammography reports—may eventually offer some clues to solve this riddle. So will the National Surgical Adjuvant Breast Project's trials, because one-third of the women are having only lumpectomies and axillary dissections, with no irradiation to their breasts. If the Gallager-Martin data are valid, about half of this group of women should have recurrences in their preserved breasts. But the outcomes of both of these long-term studies will take years. We need the marker now.

Work to find "prognostic indicators" or markers of high-recurrence-risk has long been underway in many universities and hospitals. By identifying virulent vs. sluggish cancers, breast-cancer experts hope to learn which women would benefit from adjuvant therapy immediately after surgery, even if they have no cancer in their axillary nodes. So far, the only indicator has been a woman's estrogen-receptor status: ER + women seem to do better than do women whose cancers are ER −, no matter what treatment is given. This test result plus the number of axillary lymph nodes and the size of the tumor are the only indicators now available to help doctors predict the future prognoses of their patients. And, according to everyone I have interviewed, all of these are considered "primitive."

The search goes on to find others. Dr. Maurice Black and his colleagues in New York are following women whose tumors had certain immunological characteristics; Dr. Thomas Nealon, also in New York, is studying pathological features of various cancers. So is Dr. Edwin Fisher in Pittsburgh. Biochemically-oriented scientists, like Denver's Dr. Marvin Rich, are looking for certain sugar molecules—a vast group of enzymes called glycoproteins—for the same reason. All want to find something in the tumor that will help women's doctors know what to do next.

Dr. Sydney Salmon, a breast-cancer expert at the University of Arizona Cancer Center in Tucson is taking no chances and is giving all of his patients—including those with negative axillary nodes—some adjuvant chemotherapy.

"Almost one-third of all negative-node women will recur," he told me. "From a statistical point of view, a short period of adjuvant chemotherapy will save lives."

But Dr. Salmon is in the minority. Most oncologists and breast-cancer surgeons do not want to use adjuvant treatment of any kind unless the women are definitely at high risk of having a recurrence of disease. They want a marker as much as their patients do.

Finally, women in urgent need of a marker are those who have had surgery for their primary disease and are on adjuvant treatment. These women know they are at high risk of developing a metastasis but none has any way of knowing whether or not the drugs or other anticancer agents are working unless a second cancer is detected on an X-ray or scan. The problem is especially acute for postmenopausal women, because there have been many articles in general media reporting the possible ineffectiveness of chemotherapy for this age group. So older women have the added worry of thinking, "Is it worth it?"

The women who, according to queries to the Breast Cancer Advisory Center, need such a marker most of all are those who have *no* side effects whatsoever: those who don't suffer hair-loss or spend an instant feeling queasy. Many never miss a menstrual period, even though amenorrhea is supposed to be one of the first effects of chemotherapy.

"How can the drugs be preventing a recurrence, if I'm not bald?"

I have been asked this question again and again, and the only answer is to remind them that they are still free of disease.

There are efforts being made to find a marker for these women too. Since 1976, Dr. Dao and his associate at Roswell Park, Dr. Clement Ip, have been measuring levels of an enzyme—sialyl-transferase—in patients' blood to monitor the progress of their disease (including mine). So far, there has been a 100 percent correlation between elevations of this enzyme and recurrence. Decreases of the enzyme's level, on the other hand, have been associated with improvement; women whose serum sialyltransferase levels remain within normal limits have continued to be free of disease. Drs. David Kessel and his colleagues at the Wayne State University in Michigan, Allen Lipton at the Hershey Medical Center in Pennsylvania, and Phillip Waalkes at the Johns Hopkins Cancer Center in Baltimore have done research along the same lines: to find a marker for the early detection of a recurrence.

I must apologize to the dozens of scientists doing marker research who have not been named here: to have listed them all would have made this section a book in itself.

Monoclonal antibodies and markers are, according to my pink-paper crystal ball, the broad waves of The Future. But there are earlier ripples among these waves that will help us wait. As I said earlier, much of the research is preliminary and not yet ready to move from the laboratory to doctors' offices. But progress is being made.

A vaccination against breast cancer?

Maybe.

There are scientists working with conventional immunization ideas using the murine mammary tumor virus (MMuTV) I referred to when I talked about monoclonal antibodies. This would be a smallpox- or polio-type technique involving killed or weakened mouse-cancer cells. Theoretically, young women immunized against the particular type of human breast cancer that appears to be similar to murine cancer would never get the disease. Aside from the ethical problem of giving a healthy woman an unknown substance that may be carcinogenic, there is little evidence that human breast cancer is caused by this strain of cells.

Prevention by other methods?

Maybe.

There is considerable epidemiological evidence linking dietary fats, animal and vegetable, to breast cancer, although much of the necessary laboratory data are still missing. So far, there is a definite "link" between fats, hormones, and breast cancer, but no one has identified what the link is. Evidence clearly indicates, however, that a high-fat diet is high risk. So changing eating habits may cut down women's breast-cancer incidence and weight. Surprisingly, there also appears to be some evidence that trace elements like selenium, zinc, and tin may somehow be involved in preventing breast-cancer and vitamins A (*not* as the drugstore-shelf substance, but as retinoids—an important difference!), C, E, and some of the B vitamins are being studied as "chemo-preventors."

Epidemiological evidence that certain groups of women (e.g., Japanese, African, American Indian) have lower incidences of breast cancer and higher levels of serum estriol—another female hormone—have led some scientists to believe that the addition of this substance may be protective. Another epidemiological finding, that early age-at-first-birth is protective, has spurred some scientists into looking for ways to artificially imitate a woman's hormonal status after childbirth. Again theoretically, if this postpartum condition can be created in young women, it may confer some kind of protection.

Some kind of protection will certainly be needed. When I was in my childbearing years, anyone who had not yet had a baby by age twenty-five was considered "barren." Now, the average age-at-first-birth in the United States is well over thirty, according to the Population Reference Bureau. If this epidemiological factor is reliable, our country may well be on the doorstep of a major breast-cancer epidemic. Imitating pregnancy may be the only way to avoid this kind of catastrophe.

The NCI is, of course, pursuing all avenues of basic research, including nutrition, to find links between virtually everything and all cancers. This covers much territory and crosses the boundaries of all disciplines. For example, a deficiency of vitamin C may not only suppress the immune system but may also interfere with a substance, fibronectin, that is responsible for the strength of collagen—the basic stuff holding our bodies together. Certain substances have, in the laboratory, been able to turn malignant cells back to health, and reconversion of transformed cells is a popular basic research field in many universities and hospitals. So far, the work has been done only with lower animals, but it seems to be promising. If we could return a man from the moon, why not return a cancer cell to health?

Much information is being learned from breast-cancer patients whose families have strong histories of cancer, not only of breast cancer. At the NCI and other institutions, such women are being asked to participate in various studies (*not* experiments! They only donate blood and urine) to see if there are any factors that all have in common—factors that might help identify other high-risk young women.

But early detection of breast cancer is still the only weapon we women can rely upon to try to save our breasts as well as our lives, and mammography is still the most reliable technique. Thanks to improved technological know-how, radiation-exposure dosages have been reduced while the quality of imaging has gone up. I have been told that a still-unrefined X-ray technique known as Xonics will, when perfected, be able to obtain excellent and clear images using a total radiation dosage of less than half of one rad. But it is not perfected yet.

Mammography (reproduced by a Xerox machine as xerography) may also be valuable to women by classifying us into certain risk groups, according to criteria established by Dr. John Wolfe, Jr. of the Hutzel Hospital in Detroit. Based on analyses of thousands of xerograms of breast-cancer patients, Dr. Wolfe has found a high degree of correlation between groups he has categorized as N1, P1, P2, and DY. Many researchers are following some of the 280,000 women enrolled in the NCI/ACS Breast Cancer Detection Demonstration Projects to see if the Wolfe criteria are indeed reliable. If so, these ductal patterns (women with prominent ducts, according to Wolfe, are at higher risk) could be considered a new kind of "marker."

There will be no shortage of new and expensive machinery for women who have the money and the time to take advantage of them. Ultrasound is becoming more reliable, popular, and convenient. New designs and computerization have improved their reliability, especially for women under age 50 whose dense breasts should not be mammographed. (In Japan, by the way, ultrasonography [echograms] is the diagnostic modality most breast-cancer surgeons use.)

Thermography is also in a controversial category, because interpreting heat-retention photographs is so subjective and dependent on the training and experience of the person doing the interpretation. However, Dr. JoAnn Haberman, a long-time thermographer in Oklahoma, has been working with the Minneapolis Honeywell Corporation to computerize the technique and take a great deal of the subjectivity out of it. In other countries, especially in France, thermography is highly regarded, so the technique may be the victim of one of those vicious circles: because few people are well-trained in reading thermograms, the entire field suffers a bad reputation. Naturally, this means few people will bother to learn how to interpret them well.

What does the pink-paper ball say about treatment?

Nothing about surgery. Researchers do not seem to consider breast-cancer surgery worthy of grant applications, so I will have to rely on reports to the Breast Cancer Advisory Center, instead. Since June 5, 1979, the two-stage procedure has, to my great surprise, become the rule where it was the glaring exception on June 4. Women calling the Center from towns and villages throughout our country have reported a 180 degree spin-around in surgical opinion since the NIH Consensus Development Conference. Nor have I heard from any woman who had a Halsted radical mastectomy since that historic date.

Even more important, women are now being permitted to choose lesser surgeries, usually followed by irradiation of the breast, by doctors who would never have dreamed of doing so when my first book was written in 1974. Surgeons no longer seem to be afraid to say, "I don't know what's best."

Perhaps the most significant improvement to women is the fact that two states have enacted legislation making it a violation of the law for any surgeon to railroad a woman through a mastectomy without giving her a description of alternative treatments first. At this time, this milestone governmental consumer-protection is on the lawbooks in Massachusetts (since May 1979) and in California (since September 1980). It is also being considered in Connecticut, and—I have been told—will probably be passed in an upcoming session. Other states have similar bills in committee or in other stages of pre-passage evolution.

I agree with the medical profession that it is a shame government intervention is needed to see to it that the barbaric practices of the past are abolished. It is also a shame that we need an FDA to supervise the processing of foods and the production of drugs and cosmetics. The Bureau of Radiological Health should be unnecessary too, because all manufacturers and users of radiation equipment should police themselves.

As a taxpayer, I object to the expenditure of my tax dollars to protect me from over-zealous surgeons. But there would be no such laws if there were no need for them.

The NSABP and NCI clinical trials, I am confident, will complete the full recruitment of patients to get those significant data so vitally important to statisticians. Once all of the women are enrolled, we will have to wait ten years to have the survival data necessary to see if segmental surgery plus X-ray of the preserved breast is "as good as" mastectomy. I am sure this comparison (not based on hunches or pink-sheets but on existing results from nonrandomized trials) will show that mastectomies belong on the medical-museum shelf with mastoidectomies.

I am especially anxious to know whether the nonirradiated group in the NSABP trial will have different results. When I asked Dr. Bernard Fisher for the current results of this section of the trial, he said only, "We have had no reason to abandon this part of the study." It is illegal to continue any trial, in the United States, if its data show patients are not doing as well as they would receiving standard treatment.

So, I infer that the survival and recurrence rates of the nonirradiated women are identical with the other two groups. However, I cannot even make an educated guess about the final results.

If staging and wider use of the estrogen-receptor assay may be considered parts of treatment, both will be more prevalent in the near future. Wall Street has put medical advances on the front page (most pharmaceutical firms now have Marker Divisions!), and the technological know-how to detect occult micrometastases will certainly make their yield go up. This, along with the delay of the two-stage procedure, should make presurgical examinations routine. Private industry's promotion of the ERA, tamoxifen and aminoglutethemide will also affect the test's use as an indicator for endocrine manipulation instead of, or in addition to, cytotoxic drugs.

Cytotoxic drugs, I am sure, will be improved so they are more effective with less toxicity. In addition, there will soon be "radio-enhancers" and "radioprotectors," drugs that—when given along with radiation—will be able to do one of two things: 1) permit radiotherapy to do its job better with smaller dosages, and 2) prevent healthy tissue from being harmed by the ionizing radiation.

While the first group of drugs were the result of specific research to increase the effects of medical radiotherapy, protective agents are, once again, fall-out from the Pentagon. Because of the possible dangers of being involved in a nuclear disaster, the Department of Defense ordered its scientists to develop substances that could protect U.S. troops from an enemy's radiation weapons. One of the most successful radioprotectors has been named WR- (for Walter Reed Army Medical Center) 2721, a powerful sulfur-based cell-protecting drug. According to *Medical World News,* radiation therapists at the University of Pennsylvania have conducted human trials of the substance with great success.

Dr. Eli Glatstein, chief of the NCI's Radiation Oncology Branch told me the drug's development grew out of army research done in the 1960s.

"There have been many studies showing that WR-2721 and other drugs like it will permit us to give several times the normal doses of whole-body X-ray than we could before," he explained. "This means we'll be able to get really curative quantities to tumors we usually couldn't treat because of the toxicities involved."

Since primary breast cancer is not a deep-seated cancer, radioprotectors would only be useful to treat metastatic disease that might have spread to other organs.

Radiation therapy is also being tried intra-operatively in cases where a breast tumor is so large it cannot be removed. I knew this technique has been used in Japan for some time, but it is apparently a novel procedure here. Perhaps our early-detection programs have succeeded in getting women to the operating room before their cancers require such treatment, and it is not needed in the United States.

Hyperthermia—heating a cancer to death by microwaves, electricity, or electronic devices—has not been effective against mammary carcinoma so far, although it holds promise for other malignancies.

Of course, the NCI supports research to test virtually everything on earth and in the seas to see if there is antitumor activity. This applies to marine animals, plants—domestic and exotic—and complex mixtures of chemicals. At this time, however, there are fewer than ten drugs and hormones that have been proven to be effective against breast cancer. The experimental and clinical-trial activity revolves around giving these in varying dosages, in different combinations, on different schedules and—like intra-operative radiotherapy—beginning drug treatment in the operating room during surgery.

Foremost on the list of new anticancer agents are biological-response modifiers. In Chapter 12, I detailed how the body's own defense mechanism—the immune system—is able to prevent and also treat cancer. Exploiting this ability is now the new pharmacological frontier in the continuing war on the disease. I have already described BCG and *C. Parvum* as "non-specific" immune boosters given to stimulate a woman's own weakened system. There are others being tested, substances that are still known only by cryptic numbers and letters but whose purpose is the same: to strengthen women's self-defense mechanism so their bodies can fight the malignant invaders themselves. Interferons of all kinds, of course, are lymphokines—also biological-response-modifiers, even though magazines and newspapers have described them as new wonder drugs. Data from trials using pure, cloned IF are not available at the time of this writing. Past trials, as I wrote earlier, showed interferons to be less effective against breast cancer than existing agents.

The most recent addition to the arsenal of naturally produced substances is thymosin, a "new" anticancer agent that was first discovered in 1965 by Dr. Allan L. Goldstein, chairman of biochemistry at the George Washington University in Washington, D.C. The reason for the "newness" of this weapon is that researchers at Hoffman-LaRoche have manufactured a fraction of this thymus-gland hormone and have named it Alpha-1. The "old" thymic hormone, thymosin-5, was tried by Dr. Goldstein in 1966, along with chemotherapy, to treat patients with inoperable lung cancer. Even though it prolonged disease-free periods and increased survival, it was abandoned. Now, many old-timers are being revived as biological-response-modifiers, and thymosin and thymosin-related extracts and fractions are part of the movement.

The body's own defense components have been neglected for so many years because of the vagaries of human nature in general. When anticancer drugs were developed and were shown to be so successful by themselves, scientists believed there was no longer any reason to try to stimulate the body's defenses.

"Don't forget," Dr. John Macdonald, the NCI's associate director for cancer therapy, told me, "when cytotoxic agents were first used, they were enormously successful against fast-growing diseases like leukemia and Hodgkins. Now, we're dealing with more stubborn cancers like breast, lung, and colorectal disease, and there's just so far that you can go with cytotoxic drugs. Every one of them also kills healthy cells, and there's a limit as to how much they can be used alone, without somehow strengthening the body, too."

Dr. Macdonald also pointed out that not as much was known a decade or more ago about the powerful components of the immune system and how they could be enhanced and stimulated to counter the weakening effects of chemo- and radiotherapy.

"In those years, we knew nothing about natural killer cells, suppressor cells, or most of what we know now," he said. "So we didn't have much to go on in the understanding of how to use T-cells, B-cells, and macrophages. It's not a case of giving a new name to old agents; it's really new. We think we're really finding a way to get the body able to do its own fighting."

As Hoffman-LaRoche's research shows, private industry is now working closely with cancer researchers, a situation that did not always exist. At a recent meeting of the NCAB, I was astonished to hear that anticancer agents were "orphan drugs" not too long ago. Having been involved in NCI activities only since 1974, when adjuvant chemotherapy was already under way, I did not know that drugs had been used so rarely that pharmaceutical firms had not wanted to invest in such unprofitable ventures. Times have certainly changed in the drugstore. A glance at the financial pages quickly shows that stock in firms prominent in antineoplastic agents keep going up and up. Research & Development in the private drug sector do not show up in my pink-paper ball, but I can still glimpse a bit of what is happening.

Not only is the private sector eager to investigate and invest in anticancer agents, but scientists are now willing to work closely with them, because government can no longer be relied on to support expensive laboratories. Investigators who need hundreds of thousands of dollars for sophisticated equipment and salaries for highly skilled technical personnel must look elsewhere for their funding. As a result, the latest trend is for scientists to turn to pharmaceutical companies for development money after NCI resources are exhausted.

For example, the clonogenic stem-cell assay I described in Chapter 11 will soon be available commercially. This technique for custom-tailoring chemotherapy, just as antibiotics are chosen for specific organisms, will revolutionize cancer treatment. Drugs will be tested first against a patient's cancer cells in a test tube or Petri dish, sparing him or her the possible side effects of an ineffective substance. Many of the markers we need so desperately will also be developed by private pharmaceutical firms, and the profit-motive (read economic incentive) should speed progress considerably.

In addition, the specialty of oncology has exploded. When I wrote *Breast Cancer* in 1974, medical oncology had been recognized as a specialty for only a little more than two years. By 1979, there were 1,788 certified oncologists in the United States, and now there are almost 3,000. According to Dr. Emil Frei III, director of the Sidney Farber Cancer Center in Boston, the growth of medical oncology has contributed to a dramatic decrease in cancer mortality.

"In subjects under the age of 45," he said, "there has been a greater than 20 per cent decline in mortality from cancer. The incidence . . . in these age groups has not changed during this time period. Therefore, this decrease has resulted from improved treatment."

In *Breast Cancer*, the last chapter was also The Future, and I interviewed Dr. Erwin Vollmer—then recently retired—for his opinions. I wrote: "I've seen great new ideas come and go for more years than I like to think about," the graying, battle-scarred veteran of the war against cancer told me.

Dr. Vollmer was the chief of the Breast Cancer Project's Coordinating Branch at the National Cancer Institute for years. But he began his career as a working endocrinologist, "back in the years when hormones were 'it'," he explained, smiling. "After a while," he continued, "we found out hormones alone weren't it, at all. They weren't the whole answer to breast cancer—just another clue."

He shook his head. "Then, after the A-bomb was developed, we were sure that somehow nuclear medicine would have an answer for curing breast cancer. But no soap. Radioisotopes and supervoltage X-ray just became extra tools, not cures. Then it was chemotherapy, and I guess it still is," Dr. Vollmer went on. "Certainly, some day soon, I hope, a tumorcidal drug will be found that doesn't have to kill the patient to cure the cancer.

"After Joe Bittner discovered the mouse mammary-tumor virus, back in '36, the big push was to find a human virus. Now all the younger research people think immunology is 'it'." He smiled. "As soon as they find the little bug, they're positive they'll be able to put together some kind of vaccine to prevent breast cancer or a serum to cure it."

A slender, slight man, Dr. Vollmer stared above my head at nothing, his Paul-Newman-blue eyes looking, perhaps, to the future. "I hope they're right. In all these years, after spending so much money, it's incredible that we're still losing as many women from breast cancer as we did forty years ago. There has just got to be a breakthrough soon."

I called on Dr. Vollmer again for his opinion about the state of breast cancer affairs at the beginning of a new decade.

"What did I say last time?" he asked.

After I read the paragraphs to him, he laughed. "Well, I don't know about those Paul-Newman blue eyes," he said. "Colors fade with age you know."

There was a long silence, and I could imagine him making a mental account of what has happened since 1974. Finally, his voice came back.

"I wouldn't be so pessimistic now. I think we're on the brink of exciting times. We've got tremendous new tools for detection and treatment, and I am very impressed with the plans they're making to use naturally produced substances to fight cancer. No, I wouldn't be so pessimistic at all now; we're finally saving women's lives."

Appendix

UNDERSTANDING CANCER

In June 1981, Senator Paula Hawkins of Florida held a subcommittee hearing to find out why—after ten years—the National Cancer Institute had not yet been able to find a way to prevent or cure cancer. Although none of the senators mentioned the hackneyed phrase, "If we could get a man to walk on the moon . . . ," the question was in the air for everyone to breathe.

Why, indeed, has the Conquest of Cancer Act—passed with such passion and zeal by Congress in 1971—failed to eradicate this most dreaded disease? Why did cancer not succumb to a massive American attack as polio and other infectious diseases did . . . and with far less money?

The answer is that no prevention or cure is possible without knowing the cause of a disease, and learning why a healthy and normal cell suddenly goes haywire is learning the mysteries of life itself. And all life—plant and animal—begins with a microscopic collection of complex molecules: the cell.

To understand cancer, it is important to know a little about a normal cell and how it works. Cells—all cells—are microscopic bits of a jellolike material called protoplasm or cytoplasm. Inside the cell is a structure called the nucleus, and around the outside of the cell is a membrane that filters certain materials in and others out. Scattered through the cell are various microscopic factories that extract whatever they need from the nutrients that are sieved through the membrane from the bloodstream. The most important work of cells is to produce energy to support the functions of the particular organ in which a cell is situated and—except for muscle and nerve cells—to reproduce themselves, by mitosis (or division). (Nerve and muscle cells—including those of the heart—do not reproduce; when we are born, we have all of them we will ever have.)

Cells reproduce at different intervals. Those of the blood, marrow, and skin, for example, reproduce rapidly; liver cells very slowly. But they all reproduce by the same technique—mitosis.

Inside the nucleus of every cell of every animal is a certain number of chromosomes, arranged in strands. Every organism has a different number; humans normally have forty-six, twenty-three inherited from each parent. At specified, regulated periods in every cell's life, the strands of chromosomes begin to duplicate themselves, in a process called twinning. When a double set of "daughter" chromosomes has developed, the two strands separate from each other and move toward opposite sides of the cell. The two sets of daughter chromosomes will be parts of the nuclei of two new daughter cells by the time the cell division is completed.

Meanwhile, the outer membrane of the cell has developed a barely perceptible waistline, which indents quickly into a wasp waist, once the daughter chromosomes are in place. The "cleavage"—the last stage of mitosis—occurs when the parent cell breaks apart at the waistline into two daughter cells.

After resting for whatever length of time their biological stopwatches have decreed they should, the daughter cells begin the reproductive cycle again.

Until the electron microscope was invented, the existence of this stopwatch was theory, not fact. How a cell knew what to do, and when, was one of the big mysteries of life. Now scientists have unraveled enough about the computer-tape-like chromosomes to know that they are winding strips of complex molecules called deoxyribonucleic acid—DNA, or "genes." Everyone knew about the genes, those bits of matter on the chromosomes that somehow pass along parental traits and characteristics. But it took the electron microscope to show that the bits are not just passengers on the chains, but are actually segments of DNA, hooked together in two linked spirals—the "double helix."

DNA strands separate and produce a "messenger" known as RNA (ribonucleic acid) that carries the information from the genes out of the nucleus and into the cytoplasm where it tells the cell's protein-making machinery what has to be done next to keep that particular piece of the body's tissue working properly.

If all goes well and the chromosomes duplicate and split identically, without an error, or mutation, the daughter cells will look and behave exactly like the parent—down to having the same stopwatch, for instance.

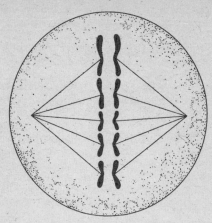

Chromosomes Twinning

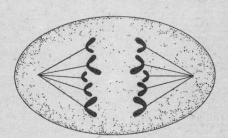

"Daughter" Chromosomes Moving Apart

But there are those mutations.

Serious mutations happen rarely. Considering that DNA consists of thousands of units of four different substances arranged in a very precise order, it is a marvel that mistakes are not more frequent. For example, the same two substances must always be paired directly opposite each other on the twisting chains. If for some reason just two units on a chain are switched, this pairing would not occur. In addition, adjacent pairings of the other two substances would also be mutated.

Sometimes the mutation is so damaging that the cell dies altogether. But most errors are not so severe; they just change the way one particular gene behaves. If the mutation is in the gene

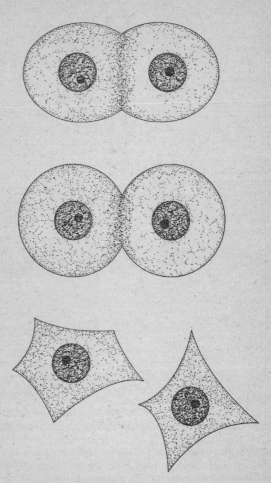

Cleavage of a Cell into Two New "Daughter" Cells

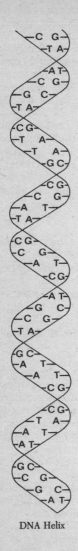

DNA Helix

Diagram of Part of a DNA Molecule

that regulates iron absorption, for example, that one cell's daughter cells and their descendants will not use this mineral normally. However, the end result of this kind of mutation is unlikely to affect the overall functioning of the organ very seriously.

On the other hand, if the mutation is in the gene that regulates the growth and reproduction of the cell itself, the result could be cancer. This is how all cancers begin: one cell loses control over its own reproductive machinery, and a neoplasm—a malignant tumor—is born.

Before going on, I must emphasize that the cellular reproduction under discussion here is *not* the kind of reproduction that results in a baby. Gamete reproduction—both the sperm and the egg are gametes—is a unique and different process. (Mutations can occur in the genes of the sperm or the egg, or in the developing baby during pregnancy—mutations that could cause albinism, a different color in each eye, physical malformation, and some diseases. Also, there are some neonatal cancers—for example, Wilms' tumor, a kidney malignancy.)

Most of us think of genes only in relation to babies. Genes are actually present in every cell of every organ in the body from fertilization onward and are constantly being duplicated by mitosis throughout the organism's lifetime. In humans, by the way, it is a random half of the forty-six chromosomes that makes up the twenty-three each parent gives to the sperm or the egg. Each sperm and each egg hold a different selection of chromosomes from the father and mother. (Only identical twins, the result of a freakish separation of the fertilized egg, have the same sets of chromosomes.)

Returning to mutations that affect cellular reproduction, one way this function can be altered is by a chance or accidental disarrangement in the gene governing growth and reproduction. Other suspects are chemicals that get into our tissues one way or another. In the case of some neoplasms—including some of the breast cancers—viruses may be the causative agents. Irradiation from the sun's rays, from X-rays, and from nuclear particles can also affect that important dot of DNA and cause a cell to "transform" from being healthy to being cancerous.

So far, nothing has been targeted as a single cause of malignancy in the cells of the breast, although there are many theories. The process is known, however. For a healthy cell to become malignant, its growth-and-reproduction gene must be changed during the brief period when the chromosomes are twinning. Whatever the cause of the cancer may be, the basic mechanism is the same: a foul-up during the duplication of the gene that computer-programs how much a cell will grow, how rapidly it will divide, and how long it will continue to reproduce.

Just think, if the cells of the body did not have such a preordained brake on their growth and reproduction, we would have a world filled with giants; all of us would be eternally growing children who never reached adulthood. Luckily, there is a built-in stop light, and cells eventually reach a point at which they reproduce exactly the number required to replace those that die off, but no more.

If they are normal cells, that is. Cancer cells never stop reproducing.

Understanding the role of DNA and mutations clarified how cancer begins, but it did not help me understand the step-by-step transformation of a normal cell to a malignant one. I asked a research professor I was interviewing for a simple explanation.

"Something occurs in the growth gene during the twinning process," he explained. "This can best be described by showing you a very simplified diagram of the life cycle of a cell."

I studied the diagram while he continued his professional lecture. "The life cycle of a normal cell can be divided into four periods. There is D—it stands for division—the period during which actual separation into two cells occurs.* This is followed by a stage called the G-1—meaning Gap 1—period, which begins as soon as the previous mitosis has been completed and lasts until the beginning of the next cycle of DNA duplication. That is the S—for synthesis—period, when the DNA molecules—those forty-six chromosomes in the human—manufacture their identical twins. The G-2 period is the interval during which the two sets of chromosomes move apart and the parent cell prepares to break into two daughter cells.

"While the length of the G-1 period varies from organ to organ, the other phases are the same in all cells. The G-2 period lasts two hours, D takes forty minutes, and S seven hours."

"The single gene, or segment of DNA, in every cell that is preprogramed to control growth and reproduction knows exactly how frequently that particular cell should divide," the professor went on. "The gene also knows when the cell should stop reproducing altogether and just stay dormant, remaining so until the tissue of which it is a part needs new cells to replace those that have died. This resting phase occurs during the G-1 period in every healthy cell, but different kinds of cells have different dormant times."

---

*Many scientists call this the M period—for mitosis, the technical term for cell division.

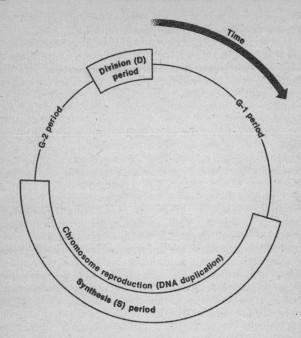

Life Cycle of a Cell

He reminded me that nerve and muscle cells are arrested in the G-1 period when the organism is born and never reproduce again. Blood, marrow, and skin cells, on the other hand, have very short G-1 periods and are always making new daughters.

Then the professor gave me a list of books to read for more information about transformation—the process by which a normal cell becomes malignant.

Using as my mental guide an accidental switch in the arrangement of the substances of the growth gene, transformation was not too hard to understand.

During the S period of the cell, while the chromosomes are twinning, that accidental switch will be duplicated too. The chromosome carrying the altered gene will make two new chromosomes with the same mutation built into them. The two resulting daughter cells will be different from their parent cell.

Their built-in brake has been changed, and it no longer tells them when to stop growing and go into G-1 sleep, as their healthy sisters do. Instead, the mutated daughter cells keep dividing and making new daughters quite madly, on their own new preprogramed schedule.

In normal breast tissue, for example, cells generally go to sleep after twenty or thirty divisions and stay in G-1 until the breast signals that it needs some replacement parts. The cells then wake up and go through just enough "passages" to fill the order, before they return again to their dormant G-1 period. Their transformed sisters, however, keep on reproducing themselves long after the need for new cells has passed. They have become cancer.

Since the beginning of medical history, doctors and scientists have been fascinated with the craft of alchemy—the trick of turning base metal into gold. In the late 1970s, researchers at several of the world's medical schools reported the possibility of an even more miraculous kind of alchemy—returning cancer cells to health. The magic elixir is known as DHEA, dehydroisoandrostenone. Success has been too meager to have even been reported in weekly tabloids. Yet there is no question that DHEA has been able, somehow, to halt the inevitable process from normal to malignant and to reverse the process in some cells.

Alchemy may, someday, become the "magic bullet" everyone has been looking for for centuries.

Index